Epilepsy Surgery: Paradigm Shifts

Editors

R. MARK RICHARDSON
JIMMY C. YANG

NEUROSURGERY
CLINICS OF NORTH AMERICA

www.neurosurgery.theclinics.com

Consulting Editors
RUSSELL R. LONSER
DANIEL K. RESNICK

January 2024 • Volume 35 • Number 1

ELSEVIER

1600 John F. Kennedy Boulevard • Suite 1800 • Philadelphia, Pennsylvania, 19103-2899

http://www.theclinics.com

NEUROSURGERY CLINICS OF NORTH AMERICA Volume 35, Number 1
January 2024 ISSN 1042-3680, ISBN-13: 978-0-443-13167-7

Editor: Stacy Eastman
Developmental Editor: Akshay Samson

Neurosurgery Clinics of North America (ISSN 1042-3680) is published quarterly by Elsevier Inc., 360 Park Avenue South, New York, NY 10010-1710. Months of issue are January, April, July, and October. Business and Editorial Offices: 1600 John F. Kennedy Blvd., Suite 1800, Philadelphia, PA 19103-2899. Customer Service Office: 11830 Westline Industrial Drive, St. Louis, MO 63146. Periodicals postage paid at New York, NY, and additional mailing offices. Subscription prices are $465.00 per year (US individuals), $499.00 per year (Canadian individuals), $579.00 per year (international individuals), $100.00 per year (US students), $255.00 per year (international students), and $100.00 per year (Canadian students). For institutional access pricing please contact Customer Service via the contact information below. International air speed delivery is included in all *Clinics* subscription prices. All prices are subject to change without notice. **POSTMASTER:** Send address changes to *Neurosurgery Clinics of North America*, Elsevier Periodicals Customer Service, 11830 Westline Industrial Drive, St. Louis, MO 63146. **Customer Service: 1-800-654-2452 (US and Canada). From outside the US and Canada, call: 1-314-453-7041. Fax: 1-314-453-5170. E-mail: JournalsCustomerService-usa@elsevier.com (for print support) and journalsonlinesupport-usa@elsevier.com (for online support).**

Reprints. For copies of 100 or more, of articles in this publication, please contact the Commercial Reprints Department, Elsevier Inc., 360 Park Avenue South, New York, NY 10010-1710. Tel. 212-633-3874; Fax: 212-633-3820; E-mail: reprints@elsevier.com.

Neurosurgery Clinics of North America is covered in *MEDLINE/PubMed (Index Medicus), EMBASE/Excerpta Medica, and Current Contents/Clinical Medicine (CC/CM).*

Contributors

CONSULTING EDITORS

RUSSELL R. LONSER, MD
Professor and Chair, Department of Neurological Surgery, The Ohio State University Wexner Medical Center, Columbus, Ohio, USA

DANIEL K. RESNICK, MD, MS
Professor and Vice Chairman, Program Director, Department of Neurosurgery, University of Wisconsin-Madison School of Medicine and Public Health, Madison, Wisconsin, USA

EDITORS

R. MARK RICHARDSON, MD, PhD
Director of Functional Neurosurgery, Department of Neurosurgery, Massachusetts General Hospital, Charles Pappas Associate Professor of Neurosciences, Harvard Medical School, Visiting Associate Professor of Brain and Cognitive Sciences, Massachusetts Institute of Technology, Boston, Massachusetts, USA

JIMMY C. YANG, MD
Assistant Professor, Department of Neurological Surgery, The Ohio State University College of Medicine, Columbus, Ohio, USA; Department of Neurosurgery, Emory University School of Medicine, Atlanta, Georgia, USA

AUTHORS

VIVEK P. BUCH, MD
Assistant Professor of Neurosurgery, Department of Neurosurgery, Stanford University, Palo Alto, California, USA

SYDNEY S. CASH, MD, PhD
Associate Professor, Department of Neurology, Center for Neurotechnology and Neurorecovery, Massachusetts General Hospital, Harvard Medical School, Boston, Massachusetts, USA

CATHERINE J. CHU, MD, MA, MMSc
Associate Professor, Department of Neurology, Massachusetts General Hospital, Harvard Medical School, Boston, Massachusetts, USA

MELISSA M.J CHUA, MD
Clinical Fellow, Department of Neurosurgery, Brigham and Women's Hospital, Harvard Medical School, Boston, Massachusetts, USA

DEREK J. DOSS, BE
MD/PhD Candidate, Department of Biomedical Engineering, Vanderbilt University, Vanderbilt University Institute of Imaging Science (VUIIS), Vanderbilt Institute for Surgery and Engineering (VISE), Nashville, Tennessee, USA

DARIO J. ENGLOT, MD, PhD
Associate Professor of Neurological Surgery, Neurology, Radiology and Radiological Sciences, Department of Biomedical Engineering, Department of Electrical and Computer Engineering, Vanderbilt University, Vanderbilt University Institute of Imaging Science (VUIIS), Vanderbilt Institute for Surgery and Engineering (VISE), Department of Neurological Surgery, Department of Radiological Sciences, Vanderbilt University Medical Center, Nashville, Tennessee, USA

ROBERT E. GROSS, MD, PhD
Professor, Departments of Neurosurgery and
Neurology, Emory University School of
Medicine, Atlanta, Georgia, USA

SAADI GHATAN, MD
Professor, Neurological Surgery and Pediatrics
Icahn School of Medicine at Mt Sinai, New
York, New York, USA

JIE HU, MD, PhD
Chief of Functional, Neurosurgical Group,
Professor, Department of Neurosurgery,
Huashan Hospital, Fudan University, Shanghai,
China

GEORGE M. IBRAHIM, MD, PhD
Paediatric Neurosurgeon, Division of
Neurosurgery, Hospital for Sick Children,
University of Toronto, Ontario, Canada

SHIZE JIANG, MD
Attending Physician, Department of
Neurosurgery, Huashan Hospital, Fudan
University, Shanghai, China

GRAHAM W. JOHNSON, PhD
MD/PhD Candidate, Department of Biomedical
Engineering, Vanderbilt University, Vanderbilt
University Institute of Imaging Science (VUIIS),
Vanderbilt Institute for Surgery and Engineering
(VISE), Nashville, Tennessee, USA

KRISTOPHER T. KAHLE, MD, PhD
Nicholas T. Zervas Endowed Chair and
Associate Professor, Harvard Medical School,
Department of Neurosurgery, Director of
Pediatric Neurosurgery, Massachusetts
General Hospital, Boston, Massachusetts,
USA

ANKIT N. KHAMBHATI, PhD
Assistant Professional Researcher,
Department of Neurosurgery, Weill Institute for
Neurosciences, University of California, San
Francisco, San Francisco, California, USA

**VASILEIOS KOKKINOS, CNIM, NA-CLTM,
PhD, PhD, PhD, FACNS**
Assistant Professor of Neurology,
Comprehensive Epilepsy Center, Northwestern
Memorial Hospital, Chicago, Illinois, USA

LUMING LI, PhD
Professor, National Engineering Research
Center of Neuromodulation, School of

Aerospace Engineering, Tsinghua University,
IDG/McGovern Institute for Brain Research at
Tsinghua University, Beijing, China

JOHN R. MCLAREN, MD
Department of Neurology, Massachusetts
General Hospital, Harvard Medical School,
Boston, Massachusetts, USA

PRANAV NANDA, MD, MPhil
Clinical Fellow, Department of Neurosurgery,
Massachusetts General Hospital, Department
of Neurosurgery, Harvard Medical School,
Boston, Massachusetts, USA

JOSEF PARVIZI, MD, PhD
Professor of Neurology, Stanford University,
Palo Alto, California, USA

ANGELIQUE C. PAULK, PhD
Instructor, Department of Neurology, Center
for Neurotechnology and Neurorecovery,
Massachusetts General Hospital, Harvard
Medical School, Boston, Massachusetts, USA

RORY J. PIPER, MRCS
Neurosurgery Registrar, Developmental
Neurosciences, UCL Great Ormond Street
Institute of Child Health, Department of
Neurosurgery, Great Ormond Street Hospital,
London, United Kingdom

XIAOYA QIN, PhD
Precision Medicine and Healthcare Research
Center, Tsinghua-Berkeley Shenzhen Institute,
Tsinghua University, Shenzhen, China; National
Engineering Research Center of
Neuromodulation, School of Aerospace
Engineering, Tsinghua University, Beijing, China

R. MARK RICHARDSON, MD, PhD
Director of Functional Neurosurgery,
Department of Neurosurgery, Massachusetts
General Hospital, Charles Pappas Associate
Professor of Neurosciences, Harvard Medical
School, Visiting Associate Professor of Brain
and Cognitive Sciences, Massachusetts
Institute of Technology, Boston,
Massachusetts, USA

JOHN D. ROLSTON, MD, PhD
Associate Professor, Department of
Neurosurgery, Brigham and Women's

Hospital, Harvard Medical School, Boston, Massachusetts, USA

PARIYA SALAMI, PhD
Instructor, Department of Neurology, Center for Neurotechnology and Neurorecovery, Massachusetts General Hospital, Harvard Medical School, Boston, Massachusetts, USA

HARGUNBIR SINGH, MBBS
Research Fellow, Department of Neurosurgery, Brigham and Women's Hospital, Harvard Medical School, Boston, Massachusetts, USA

DEREK G. SOUTHWELL, MD, PhD
Assistant Professor, Department of Neurosurgery, Graduate Program in Neurobiology, Duke University, Durham, North Carolina, USA

MICHAELA A. STAMM, MS
Research Assistant, Department of Neurosurgery, Brigham and Women's Hospital, Harvard Medical School, Boston, Massachusetts, USA

MARTIN M. TISDALL, FRCS(SN), MD
Consultant Neurosurgeon and Chief of Service, Brain Directorate, Developmental Neurosciences, UCL Great Ormond Street Institute of Child Health, Department of Neurosurgery, Great Ormond Street Hospital, London, United Kingdom

STEVEN TOBOCHNIK, MD
Instructor, Department of Neurology, Brigham and Women's Hospital, Harvard Medical School, Massachusetts, Boston, USA

AARON E.L. WARREN, PhD
Research Fellow, Department of Neurosurgery, Brigham and Women's Hospital, Harvard Medical School, Boston, Massachusetts, USA

ANDREW I. YANG, MD
Clinical Fellow, Department of Neurosurgery, Emory University School of Medicine, Atlanta, Georgia, USA

JIMMY C. YANG, MD
Assistant Professor, Department of Neurological Surgery, The Ohio State University College of Medicine, Columbus, Ohio, USA; Department of Neurosurgery, Emory University School of Medicine, Atlanta, Georgia, USA

YI YAO, M.Med
Director, Department of Functional Neurosurgery, Xiamen Humanity Hospital Affiliated to Fujian Medical University, Fujian, China; Surgery Division, Epilepsy Center, Shenzhen Children's Hospital, Shenzhen, Guangdong, China

HUILING YU, MD
Postdoctoral Fellow, National Engineering Research Center of Neuromodulation, School of Aerospace Engineering, Tsinghua University, Beijing, China

YUAN YUAN, PhD
Senior Engineer, Precision Medicine and Healthcare Research Center, Tsinghua-Berkeley Shenzhen Institute, Tsinghua University, Shenzhen, China; National Engineering Research Center of Neuromodulation, School of Aerospace Engineering, Tsinghua University, Beijing, China

RINA ZELMANN, PhD
Instructor, Department of Neurology, Center for Neurotechnology and Neurorecovery, Massachusetts General Hospital, Harvard Medical School, Boston, Massachusetts, USA

YANMING ZHU, MD, PhD
Candidate, Program in Speech and Hearing Bioscience and Technology, Harvard Medical School, Department of Neurosurgery, Massachusetts General Hospital, Boston, Massachusetts, USA

Contents

Section I: Focus on Quality of Life

> Since the late nineteenth century, the prevailing view of epilepsy surgery has been to identify a seizure focus in a medically refractory patient and eradicate it. Sadly, only a select number of the many who suffer from uncontrolled seizures benefit from this approach. With the development of safe, efficient stereotactic methods and targeted surgical therapies that can affect deep structures and modulate broad networks in diverse disorders, epilepsy surgery in children has undergone a paradigmatic evolutionary change. With modern diagnostic techniques such as stereo electroencephalography combined with closed loop neuromodulatory systems, pediatric epilepsy surgery can reach a much broader population of underserved patients.

> Intracranial neuromodulation is an evolving therapy for patients with drug-resistant epilepsy (DRE). Deep brain stimulation (DBS) is now available as a therapy for patients with DRE and focal-onset seizures in select health care systems; however, there remains a substantial need of efficacy data before DBS can be more widely adopted into routine clinical practice. This review and commentary focuses on a particular shifting paradigm: *DBS as a therapy for children with generalized-onset seizures.*

> Current applications of neurostimulation for generalized epilepsy use a one-target-fits-all approach that is agnostic to the specific epilepsy syndrome and seizure type being treated. The authors describe similarities and differences between the 2 "archetypes" of generalized epilepsy—Lennox-Gastaut syndrome and Idiopathic Generalized Epilepsy—and review recent neuroimaging evidence for syndrome-specific brain networks underlying seizures. Implications for stimulation targeting and programming are discussed using 5 clinical questions: What epilepsy syndrome does the patient have? What brain networks are involved? What is the optimal stimulation target? What is the optimal stimulation paradigm? What is the plan for adjusting stimulation over time?

Epileptic encephalopathies are defined by the presence of frequent epileptiform activity that causes neurodevelopmental slowing or regression. Here, we review evidence that epilepsy surgery improves neurodevelopment in children with epileptic encephalopathies. We describe an example patient with epileptic encephalopathy without drug refractory seizures, who underwent successful diagnostic and therapeutic surgeries. In patients with epileptic encephalopathy, cognitive improvement alone is a sufficient indication to recommend surgical intervention in experienced centers.

Section II: Network Surgery and the Evolution of Stereoelectroencephalography (SEEG)

Epilepsy surgery is a potentially curative treatment of drug-resistant epilepsy that has remained underutilized both due to inadequate referrals and incomplete localization hypotheses. The complexity of patients evaluated for epilepsy surgery has increased, thus new approaches are necessary to treat these patients. The paradigm of epilepsy surgery has evolved to match this challenge, now considering the entire seizure network with the goal of disrupting it through resection, ablation, neuromodulation, or a combination. The network paradigm has the potential to aid in identification of the seizure network as well as treatment selection.

Understanding and discriminating the normal and abnormal elements of the intracranial electroencephalogram (iEEG) is essential in decision-making for epilepsy surgery. The hippocampus is widely acknowledged as a key structure in decision-making processes for surgical treatment in temporal lobe epilepsy and epilepsies that involve the mesial temporal structures. This review will provide a summary of the current state of our knowledge and understanding regarding normal and abnormal features of the iEEG of the human hippocampus.

Overall stereoelectroencephalography (SEEG) has a favorable risk profile, patient tolerability, and superior investigative capability of individualized 3-dimensional seizure onset activity over subdural electrodes. Further, our recent surgical approach to safely enable multinuclear thalamic propagation mapping can only be performed with SEEG. For these reasons, SEEG has become the gold standard of phase II monitoring at our institution, and believe the ability to develop precision network-centric approaches to therapy will be critical to enhance our ability to care for medically refractory, and importantly, even complex multifocal, generalized, or surgically refractory epilepsy patients.

The practice of invasive monitoring for presurgical epilepsy workup has evolved at Massachusetts General Hospital (MGH) in parallel to the evolution in the field's understanding of epilepsy as a network disorder. Implantations have shifted from an emphasis on singularly finding single foci for the purpose of resection to a network-hypothesis–driven approach aiming to delineate patients' seizure networks with the goal of developing surgical interventions that disrupt critical nodes of these networks. Here, the authors review all invasive monitoring cases at MGH from April 2016 through June 2023 to describe how this paradigm shift has taken form.

Temporal lobe epilepsy (TLE) is one of the most common drug-refractory epilepsies. However, the diagnosis and treatment of TLE may be improved by better understanding its complex network. In this article, the authors summarize their experience with TLE and discuss their process for using stereo-electroencephalography (SEEG) as part of presurgical evaluation in the past 10 years. The authors demonstrate the value of SEEG in different types of TLE and discuss how their findings have impacted treatment options. Ultimately, the authors' experience will help other centers in addressing TLE cases.

As the pathophysiological mechanisms of vagus nerve stimulation (VNS) causing individual differences in the vagal ascending network remains unclear, stereoelectroencephalography (SEEG) provides a unique platform to explore the brain networks affected by VNS and helps to understand the anti-seizure mechanism of VNS more comprehensively. This study presents a preliminary exploration of the acute effect of VNS. SEEG signals were collected to assess the acute effect of VNS on neural synchronization in patients with drug-resistant epilepsy, especially in epileptogenic networks. The results show that the better the efficacy of VNS, the wider the spread of desynchronization assessed by weighted phase lag index at a high frequency band caused by VNS. Future studies should focus on the association between the change in synchronization and the efficacy of VNS, exploring the possibility of synchronization as a biomarker for patient screening and parameter programming.

Section III: Cutting Edge Technologies

Deep brain stimulation has demonstrated efficacy in reducing seizure frequency in patients with drug-resistant epilepsy who may otherwise not be candidates for other surgical procedures. Recently, a clinical device that can monitor neural activity in the form of local field potentials around the deep brain stimulator lead implant site has been introduced. While this technology has been clinically adopted in other disorders treated with deep brain stimulation, such as Parkinson's disease, its application in epilepsy remains unclear. Previous research using investigational devices has suggested that specific frequency bands may correlate with clinical response to deep brain stimulation in epilepsy, but features of the clinical device may prevent its use. The authors present their experience with using this technology in epilepsy patients and describe some of its limitations. Ultimately, novel biomarkers will need to be identified to elucidate how neural activity at deep brain stimulation sites may change with clinical response.

Responsive neurostimulation (RNS) therapy is an effective treatment for reducing seizures in some patients with focal epilepsy. Utilizing a chronically implanted device, RNS involves monitoring brain activity signals for user-defined patterns of seizure activity and delivering electrical stimulation in response. Devices store chronic data including counts of detected activity patterns and brief recordings of intracranial electroencephalography signals. Data platforms for reviewing stored chronic data retrospectively may be used to evaluate therapy performance and to fine-tune detection and stimulation settings. New frontiers in RNS research can leverage raw chronic data to reverse engineer neurostimulation mechanisms and improve therapy effectiveness.

Recording neural activity has been a critical aspect in the diagnosis and treatment of patients with epilepsy. For those with intractable epilepsy, intracranial neural monitoring has been of substantial importance. Clinically, however, methods for recording neural information have remained essentially unchanged for decades. Over the last decade or so, rapid advances in electrode technology have begun to change this landscape. New systems allow for the observation of neural activity with high spatial resolution and, in some cases, at the level of the activity of individual neurons. These new tools have contributed greatly to our understanding of brain function and dysfunction. Here, the authors review the primary technologies currently in use in humans. The authors discuss other possible systems, some of the challenges which come along with these devices, and how they will become incorporated into the clinical workflow. Ultimately, the expectation is that these new, high-density, high-spatial-resolution recording systems will become a valuable part of the clinical arsenal used in the diagnosis and surgical management of epilepsy.

Current epilepsy surgical techniques, such as brain resection, laser ablation, and neurostimulation, target seizure networks macroscopically, and they may yield an unfavorable balance between seizure reduction, procedural invasiveness, and neurologic morbidity. The transplantation of GABAergic interneurons is a regenerative technique for altering neural inhibition in cortical circuits, with potential as an alternative and minimally invasive approach to epilepsy treatment. This article (1) reviews some of the preclinical evidence supporting interneuron transplantation as an epilepsy therapy, (2) describes a first-in-human study of interneuron transplantation for epilepsy, and (3) considers knowledge gaps that stand before the effective clinical application of this novel treatment.

NEUROSURGERY CLINICS OF NORTH AMERICA

SERIES OF RELATED INTEREST

Neurologic Clinics
https://www.neurologic.theclinics.com/
Neuroimaging Clinics
https://www.neuroimaging.theclinics.com/

THE CLINICS ARE AVAILABLE ONLINE!
Access your subscription at:
www.theclinics.com

Preface

Evolution in Epilepsy Surgery and the Need to Address a Public Health Crisis of Underutilization

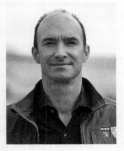
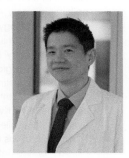

R. Mark Richardson, MD, PhD   Jimmy C. Yang, MD

Editors

In patients with drug-resistant epilepsy, surgery is an effective option that can lead to seizure freedom in a majority of children and adults.[1] However, despite publication of a practice parameter in 2003 that recommended referral of patients with drug-resistant epilepsy to a surgical epilepsy center,[2] subsequent studies showed that the needle did not move, with the average time to surgical referral hovering around 18 years.[3,4] The International League Against Epilepsy continues to support surgical referral of patients with drug-resistant epilepsy, recently publishing consensus recommendations that a surgical evaluation should be offered to every patient with drug-resistant epilepsy up to 70 years of age, as soon as drug resistance is ascertained, regardless of epilepsy duration, sex, socioeconomic status, seizure type, epilepsy type (including epileptic encephalopathies), localization, and comorbidities.[5] Given that ~1.2 million Americans with epilepsy remain surgical candidates, underutilization of epilepsy surgery is a public health crisis.[6]

The reasons behind underutilization of epilepsy surgery are diverse, spanning patient and provider education, technological factors, and system-based limitations.[7] For instance, patients may be hesitant to pursue epilepsy surgery due to impressions regarding the risks, even if surgery could lead to seizure freedom.[8] Similarly, those who care for patients with epilepsy may have outdated views on the roles and risks of surgery.[9] Strategies for improving these gaps include efforts focused on raising awareness and educational interventions for both patients and providers.[10] Ultimately, with ongoing evolution in the surgical treatments available to patients, including laser ablation and neuromodulation, the number of patients who are good candidates for epilepsy surgery will continue to expand.

Recent work in the fields of natural language processing and artificial intelligence has highlighted ways in which new technologies may be able to identify epilepsy surgery candidates and facilitate their referral for surgical workup.[11] For example, a recent randomized clinical trial used machine learning to provide alerts to providers regarding epilepsy surgery referral, ultimately leading to increased numbers of referrals for appropriate candidates.[12] Although not highlighted in this issue, these new technologies should facilitate patients' access to epilepsy surgery options.

The articles in this issue of *Neurosurgery Clinics of North America* provide diverse examples of how recent paradigm shifts have evolved the field of epilepsy surgery. The first group of articles highlight the shift in recognizing a positive quality-of-life impact from surgery rather than using seizure freedom as the sole surgical goal. This shift has

Neurosurg Clin N Am 35 (2024) xiii–xiv
https://doi.org/10.1016/j.nec.2023.09.009
1042-3680/24/© 2023 Published by Elsevier Inc.

been evident in the use of surgical therapies for expanded indications, such as generalized epilepsy and epileptic encephalopathy. Patients with these nontraditional indications are increasingly experiencing significant quality-of-life improvements as a result of adapting current technologies and strategies for treating these disease-specific epilepsy networks.

The second group of articles highlight the shift from focus-oriented to network-oriented approaches to epilepsy surgery,[13] demonstrating how surgical strategies have evolved along with the increasing use of stereoelectroencephalography (SEEG), including how the advent of responsive neurostimulation therapy has caused SEEG itself to evolve. The last group of articles highlight how new technologies are creating additional paradigm shifts, across both device-based and biologic therapies, which promise a continued and exciting evolution in the field of epilepsy surgery. We hope that increasing recognition of the positive benefits of these paradigm shifts by patients, patient-advocates, general practitioners, neurologists, and neurosurgeons will help bring epilepsy surgery to more patients who need it.

R. Mark Richardson, MD, PhD
Department of Neurosurgery
Massachusetts General Hospital
55 Fruit Street
Boston, MA 02114, USA

Jimmy C. Yang, MD
Department of Neurological Surgery
The Ohio State University College of Medicine
480 Medical Center Drive
Columbus, OH 43210, USA

E-mail addresses:
mark.richardson@mgh.harvard.edu
(R.M. Richardson)
jimmy.yang@osumc.edu (J.C. Yang)

REFERENCES

1. Lamberink HJ, Otte WM, Blümcke I, et al. Seizure outcome and use of antiepileptic drugs after epilepsy surgery according to histopathological diagnosis: a retrospective multicentre cohort study. Lancet Neurol 2020;19(9):748–57.

2. Engel J, Wiebe S, French J, et al. Practice parameter: temporal lobe and localized neocortical resections for epilepsy. Report of the Quality Standards Subcommittee of the American Academy of Neurology, in Association with the American Epilepsy Society and the American Association of Neurological Surgeons. Neurology 2003;60(4):538–47.

3. Haneef Z, Stern J, Dewar S, et al. Referral pattern for epilepsy surgery after evidence-based recommendations. Neurology 2010;75(8):699–704.

4. Eriksson MH, Whitaker KJ, Booth J, et al. Pediatric epilepsy surgery from 2000 to 2018: changes in referral and surgical volumes, patient characteristics, genetic testing, and post-surgical outcomes. Epilepsia 2023. https://doi.org/10.1111/epi.17670.

5. Jehi L, Jette N, Kwon C, et al. Timing of referral to evaluate for epilepsy surgery: expert consensus recommendations from the Surgical Therapies Commission of the International League Against Epilepsy. Epilepsia 2022;63(10):2491–506.

6. Richardson RM. Closed-loop brain stimulation and paradigm shifts in epilepsy surgery. Neurol Clin 2022;40(2):355–73.

7. Samanta D, Ostendorf AP, Willis E, et al. Underutilization of epilepsy surgery: part I: a scoping review of barriers. Epilepsy Behav 2021;117:107837.

8. Prus N, Grant AC. Patient beliefs about epilepsy and brain surgery in a multicultural urban population. Epilepsy Behav 2010;17(1):46–9.

9. Erba G, Moja L, Beghi E, et al. Barriers toward epilepsy surgery. A survey among practicing neurologists. Epilepsia 2012;53(1):35–43.

10. Samanta D, Singh R, Gedela S, et al. Underutilization of epilepsy surgery: part II: strategies to overcome barriers. Epilepsy Behav 2021;117:107853.

11. Tan S, Tang C, Ng JS, et al. Identifying epilepsy surgery candidates with natural language processing: a systematic review. J Clin Neurosci 2023;114:104–9.

12. Wissel BD, Greiner HM, Glauser TA, et al. Automated, machine learning–based alerts increase epilepsy surgery referrals: a randomized controlled trial. Epilepsia 2023;64(7):1791–9.

13. Richardson RM. Decision making in epilepsy surgery. Neurosurg Clin North Am 2020;31(3):471–9.

Section I: Focus on Quality of Life

Pediatric Neurostimulation and Practice Evolution

Saadi Ghatan, MD[1]

KEYWORDS

- Neuromodulation • Childhood • Adolescent • Network • Connectome • Seizure • Epileptogenic

KEY POINTS

- Refractory pediatric epilepsy presents a lifelong challenge for patients and their families.
- Some of the challenges faced are dependence on antiseizure medicines, lost control of developmental potential, social isolation, and a future with dependence on others.
- When two medications fail, referral to a designated epilepsy center and consideration for surgical management should be made.
- Modern epilepsy surgery can be curative in some cases and helpful in most cases, reaching a broader population of children whose refractory epilepsies can be more challenging due to their multifocal, non-lesional, genetically associated, extratemporal, and network nature.

INTRODUCTION

Medically refractory pediatric epilepsy presents a lifelong challenge for patients and families. The prospect of dependence on antiseizure medications, lost developmental potential, social and familial isolation, and a future without independence are just some of the challenges faced. Given limited options when medications fail to control seizures, surgical evaluation must be entertained early and comprehensively. While epilepsy surgery can be curative in some cases, it can also help a broader population of refractory children whose epilepsies can be more challenging, where multifocal, non-lesional, genetically associated, extratemporal, and network epilepsies are typically encountered.

Technological advances in the past 15 years have brought about paradigm shifts[1] in epilepsy surgery, with diagnostic tools like robotic stereo-electroencephalography (sEEG), thermal ablation techniques to target epilepsies associated with deep-seated lesions, and neuromodulatory devices to treat nodal and network seizure disorders. Pediatric epilepsies are ideally suited to these advances. Herein, we will explore the factors behind a mandatory evolution toward neurostimulation and neuromodulatory approaches in pediatric epilepsy surgery, to help overcome the limitations of historical ablative and resective strategies, and ultimately reach a broader audience to make a safe and lasting impact on this vulnerable and underserved population.

Pediatric Epilepsy and Epilepsy Surgery: The Stakes

The burden of epilepsy is magnified beyond the suffering experienced by the patient: the loss of independence, uncertainty of future direction, and ongoing risk to physical and psychiatric health and wellness are well recognized by the individual, but family, caregivers, and society at large shoulder the weight of this disease. The gravity of this disorder is intensified in medically refractory epilepsy in children, where most seizures disorders will not be "outgrown," developmental potential will be lost, and a lifetime of dependence on family, social services, and the health care system will be seemingly inevitable. The psychological burden of living with a chronic disease is borne by the individual and family alike.

Dysregulated electrical activity in the form of seizures has myriad consequences in the developing

Neurological Surgery Icahn School of Medicine at Mt Sinai, New York, NY 10128, USA
[1] Present address: 1000 10th Avenue, Suite 10G, New York, NY 10019, USA
E-mail address: saadi.ghatan@mountsinai.org

Neurosurg Clin N Am 35 (2024) 1–15
https://doi.org/10.1016/j.nec.2023.09.006
1042-3680/24/© 2023 Elsevier Inc. All rights reserved.

brain. Repeated seizures put cognitive and sensori-motor development at risk: intellectual dysfunction can directly correlate with severity of epilepsy, particularly during the first few years of life.[2–5] As with cognition, global motor development can be delayed because of severe epilepsy in childhood, and focal sensorimotor dysfunction due to lateral-ized or regionalized epilepsy is a well-recognized phenomenon among pediatric epilepsy specialists. While side effects of antiseizure medications (ASMs) have been greatly reduced, early and more modern antiseizure medications can adversely affect sys-tems that include but are not limited to cognitive, vi-sual, hematopoietic, dermatologic, immune, and reproductive, to say nothing of the financial burden that some families must bear over the course of a child's life.[6,7]

Social, behavioral, and communication skills can be adversely affected by epilepsy: uncontrolled seizures are synonymous with poor school perfor-mance that ultimately restricts employment and economic productivity. Children with epilepsy are less likely to develop normal social relationships and ultimately marry,[8] and children with epilepsy will be more likely to be targeted by and suffer at the hands of emotional and sexual abuse than their counterparts without epilepsy.[9–11] Autism Spec-trum Disorder (ASD) and epilepsy are commonly linked, and the former's severity is exacerbated by the latter.[12–14] Psychiatric comorbidities of attention-deficit/hyperactivity disorder, anxiety, and depression are well known to occur in children with epilepsy.[15]

More rare but an omnipresent concern among families of children with epilepsy, mortality risk is 90-fold higher in children with medically intrac-table epilepsy in comparison to their healthy counterparts, and epilepsy is the most common cause of sudden death in children.[16,17] Sudden unexpected death in epilepsy (SUDEP) as well as traumatic injury and drowning due to seizures are difficult subjects to discuss with parents but must be acknowledged in the pediatric popula-tion. Over the course of a child's upbringing and adolescence, the risk is cumulative and substan-tial (10% over 20 years) and must be carefully weighed in medical and surgical decision-making.[16,18]

Pediatric Epilepsy: Non-surgical Therapeutics Options

While natural history and ASMs allow for about two-third of all patients with seizure disorders to become seizure free,[19,20] over one-third of pediat-ric patients will remain medically refractory.[21] Further non-surgical interventions are limited but include dietary changes and *repetitive Transcranial Magnetic Stimulation* (rTMS).

A well-documented response of seizure control to dietary changes has been established over a century of observation, more recently with ran-domized controlled trials (RCTs) that demonstrate that diets low in carbohydrates can provide better control when medication has failed.[22–24] In order of an increasing percentage of carbohydrates and protein from a bare minimum, the *ketogenic diet* , *modified Atkins Diet*, *Low Glycemic Index Diet*, and the *Medium Chain Triglyceride Diet* are variations on caloric intake that appear to work by multifactorial reduction in cortical hyperexcit-ability, with decreased glucose and increased ketone bodies having a beneficial effect on synap-tic stabilization and excitatory neurotransmitter decrease.[25] However, adherence and sustained compliance with these strict dietary regimes can be difficult to maintain[26] with about half of families being able to adhere to the strict diet at 1 year, directly correlating with seizure control. Parental stress in food preparation and strict adherence in the setting of refractory epilepsy no doubt plays a role in failed compliance in the long term.[27]

rTMS has shown some utility in the treatment of pediatric neurologic disorders such as depression, autism, tics, and hemiparesis due to early stroke, as well as adult migraine and depression. rTMS uses electromagnetic coils to inhibit neurons when given in low amplitude repetitive pulses that in theory could diminish cortical hyperexcit-ability. Nevertheless, its effectiveness in the treat-ment of epilepsy has not been established.[28] While TMS is a valuable experimental tool, that for example, can measure ASM effects on cortical hy-perexcitability, mixed results of its efficacy in sup-pressing ictal and interictal discharges has limited its widespread use.[29] Variability in coil structure and unstandardized stimulation paradigms used across studies has made it difficult to adopt rTMS on a large scale for the treatment of epilepsy in children, and a single RCT failed to show a sta-tistically beneficial effect.[30]

Pediatric Epilepsy Surgery: Concerns and Considerations

Sadly, when medical and non surgical options fail to adequately control seizures in children, further medication trials are the norm and lead to a delay in more definitive treatment, potentially exacer-bating the patient's epilepsy and causing further deterioration in quality of life and cognition.[31] The criterion for which children are considered medi-cally intractable is the same as that in adults: addi-tional medical therapies are unlikely to succeed in controlling seizures if epilepsy is refractory to 2 or more medications[19,21,32,33]. Expeditious referral to a comprehensive epilepsy center is critical to facilitate full evaluation and a discussion of diagnostic and therapeutic surgical options.

While all surgical decision-making should be made with advocacy, a critical aspect distinguishing pediatric epilepsy surgery from its adult counterpart is that treatment decisions are made by parents or guardians on behalf of the child in their care, and not by the surgical candidates themselves. In the past decade, narrative medicine has shed light on a major determinant of access to epilepsy surgery, which has historically been notoriously limited. Baca and colleagues[34] elegantly documented the journey to epilepsy surgery taken by parents as a "trip around the world," through video narratives. These recordings showed thematic consistencies as follows (1). A realization that epilepsy was a problem was followed by (2). A baffling, circuitous journey with multiple barriers including insurance obstacles to find a surgeon and center, and then (3). Accepting that surgery was not a catastrophic last resort, but rather a safer and less invasive option compared to suffering through years of seizures. Ultimately, (4). Parents were deeply satisfied with their decision and wanted to give back to other parents and families.

Another common concern among families of pediatric epilepsy surgery candidates is the child's ability to tolerate the hospital stay, especially if intracranial monitoring is involved. The stress associated with surgery and invasive monitoring is particularly worrisome for children with a history of behavioral issues or those who are too young or cognitively disabled to provide assent and cooperate with treatment. Pediatric epilepsy surgery candidates also have an increased incidence of neurodevelopmental conditions, most notably ASD, which can present a behavioral challenge during the hospital stay. Such cases can sometimes require additional medical and safety measures, and they are best managed at a specialized pediatric comprehensive epilepsy center by a multidisciplinary pediatric team of physicians, nurses, and other health care professionals.[14,35] A child-friendly environment allowing for family involvement during all stages of the hospital stay is crucial to the overall success of surgery. In the setting of invasive monitoring, ironically, epilepsy surgery becomes a safer and simpler undertaking: general anesthesia accompanies both diagnostic and therapeutic surgical interventions, allowing both intracranial and extracranial monitoring to be instituted without discomfort or anxiety to a patient who would otherwise be unable to cooperate.

But impediments to successful pediatric epilepsy surgery are not only referable to patient/family and/or referring provider attitudes: the myriad complexities of modern health care can be prohibitive to even the most enabled families. The journey toward pediatric epilepsy surgery, once embarked upon, has been described as "5 years of hell" in a well-documented analysis of parental experience.[36] This narrative experience underscores the need for a "champion" to act as an advocate and guide on behalf of the patient and family. A nurse navigator has been used by other centers[37,38] and the author's to provide advocacy in the navigation of health insurance challenges, treatment options, second and third opinions, and peer-support.

For parents and caregivers, holistic, team-based care in a comprehensive epilepsy center is the best way to overcome fear of any intervention, especially ablative, resective, or disconnective procedures that may have uncertain success rates immediate and remote, over the course of the child's life. Parents who are raising children with a chronic condition are an invaluable resource for other parents whose referral for surgery is being delayed by fear[34,39]

As this article highlights, epilepsy surgery through neurostimulation has evolved to ease many prior concerns accompanied ablative techniques. More novel neuromodulatory approaches implicitly bypass these fears because the treatments are less invasive, modulatory rather than destructive, and reversible if parental or patient satisfaction wanes.[40–42] Moreover, successful seizure control through neuromodulation can be built upon over the course of a child's development with inherent capitalization on the developing brain's plasticity. The safety of a closed loop system that is responsive rather than tonic obviates cognitive and mood concerns that accompany open loop devices and duty cycles in the developing brain.[43] Most importantly, a parent or patient advocate will be more likely to select a neuromodulatory approach over an ablative or resective strategy if there is clinical equipoise. The promise of technological advance in improving efficacy without added invasiveness has prompted multiple groups to use responsive neuromodulatory strategies off-label in children in the past 5 years, more of which will be discussed later.[40–42,44–53]

SURGICAL APPROACHES: DIAGNOSTIC

As with any medically refractory epilepsy patient, the surgical approach to the pediatric patient with epilepsy depends on the hypothesis formulated during presurgical evaluation. The goals of the operation, from cure to an improvement in quality of life,[1] are made clear in discussions with parents and caregivers, and single or staged approaches are undertaken depending on the findings. The surgical team's endeavor is the identification and understanding of epileptogenic networks and their disruption, whether this involves a discrete focus, zone of onset, a regionalized network, multifocal nodes, and even bilateral onsets. Later, an overview of the 3 main facets of pediatric epilepsy surgery are outlined (Diagnostic, Resective, and Neuromodulatory procedures), with reference to the more common etiologic conditions encountered, to provide a framework for application in specific cases.

The author considers stereo-Electroencephalography (sEEG) and Subdural Electrode techniques for intracranial electroclinical diagnosis, and therapeutic strategies such as Resective/Ablative/Disconnective approaches, with Neuromodulatory techniques together to demonstrate the utility of being facile with all modalities. Multiple diagnostic and therapeutic surgical options, employed appropriately, should increase utilization and early referral for surgery, and positively influence diagnostic and treatment goals. Implicit in each surgical choice is the understanding that no 1 approach to epilepsy should be considered exclusive: each technique can be used in combination to minimize invasiveness and side effects, as weapons in an armamentarium against epilepsy. Furthermore, specific epilepsy syndromes that frequently occur in the pediatric population are considered during discussions of technique, to emphasize that 1 treatment does not fit all etiologies, nor does 1 etiology necessarily have to depend on a single treatment.

Stereo-Electroencephalography

Robotic-assisted stereotactic navigation has transformed epilepsy monitoring due to its safety, minimally invasive nature, and utility in electroclinical diagnosis.[54,55] This well-developed technique using multiple-depth electrodes can determine laterality, regionalize, potentially localize the epileptogenic zone,[56,57] and ultimately provide insights into epileptogenic networks that can be targeted through neuromodulatory therapies[41] (Fig. 1).

The author frequently uses symmetric bilateral implantation strategies with bilateral thalamic sEEG leads[58,59] in cases where anatomicoelectroclinical data are not concordant, and in cases where the author hypothesizes that a neuromodulatory approach will be favored over an ablative/disconnective therapy, such as a "network epilepsy" like Lennox Gastaut Syndrome (LGS) or Tuberous Sclerosis (TS), genetic, and multifocal

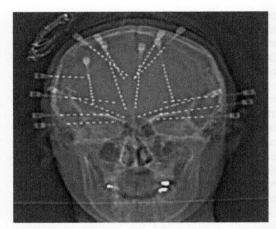

Fig. 1. Bilateral stereo-electroencephalography (sEEG) to investigate network epilepsy in a child.

non-lesional epilepsies. Rather than be dismissed as a "fishing expedition," symmetric bilateral implantations are meant to increase the utilization of epilepsy surgery for populations of children and adults who would have previously not been considered candidates for therapeutic approaches with responsive or deep brain neurostimulation. Furthermore, stimulation mapping through the electrodes can be performed in an attempt to map eloquent cortical areas, and to reproduce a child's seizures and to confirm localization of a seizure focus.[60] With pre-operative planning using volumetric contrast MRI and stereotactic guidance (frame-based, frameless, robotic, intraoperative MRI [iMRI]), hypotheses developed based strongly on semiology, the EEG, and MRI are used to guide depth electrode placement through multiple millimeter-sized twist drill holes, followed by long-term monitoring in the epilepsy monitoring unit. The efficiency, safety, efficacy, and tolerability of this approach have been well established, and current advances in imaging and robotic guidance have made this a popular approach among practitioners and families.[54,55,61–64]

Grid, Strip, and Depth Electrodes

Despite the enhanced safety, comfort, and ability to map networks across both hemispheres that sEEG affords, subdural electrode placement is still occasionally performed.[65] The safety of this technique has been well established,[66] and its main benefit appears to derive from the ability to perform extraoperative functional mapping. The capture and mapping of seizures occurs in the pediatric intensive care unit and epilepsy monitoring unit. Comprehensive motor, sensory, and language mapping can be performed extraoperatively in this population that is felt to be less likely to tolerate an awake craniotomy, even though it is safe, feasible, and well-tolerated but underutilized due to assumptions of greater vulnerability and fragility.[67,68] A second-stage operation is undertaken up to 1 to 2 weeks later, with the removal of electrodes and resection or disconnection of the epileptogenic zone as established through invasive mapping.

SURGICAL APPROACHES: THERAPEUTIC

Clear class 1 evidence demonstrating the effectiveness of epilepsy surgery over medical therapy in refractory cases exists for both pediatric and adult patients. The RCT by *Wiebe*[69] and Engel's study done early in the course of epilepsy[70] are now accompanied by an RCT in pediatric epilepsy surgery by Dwivedi,[71] revealing similar results, despite less defined epilepsy networks and more extratemporal and multifocal cases encountered in children. In this series, lesional, focal epilepsies were safely and effectively treated with resective epilepsy surgeries, with better rates of seizure control than their medically treated counterparts.[71] A prospective population-based longitudinal study found lasting seizure freedom and many children being weaned from antiseizure medications when referred early in the course of their epilepsy.[72] A recent systematic review further corroborated these results in children, albeit with a shrinking success rate in terms of seizure freedom at 10 years' follow-up.[73,74]

But even with RCTs demonstrating its efficacy, epilepsy surgery has remained woefully underutilized with myriad barriers as described earlier.[75] And as rates of diagnostic epilepsy surgeries have risen in the era of robotic sEEG-guided operations, therapeutic procedures have declined.[76] To understand why, we must examine the strengths and limitations of the traditional view of epilepsy surgery that revolves around identification and eradication of a focus. When we consider evolution toward network epilepsies, we see the ability to reach the larger population of potential surgical candidates.

Focal Resection/Ablation: The Limitations

Presently, the most commonly identified surgically remediable epilepsies in children occur with structural abnormalities, even though they are not representative of the majority of medically refractory epilepsy patients. Such patients can occasionally have epileptogenic foci targeted through single-stage approaches. The classic example of this encountered in pediatrics is the *Hypothalamic Hamartoma* causing gelastic seizures, effectively treated via stereotactically guided selective laser ablation (Laser Interstitial Thermal Therapy or LITT),[77,78] minimally invasive endoscopic,[79,80] and transcallosal/transventricular approaches.[81] Preliminary results for LITT in focal epilepsy from other less common sources in children, such as *mesial temporal sclerosis*, are variable,[82–85] and now more multicenter and metanalytical data demonstrating its safety and efficacy in children exist.[86–90] The author and others have used LITT with good results for *periventricular nodular heterotopias* in children, where access to dominant temporal or periatrial onset zones would be prohibitively invasive.[91]

Targeted resection or ablation of certain focal cortical dysplasias (FCDs) can achieve success with seizure freedom. In simple cases, where there is concordance between electroclinical characteristics and structural pathology, surgical cure rates can approach 75% in short-term follow-up.[73] Most commonly, well-localized seizures secondary to *type II cortical dysplasias* can be approached via a single-stage craniotomy and excision of the epileptogenic zone, when separate from eloquent cortical areas. Successful seizure control correlates with extent of resection of the radiographically apparent dysplastic region.[92–94] With proximity to functional cortical zones such as language, sensorimotor function, cognition, and visual function, this more comprehensive resective strategy is limited.

Type I dysplasia are generally diffuse, multilobar, and magnetic resonance (MR) negative, and surgery is associated with poorer outcomes by standard neurosurgical methods of excision, disconnection, or ablation.[94] In these cases, depending upon electroclinical diagnosis, a neuromodulatory approach can be considered, and is discussed later. *Type III FCDs* represent pathologic changes associated with structural abnormalities such as benign tumors, vascular malformations, or inflammatory changes.[95] Long-standing seizures secondary to cavernous malformations, tubers, low-grade tumors,[96,97] and other developmental epileptogenic lesions, such as *dysembryoplastic neuroepithelial tumors*, can be treated more effectively with staged approaches (eg, sEEG, subdural electrodes), depending on semiology and video-EEG characteristics, to comprehensively remove not only the MR-visibile abnormality but also the epileptogenic cortex surrounding the lesion. Some pediatric epilepsy surgery centers favor intraoperative electrocorticography to guide resection in single-stage approaches.[98] In simple cases, where there is concordance between electroclinical characteristics and structural pathology, surgical cure rates and complete seizure freedom can approach 75%

in short-term follow-up,[73] but reduce over 10 years to about 60% of patients having long-term seizure control.[74] Again, proximity to functional cortical areas can limit resection zones and negatively influence seizure control outcomes.

In *TS*, a common disorder seen in pediatric epilepsy surgical series, children develop tubers that developmentally and histologically resemble type 2 FCDs.[95] Stereo-EEG is an ideal tool for intracranial monitoring in patients with multiple tubers, given that both hemispheres and multiple targets can be safely interrogated with this technique. Surgical resection of a single or multiple epileptogenic tubers is an established and effective treatment of children with TS and medically refractory seizures,[99,100] but seizure recurrence after resection is common.[101] Limited experience with LITT has been compiled for treatment of tubers with mixed results and follow-up times are limited in those patients who have had beneficial outcomes, which are still in the minority among the few dozen patients accumulated.[82–84]

Other structural etiologies amenable to focal resection include vascular lesions, with *cavernous malformations*, *arteriovenous malformations*, and gliotic injury caused by *early childhood stroke*, and all can lead to potential cures with surgical intervention through similar single or staged approaches. Although children are rarely affected by ischemic, embolic, or hemorrhagic cerebrovascular accidents, up to two-thirds may develop epilepsy after perinatal strokes and hypoxic or ischemic injury, and 25% of those will develop intractable epilepsy. In this population, treatment options range from focal to multilobar resections, disconnections and even hemispherotomies, most effectively guided by intracranial electrode monitoring.[102]

Epilepsy associated with *cavernous malformations* is more common when the cavernoma is cortical rather than subcortical. Other risk factors for epilepsy include temporal localization, multiple cavernomas, volume of the cavernoma, volume of the hemosiderin ring, and male sex. Surgical decision-making can be guided by correlating semiology with electrodiagnostic findings, and removal of the lesion and the hemosiderin ring and early intervention are advocated based upon safety and expected efficacy.[103] The author feels that the use of adjunctive invasive monitoring should be used in cases of long-standing intractability, since adjacent cortical and allocortical structures can often, independently, become epileptogenic,[104] although extended resection compared to lesionectomy alone has been called into question in a recent meta-analysis[105] and more recent series[106,] and again, proximity to

eloquent cortical and subcortical areas can limit resection or ablation of the associated epileptogenic zone.

Hemispherotomy/Disconnections

The classical paradigm of balancing seizure management and the loss of developmental potential is represented in the hemispheric epilepsies of childhood. Disorders like *Rasmussen Encephalitis (RE)*, *hemimegalencephaly*, and *Sturge–Weber Syndrome* are rare overall but well known in pediatric epilepsy centers, and present disabling and functionally damaging refractory seizures in childhood which have warranted epilepsy surgery in its most extreme form: *hemispheric disconnection*. This "gold standard"[107] treatment of hemispherotomy puts function associated with the hemisphere at risk of permanent loss but is justified given the risk of functional loss inextricably linked with ongoing seizures. The plasticity of the pediatric brain to compensate for such a comprehensive disconnection, when sustained early in childhood, justifies the invasiveness of the approach. Nevertheless, the long-term consequences of hemispherotomy must be carefully considered.

Multiple single center[107–109] and multicenter systematic reviews and meta-analyses[74,110–112,] show seizure freedom rates in over two-thirds of the patients but significant rates of functional loss and language difficulties when the dominant hemisphere is targeted.[113,114] Nahum and Liegois[115] performed a systematic review of language outcomes after left and right hemispherectomy in childhood with 1 to 15 years of follow-up, and found that for left hemispheric disconnections, all language skills were impaired except those for reading comprehension. Overall, these analyses reveal that the further removed from surgery a child advances, the lower the seizure freedom rate, and the greater the consequences of having lost language and cognitive skills, calling into question the dogma that hemispherotomy is a "gold standard" for pediatric hemispheric epilepsy in all cases. A measured approach taking into account developmental age (under or over 5), contralateral epileptiform irritability, and etiology (eg, perinatal stroke vs post meningitic epilepsy) allows for a holistic analysis of long-term risk and benefit from hemispherotomy as it concerns language development.[116]

The hemispherotomy technique involves intraventricular disruption of the descending outputs of the temporal, parietal, and frontal lobes, a frontal disconnection, complete corpus callosotomy, and insular topectomy.[117,118] Endoscopic-assisted approaches have been described recently,[119] to overcome the invasiveness and potential side effects such as hydrocephalus and superficial hemosiderosis that can be seen after larger exposures and resections.[117,118,120]

RE is a rare chronic inflammatory epilepsy and progressive disorder. The neurologic deficits are progressive and include hemiparesis, cognitive decline, and even aphasia (if the dominant hemisphere is affected.) Children with RE have severe unilateral focal epilepsy, and often *epilepsia partialis continua*. Although the MRI is often normal in the early stages of the disease, focal cortical swelling can be noted in some patients early in the disease, but the hallmark of the disease is progressive hemispheric atrophy. Surgical treatment is most commonly hemispherotomy. While effective in arresting the potentially catastrophic hemispheric epilepsies of infancy and early childhood, a recent long-term study showed only a palliative effect from hemispherotomy/hemispherectomy in RE, with only 22% seizure freedom at 10 years post-operatively, and considerable morbidity with speech and motor deficits,[109] and a quest for less invasive immunomodulatory and neuromodulatory strategies are necessary, as discussed later.

Callosotomy

First introduced by Van Wagenen in 1940,[121] this procedure is used primarily in the setting of atonic seizures, and at the author's center, division of the corpus callosum is done through a small vertex craniotomy. The author and others[122] favor the lateral position with the head tilted 45° toward vertical, to allow gravity to gently create space in the interhemispheric fissure and completely section the callosum in an extraventricular fashion, finding and maintaining the plane between the leaves of the septum pellucidum. A complete callosotomy is usually performed, with minimal long-term morbidity[123] and significant relief of atonic seizures.[124] The author has used this technique to ameliorate seizures associated with cyanosis and apnea as well. Recently, the concept of posterior callosotomy has been described to spare prefrontal connectivity with good results at 4 year follow-up,[125] and seemingly less invasive endoscopic[126] and LITT[127] approaches have recently been proposed. The most common complications include disconnection syndromes,[128] transient mutism, and weakness.[129] Whatever the methodology, the operations are irreversible and must be considered invasive given their finality and inability to ensure lasting seizure control in a pediatric population.

Toward a Neuromodulatory Strategy

The multigenerational mindset that resective surgery is superior in efficacy to neuromodulatory therapy may be true in select cases, but focal approaches to epilepsy surgery can fail and will restrict a large population of patients with refractory seizures in need of help. A neuromodulatory approach has many advantages for improving utilization of epilepsy surgery in this underserved population that includes patients with generalized, network, multifocal, and genetic epilepsies.

Overall, children represent a population that could be prime beneficiaries of a modulatory rather than ablative, resective approach. The finality and irreversibility of disconnections, resections, and ablations do not apply in neuromodulatory approaches. Rather than single therapeutic interventions that apply in cases of ablative epilepsy surgery, electrical stimulation strategies employ long-term daily therapeutic input that typically provides improvemed seizure control with time[130] in contradistinction to long-term seizure control rates after resective surgery that drop with time.[73,74] Intuitively, parents faced with the difficult decision regarding the surgical management of their child's epilepsy would more easily accept a strategy that provides safety, reversibility, and modulation with advancements in technology, all the while without threat to preservation of function. Such promise would most certainly change the utilization rates of epilepsy surgery once medical refractory epilepsy is determined.

Vagus Nerve Stimulation

Some class I evidence exists to show that Vagus Nerve Stimulation (VNS) is useful for children with generalized or multifocal epilepsy.[131] Englot and colleagues performed a systematic analysis to evaluate rates of and factors related to seizure freedom and response to VNS.[132] Factors associated with response were age of onset greater than 12 and non-lesional epilepsy, with less than 10% of patients achieving seizure freedom. A major concern of parents is the risk of SUDEP, discussed earlier, and several large-scale analyses have failed to show a benefit of VNS in reducing SUDEP risk in children.[133,134] A more recent survey of SUDEP in a parental reports cohort identified 46 cases of SUDEP, with most cases occurring in the 12 to 16 year age group, more commonly in children with neurodisabilities, and during sleep. Of note, 4 of these 46 patients had VNS at the time of death.[135]

Deep Brain Stimulation

Another neuromodulatory strategy, deep brain stimulation (DBS), has been extensively studied in adults[136] but limited data exist to highlight the experience in children.[137] Targets such as the centromedian (CM) and anterior thalamic nuclei have been chosen for most of these patients, who have mostly had generalized epilepsy, with mixed results. The author has used a directional lead in the bilateral CM with good results for a 17-year-old with multifocal epilepsy after failed temporal lobectomy, but generally has not favored an open-loop system, given the advantages of a responsive rather than tonic treatment strategy and the opportunity to obtain chronic recordings and biomarkers with Responsive Neurostimulation (RNS).

Responsive Neurostimulation

Ideally, a surgical approach that is minimally invasive, maximally effective, and modifiable with time, patient-specific needs, and technologic advances should be chosen for a child, whose developmental and epilepsy requirements may also change with time. Responsive neurostimulation (RNS) appears to fulfill this promise, but has been tested and used in an adult population to date,[130,138] and used off label by the authors' group[35,40–42,139] and others.[44–53] Seizure control results have been favorable and seem to be improving with duration of therapy in children the author has treated, with safety and tolerability in line with other implantation data for neurostimulation in the pediatric and adult population.[42,140,141]

In a near decade-long analysis, RNS has demonstrated improved results with a greater duration of stimulation,[130] suggesting a facilitation or programmed reorganization of hitherto disorganized epileptogenic networks. The immature pediatric brain is a logical therapeutic target given its inherent plasticity and potential for modulation. Furthermore, given that the technique is modulatory rather than ablative, neurostimulation allows for revision and advance with time and age. Regional networks, extratemporal localization, and temporal-plus epilepsy, which are more prevalent in children, may be better served by influencing a network rather than disconnecting or ablating tissue, as the author's preliminary evidence suggests[35,40–42,44,139,142] SUDEP rates are lower than expected in patients undergoing RNS therapy, but those data are derived from an adult population.[130,143]

Responsive Neurostimulation: Case Evolution to Guide Application

In the author's group, the evolution to using RNS was borne out of failure, with the recognition that resective and disconnective strategies were of limited benefit in certain patients[40] and populations.[14] The author first reported its use in 2 children, one of whom had undergone multiple operations including a frontal lobectomy and complete callosotomy, and a second in whose epilepsy was associated with language and Rolandic eloquent areas.[40] Both benefited, but the first patient, a traditional surgical failure, reflected a larger population of children with epilepsy and autism who, contrary to prevailing attitudes[144] did well with resective strategies when they had lesional epilepsy, but poorly when non-lesional etiologies seemed to be associated with regionality or focality.[14] The author changed his strategy in this autistic pediatric population with non-focal epilepsy, and achieved good seizure control in two-thirds and excellent seizure reduction (>90%) in a quarter of the patients.[35,41]

A larger series of children who underwent RNS placement from the author's center[42] included a patient with TS who failed multiple tuberectomies before achieving complete seizure control with an approach that incorporated sEEG and RNS with a depth lead in a dominant motor cortical tuber. Other patients included 2 with RE, for whom the author had used a combination of immunotherapy, VNS, and RNS with >90% seizure reduction, and no progression of sensorimotor or cognitive deficits at 9 and 5 years' follow-up (**Fig. 2**). Multimodal therapeutic application in this series comes from a 16 yo with a dominant temporal periventricular nodular heterotopia and good hippocampal function on that side. LITT had been applied to the periventricular nodular heterotopia and a long axis hippocampal and anterior thalamic nucleus depth electrode had been used in an attempt to control seizures while protecting memory.

Another patient in this series initially had a hemispherotomy for post meningitic epilepsy. Her seizures recurred on the contralateral, dominant

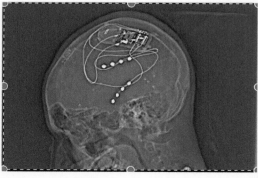

Fig. 2. Lateral Skull X-Ray of a child with Rasmussen Encephalitis and a Responsive Neurostimulator with leads over the Rolandic region and dominant temporal lobe.

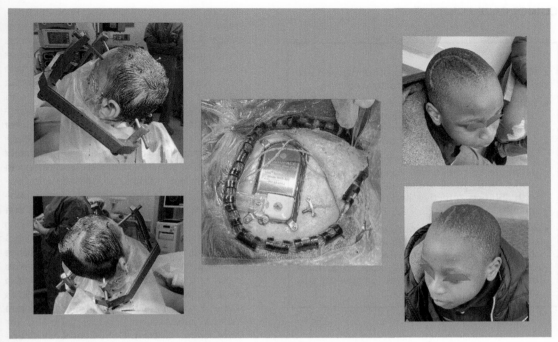

Fig. 3. Intraoperative and post operative demonstrations of Thalamic RNS placement in children.

side, and here the author eventually employed a thalamocortical RNS system in the setting of LGS epilepsy. The author had used centromedian thalamic stimulation before for LGS and autism[41] and this 'failed hemispherectomy' patient's care reflects a further evolution in the author's treatment strategies toward a neuromodulatory approach incorporating thalamic-responsive neurostimulation.[139,144]

The author has used thalamocortical and pure thalamic RNS (**Fig 3**) in 21 children with network epilepsies, and etiologies ranging from a 12 yo with generalized epilepsy and TS, to multifocal limbic epilepsy in a 14 year old with a non-lesional MRI, to a band heterotopia in a 10 year old. Overall, 8 children with thalamocortical leads appeared to fare better than the others with pure thalamic implants, thus far with 50% achieving greater than 75% seizure control and 2 children were seizure free at a mean follow-up of about 4 years. Not surprisingly, the author's preliminary connectivity analyses employing tractography to calculate the connectivity between the volume of tissue activated by the RNS and the seizure onset zone appear to show better seizure control when the seizure onset zone has higher connectivity strength to the implanted thalamic electrode's stimulated area. Such individualized strategies[145] combined with better data

analytics[146,147] can help us to achieve more comprehensive outcomes in this heretofore untreated population.

SUMMARY

Pediatric epilepsy surgery is rapidly gaining momentum as practitioners and parents realize the safety and efficacy of this discipline, when compared with the hazards posed by epilepsy to the developing brain and the long-term consequences of uncontrolled seizures as children grow to adulthood. By overcoming historical biases of the dangers of neurosurgical intervention, we have made pediatric epilepsy surgery increasingly accessible, although it is still a severely underused therapeutic modality. Minimally invasive diagnostic techniques such as sEEG, selective thermal ablation techniques like LITT, the promise of long-term monitoring and machine learning with closed-loop devices with faster time to efficacy in treatment, and the potential to mitigate epileptic encephalopathies in children through neuromodulation are rapidly being accepted. Taken together with further advances in the ability to detect epileptogenic networks and putative structural culprits through neuroimaging, pediatric epilepsy surgery remains a field with significant growth potential for rapid evolution.

CLINICS CARE POINTS

- Epilepsy surgery remains profoundly underutilized in children with refractory epilepsy.
- When children fail to achieve adequate seizure control with two medicines, referral to a comprehensive epilepsy center is necessary to consider potential surgical options.
- Stereo EEG is safe and effective for children to delineate seizure onset zones, epilepsy networks, and guide therapeutic management with ablative, resective, and neuromodulatory techniques.
- Although not yet FDA approved for use in children, Responsive Neurostimulation has been shown to be safe and effective in pediatric epilepsy and has opened the door to a much broader range of candidates for epilepsy surgery.

ACKNOWLEDGEMENT

Funder: NINDS Grant ID: 1UH3NS109557-01A1 and NINDS Grant ID: 1R61NS126776-01A1.

REFERENCES

1. Richardson RM. Closed-Loop Brain Stimulation and Paradigm Shifts in Epilepsy Surgery. Neurol Clin 2022;40(2):355–73.
2. Camfield C, Camfield P, Gordon K, et al. Outcome of childhood epilepsy: a population-based study with a simple predictive scoring system for those treated with medication. J Pediatr 1993;122:861–8.
3. Camfield C, Camfield P. Preventable and unpreventable causes of childhood-onset epilepsy plus mental retardation. Pediatrics 2007;120:e52–5.
4. Bjornaes H, Stabell K, Henriksen O, et al. The effects of refractory epilepsy on intellectual functioning in children and adults. A longitudinal study. Seizure 2001;10:250–9.
5. Berg AT, Zelko FA, Levy SR, et al. Age at onset of epilepsy, pharmacoresistance, and cognitive outcomes: a prospective cohort study. Neurology 2012;79:1384–91.
6. Canevini MP, De Sarro G, Galimberti CA, et al. Relationship between adverse effects of antiepileptic drugs, number of coprescribed drugs, and drug load in a large cohort of consecutive patients with drug-refractory epilepsy. Epilepsia 2010;51:797–804.
7. Kowski AB, Weissinger F, Gaus V, et al. Specific adverse effects of antiepileptic drugs - A true-to-life monotherapy study. Epilepsy Behav 2016;54:150–7.
8. Geerts A, Brouwer O, van Donselaar C, et al. Health perception and socioeconomic status following childhood-onset epilepsy: the Dutch study of epilepsy in childhood. Epilepsia 2011;52:2192–202.
9. Nimmo-Smith V, Brugha TS, Kerr MP, et al. Discrimination, domestic violence, abuse, and other adverse life events in people with epilepsy: Population-based study to assess the burden of these events and their contribution to psychopathology. Epilepsia 2016;57(11):1870–8.
10. Labudda K, Illies D, Herzig C, et al. Current psychiatric disorders in patients with epilepsy are predicted by maltreatment experiences during childhood. Epilepsy Res 2017;135:43–9.
11. Vederhus J, Husebye ESN, Eid K, et al. Prevalence of self-reported emotional, physical, and sexual abuse and association with fear of childbirth in pregnant women with epilepsy: The Norwegian Mother, Father, and Child Cohort Study. Epilepsia 2022;63(7):1822–34.
12. Danielsson S, Gillberg IC, Billstedt E, et al. Epilepsy in young adults with autism: a prospective population-based follow-up study of 120 individuals diagnosed in childhood. Epilepsia 2005;46:918–23.
13. Jeste SS, Tuchman R. Autism spectrum disorder and epilepsy: two sides of the same coin? J Child Neurol 2015;30:1963–71.
14. Kokoszka MA, McGoldrick PE, La Vega-Talbott M, et al. Epilepsy surgery in patients with autism. J Neurosurg Pediatr 2017;19(2):196–207.
15. Tellez-Zenteno JF, Patten SB, Jette N, et al. Psychiatric comorbidity in epilepsy: a population-based analysis. Epilepsia 2007;48:2336–44.
16. Tellez-Zenteno JF, Ronquillo LH, Wiebe S. Sudden unexpected death in epilepsy: evidence-based analysis of incidence and risk factors. Epilepsy Res 2005;65:101–15.
17. Tomson T, Nashef L, Ryvlin P. Sudden unexpected death in epilepsy: current knowledge and future directions. Lancet Neurol 2008;7:1021–31.
18. Sillanpää M, Shinnar S. SUDEP and other causes of mortality in childhood-onset epilepsy. Epilepsy Behav 2013;28(2):249–55.
19. Kwan P, Brodie MJ. Early identification of refractory epilepsy. N Engl J Med 2000;342(5):314–9.
20. Kwan P, Sperling MR. Refractory seizures: try additional antiepileptic drugs (after two have failed) or go directly to early surgery evaluation? Epilepsia 2009;50(Suppl 8):57–62.
21. Farrell K, Wirrell E, Whiting S. The definition and prediction of intractable epilepsy in children. Adv Neurol 2006;97:435–42.

22. Neal EG, Chaffe H, Schwartz RH, et al. The keto-genic diet for the treatment of childhood epilepsy: a randomised controlled trial. Lancet Neurol 2008; 7(6):500–6.

23. Sharma S, Sankhyan N, Gulati S, et al. Use of the modified Atkins diet for treatment of refractory childhood epilepsy: a randomized controlled trial. Epilepsia 2013;54(3):481–6.

24. Lambrechts DA, de Kinderen RJ, Vles JS, et al. A randomized controlled trial of the ketogenic diet in refractory childhood epilepsy. Acta Neurol Scand 2017;135(2):231–9.

25. D'Andrea Meira I, Romão TT, Pires do Prado HJ, et al. Ketogenic Diet and Epilepsy: What We Know So Far. Front Neurosci 2019;13:5.

26. Tong X, Deng Y, Liu L, et al. Clinical implementation of ketogenic diet in children with drug-resistant epilepsy: Advantages, disadvantages, and difficulties. Seizure 2022;99:75–81.

27. Operto FF, Labate A, Aiello S, et al. The Ketogenic Diet in Children with Epilepsy: A Focus on Parental Stress and Family Compliance. Nutrients 2023;15(4):1058.

28. Malone LA, Sun LR. Transcranial Magnetic Stimulation for the Treatment of Pediatric Neurological Disorders. Curr Treat Options Neurol 2019;21(11):58.

29. Tsuboyama M, Kaye HL, Rotenberg A. Review of Transcranial Magnetic Stimulation in Epilepsy. Clin Ther 2020;42(7):1155–68.

30. Cantello R, Rossi S, Varrasi C, et al. Slow repetitive TMS for drug-resistant epilepsy: clinical and EEG findings of a placebo-controlled trial. Epilepsia 2007;48(2):366–74.

31. Vasilica AM, Winsor A, Chari A, et al. The influence of disease course and surgery on quality of life in children with focal cortical dysplasia and long-term epilepsy-associated tumours: A systematic review and meta-analysis. Epilepsy Res 2023;192:107132.

32. Arts WF, Geerts AT, Brouwer OF, et al. The early prognosis of epilepsy in childhood: the prediction of a poor outcome. The Dutch study of epilepsy in childhood. Epilepsia 1999;40(6):726–34.

33. Go C, Snead OC 3rd. Pharmacologically intractable epilepsy in children: diagnosis and preoperative evaluation. Neurosurg Focus 2008;25(3):E2.

34. Baca CB, Pieters HC, Iwaki TJ, et al. "A journey around the world": Parent narratives of the journey to pediatric resective epilepsy surgery and beyond. Epilepsia 2015;56(6):822–32.

35. Fields MC, Marsh C, Eka O, et al. Responsive neurostimulation for people with drug-resistant epilepsy and autism spectrum disorder. J Clin Neurophysiol 2022. https://doi.org/10.1097/WNP.0000000000000939.

36. Pieters HC, Iwaki T, Vickrey BG, et al. "It was five years of hell": Parental experiences of navigating and processing the slow and arduous time to pediatric resective epilepsy surgery. Epilepsy Behav 2016;62:276–84.

37. Anand SK, Macki M, Culver LG, et al. Patient navigation in epilepsy care. Epilepsy Behav 2020;113: 107530.

38. Drees C, Sillau S, Brown MG, et al. Preoperative evaluation for epilepsy surgery: Process improvement. Neurol Clin Pract 2017;7(3):205–13.

39. Shilling V, Morris C, Thompson-Coon J, et al. Peer support for parents of children with chronic disabling conditions: a systematic review of quantitative and qualitative studies. Dev Med Child Neurol 2013;55:602–9.

40. Kokoszka MA, Panov F, La Vega-Talbott M, et al. Treatment of medically refractory seizures with responsive neurostimulation: 2 pediatric cases. J Neurosurg Pediatr 2018;21(4):421–7.

41. Kwon CS, Schupper AJ, Fields MC, et al. Centromedian thalamic responsive neurostimulation for Lennox-Gastaut epilepsy and autism. Ann Clin Transl Neurol 2020.

42. Panov F, Ganaha S, Haskell J, et al. Safety of responsive neurostimulation in pediatric patients with medically intractable epilepsy. J Neurosurg Pediatr 2020;26:5325–32.

43. Olaciregui Dague K, Witt JA, von Wrede R, et al. DBS of the ANT for refractory epilepsy: A single center experience of seizure reduction, side effects and neuropsychological outcomes. Front Neurol 2023;14:1106511.

44. Singhal NS, Numis AL, Lee MB, et al. Responsive neurostimulation for treatment of pediatric drug-resistant epilepsy. Epilepsy Behav Case Rep 2018;10:21–4.

45. Bercu MM, Friedman D, Silverberg A, et al. Responsive neurostimulation for refractory epilepsy in the pediatric population: A single-center experience. Epilepsy Behav 2020;112:107389.

46. Mortazavi A, Elliott RS, Phan TN, et al. Responsive neurostimulation for the treatment of medically refractory epilepsy in pediatric patients: strategies, outcomes, and technical considerations. J Neurosurg Pediatr 2021;28(1):54–61.

47. Nagahama Y, Zervos TM, Murata KK, et al. Real-World Preliminary Experience With Responsive Neurostimulation in Pediatric Epilepsy: A Multicenter Retrospective Observational Study. Neurosurgery 2021;89(6):997–1004.

48. Falls N, Arango JI, Adelson PD. Responsive neurostimulation in pediatric patients with drug-resistant epilepsy. Neurosurg Focus 2022;53(4):E9.

49. Curtis K, Hect JL, Harford E, et al. Responsive neurostimulation for pediatric patients with drug-resistant epilepsy: a case series and review of the literature. Neurosurg Focus 2022;53(4):E10.

50. Hartnett SM, Greiner HM, Arya R, et al. Responsive neurostimulation device therapy in pediatric patients with complex medically refractory epilepsy. J Neurosurg Pediatr 2022;1–8. https://doi.org/10.3171/2022.7.PEDS2281.

51. Kerezoudis P, Gyftopoulos A, Alexander AY, et al. Safety and efficacy of responsive neurostimulation in the pediatric population: Evidence from institutional review and patient-level meta-analysis. Epilepsy Behav 2022;129:108646.

52. Singh RK, Eschbach K, Samanta D, et al, PERC Surgery Registry Workgroup. Responsive Neurostimulation in Drug-Resistant Pediatric Epilepsy: Findings From the Epilepsy Surgery Subgroup of the Pediatric Epilepsy Research Consortium. Pediatr Neurol 2023;143:106–12.

53. Karakas C, Houck K, Handoko M, et al. Responsive Neurostimulation for the Treatment of Children With Drug-Resistant Epilepsy in Tuberous Sclerosis Complex. Pediatr Neurol 2023;145:97–101.

54. Cossu M, Cardinale F, Castana L, et al. Stereo-EEG in children. Childs Nerv Syst 2006;22(8):766–78.

55. McGovern RA, Knight EP, Gupta A, et al. Robot-assisted stereoelectroencephalography in children. J Neurosurg Pediatr 2018;23(3):288–96.

56. Talairach J, David M, Tournoux PL. Exploration chirurgicale stéréotaxique de lobe temporal dans L'épilepsie temporale. Paris: Masson, Libraires de l'Academie de Medecine; 1958.

57. Taussig D, Chipaux M, Lebas A, et al. Stereo-electroencephalography (SEEG) in 65 children: an effective and safe diagnostic method for presurgical diagnosis, independent of age. Epileptic Disord 2014;16(3):280–95.

58. Gadot R, Korst G, Shofty B, et al. Thalamic stereoelectroencephalography in epilepsy surgery: a scoping literature review. J Neurosurg 2022;1–16. https://doi.org/10.3171/2022.1.JNS212613.

59. Edmonds B, Miyakoshi M, Remore LG, et al. Characteristics of ictal thalamic EEG in pediatric-onset neocortical focal epilepsy. medRxiv [Preprint] 2023;23291714. https://doi.org/10.1101/2023.06.22.23291714. Update in: Clin Neurophysiol. 2023 Aug 6;154:116-125.

60. Young JJ, Coulehan K, Fields MC, et al. Language mapping using electrocorticography versus stereoelectroencephalography: A case series. Epilepsy Behav 2018;84:148–51.

61. Cossu M, Schiariti M, Francione S, et al. Stereoelectroencephalography in the presurgical evaluation of focal epilepsy in infancy and early childhood. J Neurosurg Pediatr 2012;9(3):290–300.

62. Sacino MF, Huang SS, Schreiber J, et al. Is the use of Stereotactic Electroencephalography Safe and Effective in Children? A Meta-Analysis of the use of Stereotactic Electroencephalography in Comparison to Subdural Grids for Invasive Epilepsy Monitoring in Pediatric Subjects. Neurosurgery 2019;84(6):1190–200.

63. Kim LH, Parker JJ, Ho AL, et al. Postoperative outcomes following pediatric intracranial electrode monitoring: A case for stereoelectroencephalography (SEEG). Epilepsy Behav 2020;104(Pt A):106905.

64. Triano MJ, Schupper AJ, Ghatan S, et al. Hemorrhage Rates After Implantation and Explantation of Stereotactic Electroencephalography: Reevaluating Patients' Risk. World Neurosurg 2021;151:e100–8.

65. Ghatan S. Surgery for epilepsy. Pediatr Ann 2006;35:386–93.

66. Johnston JM Jr, Mangano FT, Ojemann JG, et al. Complications of invasive subdural electrode monitoring at St. Louis Children's Hospital, 1994-2005. J Neurosurg 2006;105:343–7.

67. Lohkamp LN, Mottolese C, Szathmari A, et al. Awake brain surgery in children-review of the literature and state-of-the-art. Childs Nerv Syst 2019;35(11):2071–7.

68. Bhanja D, Sciscent BY, Daggubati LC, et al. Awake craniotomies in the pediatric population: a systematic review. J Neurosurg Pediatr 2023;1–9. https://doi.org/10.3171/2023.4.PEDS22296.

69. Wiebe S, Blume WT, Girvin JP, et al. Effectiveness and Efficiency of Surgery for Temporal Lobe Epilepsy Study Group. A randomized, controlled trial of surgery for temporal-lobe epilepsy. N Engl J Med 2001;345(5):311–8.

70. Engel J Jr, McDermott MP, Wiebe S, et al. Early Randomized Surgical Epilepsy Trial (ERSET) Study Group. Early surgical therapy for drug-resistant temporal lobe epilepsy: a randomized trial. JAMA 2012;307(9):922–30.

71. Dwivedi R, Ramanujam B, Chandra PS, et al. Surgery for Drug-Resistant Epilepsy in Children. N Engl J Med 2017 Oct 26;377(17):1639–47.

72. Reinholdson J, Olsson I, Edelvik A, et al. Long-term follow-up after epilepsy surgery in infancy and early childhood–a prospective population based observational study. Seizure 2015;30:83–9.

73. Widjaja E, Jain P, Demoe L, et al. Seizure outcome of pediatric epilepsy surgery: Systematic review and meta-analyses. Neurology 2020;94(7):311–21.

74. Harris WB, Brunette-Clement T, Wang A, et al. Long-term outcomes of pediatric epilepsy surgery: Individual participant data and study level meta-analyses. Seizure 2022;101:227–36.

75. Samanta D, Ostendorf AP, Willis E, et al. Underutilization of epilepsy surgery: part I: a scoping review of barriers. Epilepsy Behav 2021;117:107837.

76. Ostendorf AP, Ahrens SM, Lado FA, et al. United States Epilepsy Center Characteristics: A Data Analysis From the National Association of Epilepsy Centers. Neurology 2022;98(5):e449–58.

77. Curry DJ, Gowda A, McNichols RJ, et al. MR-guided stereotactic laser ablation of epileptogenic foci in children. Epilepsy Behav 2012;24:408–14.

78. Wilfong AA, Curry DJ. Hypothalamic hamartomas: optimal approach to clinical evaluation and diagnosis. Epilepsia 2013;54(suppl 9):109–14.

79. Akai T, Okamoto K, Iizuka H, et al. Treatments of hamartoma with neuroendoscopic surgery and stereotactic radiosurgery: a case report. Minim Invasive Neurosurg 2002;45:235–9.

80. Feiz-Erfan I, Horn EM, Rekate HL, et al. Surgical strategies for approaching hypothalamic hamartomas causing gelastic seizures in the pediatric population: transventricular compared with skull base approaches. J Neurosurg 2005;103:325–32.

81. Mittal S, Mittal M, Montes JL, et al. Hypothalamic hamartomas. Part 2. Surgical considerations and outcome. Neurosurg Focus 2013;34:E7.

82. Hooten KG, Werner K, Mikati MA, et al. MRI-guided laser interstitial thermal therapy in an infant with tuberous sclerosis: technical case report. J Neurosurg Pediatr 2018;23(1):92–7.

83. Stellon MA, Cobourn K, Whitehead MT, et al. "Laser and the Tuber": thermal dynamic and volumetric factors influencing seizure outcomes in pediatric subjects with tuberous sclerosis undergoing stereoencephalography-directed laser ablation of tubers. Childs Nerv Syst 2019;35(8):1333–40.

84. Tovar-Spinoza Z, Ziechmann R, Zyck S. Single and staged laser interstitial thermal therapy ablation for cortical tubers causing refractory epilepsy in pediatric patients. Neurosurg Focus 2018;45(3):E9.

85. Lewis EC, Weil AG, Duchowny M, et al. MR-guided laser interstitial thermal therapy for pediatric drug-resistant lesional epilepsy. Epilepsia 2015;56:1590–8.

86. Perry MS, Donahue DJ, Malik SI, et al. Magnetic resonance imaging-guided laser interstitial thermal therapy as treatment for intractable insular epilepsy in children. J Neurosurg Pediatr 2017;20(6):575–82.

87. Hoppe C, Helmstaedter C. Laser interstitial thermotherapy (LiTT) in pediatric epilepsy surgery. Seizure 2020;77:69–75.

88. Slingerland AL, Chua MMJ, Bolton J, et al. Stereoelectroencephalography followed by combined electrode removal and MRI-guided laser interstitial thermal therapy or open resection: a single-center series in pediatric patients with medically refractory epilepsy. J Neurosurg Pediatr 2022;31(3):206–11.

89. Arocho-Quinones EV, Lew SM, Handler MH, et al, Pediatric Stereotactic Laser Ablation Workgroup. Pediatric Stereotactic Laser Ablation Workgroup. Magnetic resonance imaging-guided stereotactic laser ablation therapy for the treatment of pediatric epilepsy: a retrospective multiinstitutional study. J Neurosurg Pediatr 2023;1–14. https://doi.org/10.3171/2022.12.PEDS22282.

90. Chen JS, Lamoureux AA, Shlobin NA, et al. Magnetic resonance-guided laser interstitial thermal therapy for drug-resistant epilepsy: A systematic review and individual participant data meta-analysis. Epilepsia 2023;64(8):1957–74.

91. Esquenazi Y, Kalamangalam GP, Slater JD, et al. Stereotactic laser ablation of epileptogenic periventricular nodular heterotopia. Epilepsy Res 2014;108(3):547–54.

92. Kloss S, Pieper T, Pannek H, et al. Epilepsy surgery in children with focal cortical dysplasia (FCD): results of long-term seizure outcome. Neuropediatrics 2002;33(1):21–6.

93. Krsek P, Maton B, Jayakar P, et al. Incomplete resection of focal cortical dysplasia is the main predictor of poor postsurgical outcome. Neurology 2009;72(3):217–23.

94. Kwon HE, Eom S, Kang HC, et al. Surgical treatment of pediatric focal cortical dysplasia: Clinical spectrum and surgical outcome. Neurology 2016; 87(9):945–51.

95. Crino PB. Focal Cortical Dysplasia. Semin Neurol 2015;35(3):201–8.

96. Berger MS, Ghatan S, Geyer JR, et al. Seizure outcome in children with hemispheric tumors and associated intractable epilepsy: the role of tumor removal combined with seizure foci resection. Pediatr Neurosurg 1991-1992;17(4):185–91.

97. Berger MS, Ghatan S, Haglund MM, et al. Low-grade gliomas associated with intractable epilepsy: Seizure outcome utilizing electrocorticography during tumor resection. J Neurosurg 1993;79:62–9.

98. Wu JY, Salamon N, Kirsch HE, et al. Noninvasive testing, early surgery, and seizure freedom in tuberous sclerosis complex. Neurology 2010;74:392–8.

99. Connolly MB, Hendson G, Steinbok P. Tuberous sclerosis complex: a review of the management of epilepsy with emphasis on surgical aspects. Childs Nerv Syst 2006;22:896–908.

100. Weiner HL, Ferraris N, LaJoie J, et al. Epilepsy surgery for children with tuberous sclerosis complex. J Child Neurol 2004;19:687–9.

101. Jansen FE, van Huffelen AC, Algra A, et al. Epilepsy surgery in tuberous sclerosis: a systematic review. Epilepsia 2007;48(8):1477–84.

102. Ghatan S, McGoldrick P, Palmese C, et al. Surgical management of medically refractory epilepsy due to early childhood stroke. J Neurosurg Pediatr 2014;14:58–67.

103. von der Brelie C, Kuczaty S, von Lehe M. Surgical management and long-term outcome of pediatric patients with different subtypes of epilepsy associated with cerebral cavernous malformations. J Neurosurg Pediatr 2014;13:699–705.

104. Schuss P, Marx J, Borger V, et al. Cavernoma-related epilepsy in cavernous malformations located within the temporal lobe: surgical management and seizure outcome. Neurosurg Focus 2020; 48(4):E6.

105. Shang-Guan HC, Wu ZY, Yao PS, et al. Is Extended Lesionectomy Needed for Patients with Cerebral Cavernous Malformations Presenting with Epilepsy? A Meta-Analysis. World Neurosurg 2018; 120:e984–90.

106. Kashida Y, Usui N, Matsuda K, et al. Is additional mesial temporal resection necessary for intractable epilepsy with cavernous malformations in the temporal neocortex? Epilepsy Behav 2019;92:145–53.

107. Bulteau C, Grosmaitre C, Save-Pédebos J, et al. Language recovery after left hemispherotomy for Rasmussen encephalitis. Epilepsy Behav 2015;53: 51–7.

108. McGovern RA, Moosa A, Jehi L, et al. Hemispherectomy in adults and adolescents: Seizure and functional outcomes in 47 patients. Epilepsia 2019;60(12):2416–27.

109. Bellamkonda N, Phillips HW, Chen JS, et al. Epilepsy surgery for Rasmussen encephalitis: the UCLA experience. J Neurosurg Pediatr 2020;26(4):389–97.

110. Hu WH, Zhang C, Zhang K, et al. Hemispheric surgery for refractory epilepsy: a systematic review and meta-analysis with emphasis on seizure predictors and outcomes. J Neurosurg 2016;124(4): 952–61.

111. Lopez AJ, Badger C, Kennedy BC. Hemispherotomy for pediatric epilepsy: a systematic review and critical analysis. Childs Nerv Syst 2021;37(7): 2153–21216cf1.

112. Weil AG, Lewis EC, Ibrahim GM, et al. Hemispherectomy Outcome Prediction Scale: Development and validation of a seizure freedom prediction tool. Epilepsia 2021;62(5):1064–73.

113. Christodoulou JA, Halverson K, Meegoda O, et al. Literacy-related skills among children after left or right hemispherectomy. Epilepsy Behav 2021; 121(Pt A):107995.

114. Borne A, Perrone-Bertolotti M, Jambaqué I, et al. Cognitive outcome after left functional hemispherectomy on dominant hemisphere in patients with Rasmussen encephalitis: beyond the myth of aphasia. Patient series. J Neurosurg Case Lessons 2022;4(22):CASE22410.

115. Nahum AS, Liégeois FJ. Language after childhood hemispherectomy: A systematic review. Neurology 2020;95(23):1043–56.

116. Lidzba K, Bürki SE, Staudt M. Predicting Language Outcome After Left Hemispherotomy: A Systematic Literature Review. Neurol Clin Pract 2021;11(2): 158–66.

117. Schramm J, Behrens E, Entzian W. Hemispherical deafferentation: an alternative to functional hemispherectomy. Neurosurgery 1995;36:509–15. discussion 515-516.

118. Villemure JG, Mascott CR. Peri-insular hemispherotomy: surgical principles and anatomy. Neurosurgery 1995;37:975–81.

119. Chandra PS, Subianto H, Bajaj J, et al. Endoscope-assisted (with robotic guidance and using a hybrid technique) interhemispheric transcallosal hemispherotomy: a comparative study with open hemispherotomy to evaluate efficacy, complications, and outcome. J Neurosurg Pediatr 2018;23(2): 187–97.

120. Peacock WJ. Hemispherectomy for the treatment of intractable seizures in childhood. Neurosurg Clin N Am 1995;6(3):549–63.

121. Van Wagenen WP, Herren RY. Surgical division of commissural pathways in the corpus callosum: relation to spread of an epileptic attack. Arch Neurol Psychiatry 1940;44:740–59.

122. Joseph JR, Viswanathan A, Yoshor D. Extraventricular corpus callosotomy. J Neurosurg 2011;114: 1698–700.

123. Passamonti C, Zamponi N, Foschi N, et al. Long-term seizure and behavioral outcomes after corpus callosotomy. Epilepsy Behav 2014;41:23–9.

124. Rolston JD, Englot DJ, Wang DD, et al. Corpus callosotomy versus vagus nerve stimulation for atonic seizures and drop attacks: a systematic review. Epilepsy Behav 2015;51:13–7.

125. Paglioli E, Martins WA, Azambuja N, et al. Selective posterior callosotomy for drop attacks: A new approach sparing prefrontal connectivity. Neurology 2016;87(19):1968–74.

126. Sood S, Asano E, Altinok D, et al. Endoscopic posterior interhemispheric complete corpus callosotomy. J Neurosurg Pediatr 2016;25(6):689–92.

127. Roland JL, Akbari SHA, Salehi A, et al. Corpus callosotomy performed with laser interstitial thermal therapy. J Neurosurg 2019;1–9.

128. Helmstaedter C, Solymosi L, Kurthen M, et al. Dr. Strangelove demystified: Disconnection of hand and language dominance explains alien-hand syndrome after corpus callosotomy. Seizure 2021;86: 147–51.

129. Chan AY, Rolston JD, Lee B, et al. Rates and predictors of seizure outcome after corpus callosotomy for drug-resistant epilepsy: a meta-analysis. J Neurosurg 2018;130(4):1193–202.

130. Nair DR, Laxer KD, Weber PB, et al, RNS System LTT Study. Nine-year prospective efficacy and safety of brain-responsive neurostimulation for focal epilepsy. Neurology 2020;95(9):e1244–56.

131. Klinkenberg S, Aalbers MW, Vles JS, et al. Vagus nerve stimulation in children with intractable epilepsy: a randomized controlled trial. Dev Med Child Neurol 2012;54(9):855–61.

132. Englot DJ, Rolston JD, Wright CW, et al. Rates and Predictors of Seizure Freedom With Vagus Nerve Stimulation for Intractable Epilepsy. Neurosurgery 2016;79(3):345–53.

133. Granbichler CA, Nashef L, Selway R, et al. Mortality and SUDEP in epilepsy patients treated with vagus nerve stimulation. Epilepsia 2015;56(2):291–6.

134. Ryvlin P, So EL, Gordon CM, et al. Long-term surveillance of SUDEP in drug-resistant epilepsy patients treated with VNS therapy. Epilepsia 2018; 59(3):562–72.

135. Craig DP, Choi YY, Hughes E, et al. Paediatric sudden unexpected death in epilepsy: A parental report cohort. Acta Neurol Scand 2020.

136. Salanova V, Witt T, Worth R, et al, SANTE Study Group. Long-term efficacy and safety of thalamic stimulation for drug-resistant partial epilepsy. Neurology 2015;84(10):1017–25.

137. Yan H, Toyota E, Anderson M, et al. A systematic review of deep brain stimulation for the treatment of drug-resistant epilepsy in childhood. J Neurosurg Pediatr 2018;23(3):274–84.

138. Heck CN, King-Stephens D, Massey AD, et al. Two-year seizure reduction in adults with medically intractable partial onset epilepsy treated with responsive neurostimulation: final results of the RNS System Pivotal trial. Epilepsia 2014;55: 432–41.

139. Fields MC, Eka O, Schreckinger C, et al. A Multicenter Retrospective Study of Patients Treated in the Thalamus with Responsive Neurostimulation. Frontiers in Neurology 2023. https://doi.org/10.3389/fneur.2023.1202631.

140. Sillay KA, Larson PS, Starr PA. Deep brain stimulator hardware-related infections: incidence and management in a large series. Neurosurgery 2008;62(2):360–6. discussion 366-7.

141. Weber PB, Kapur R, Gwinn RP, et al. Infection and Erosion Rates in Trials of a Cranially Implanted Neurostimulator Do Not Increase with Subsequent Neurostimulator Placements. Stereotact Funct Neurosurg 2017;95(5):325–9.

142. Roa JA, Abramova M, Fields M, et al. Responsive Neurostimulation of the Thalamus for the Treatment of Refractory Epilepsy. Front Hum Neurosci 2022; 16:926337.

143. Devinsky O, Friedman D, Duckrow RB, et al. Sudden unexpected death in epilepsy in patients treated with brain-responsive neurostimulation. Epilepsia 2018;59(3):555–61.

144. Sansa G, Carlson C, Doyle W, et al. Medically refractory epilepsy in autism. Epilepsia 2011;52(6): 1071–5.

145. Charlebois CM, Anderson DN, Johnson KA, et al. Patient-specific structural connectivity informs outcomes of responsive neurostimulation for temporal lobe epilepsy. Epilepsia 2022;63(8):2037–55.

146. Sisterson ND, Wozny TA, Kokkinos V, et al. A Rational Approach to Understanding and Evaluating Responsive Neurostimulation. Neuroinformatics 2020;18(3):365–75.

147. Peterson V, Kokkinos V, Ferrante E, et al. Deep net detection and onset prediction of electrographic seizure patterns in responsive neurostimulation. Epilepsia 2023;64(8):2056–69.

Deep Brain Stimulation for Children with Generalized Epilepsy

Rory J. Piper, MRCS[a,b],*, George M. Ibrahim, MD, PhD[c],
Martin M. Tisdall, FRCS(SN), MD[a,b]

KEYWORDS

• Epilepsy • Generalized epilepsy • Deep brain stimulation • Neuromodulation • Children • Pediatrics

KEY POINTS

- Bilateral centromedian nucleus of the thalamus (CMT) deep brain stimulation (DBS) shows potential as a treatment option for children with generalized epilepsy, but robust data are required to confirm this conclusion.
- DBS is available only as an off-label therapy for children (or adults) with generalized-onset seizures in our current health care systems.
- It is unclear how clinically effective CMT DBS is when compared to alternative therapies for children with drug-resistant generalized epilepsy - including vagus nerve stimulation, responsive neurostimulation, corpus callosotomy, cannabinoid therapy or ketogenic diet.
- At least two clinical trials are ongoing to prospectively evaluate the efficacy of DBS to treat generalized epilepsy in children.
- In the absence of robust Level 1 evidence, a collaborative, multicenter effort should be made to collate prospective data, with inclusion of common outcome measures.

BACKGROUND: THE CURRENT STATE OF DEEP BRAIN STIMULATION FOR TREATING DRUG-RESISTANT EPILEPSY

Epilepsy is a common neurological disorder affecting 60 million children and adults globally and predisposes those affected to have epileptic seizures—the symptoms and signs of excessive abnormal or synchronous electrical activity in the brain.[1,2] In children, epilepsy is accompanied by physical, cognitive, psychological, and social sequelae. Anti-seizure medications (ASMs) are the mainstay of therapy for patients with epilepsy, but approximately one-third of patients have drug-resistant epilepsy (DRE) and may require alternative forms of the therapy to achieve better seizure control. For those children with focal-onset seizures, surgical resection, ablation, or disconnection of the epileptogenic zone is a therapeutic option,[3] but not all patients with focal-onset seizures are suitable candidates for these surgeries. Furthermore, most of the patients with generalized-onset seizures are not suitable for surgical interventions. Pediatric epilepsy research continues, therefore, in the pursuit of effective therapeutic strategies to reduce seizure burden and improve quality of life for children affected by DRE.

Intracranial neuromodulation is developing as a treatment option for patients with DRE.[4] Intracranial neuromodulation therapies are used in DRE to stimulate specific targets within the brain to disrupt the epileptogenic network and to prevent

[a] Developmental Neurosciences, UCL Great Ormond Street Institute of Child Health, London, UK; [b] Department of Neurosurgery, Great Ormond Street Hospital, London, UK; [c] Division of Neurosurgery, Hospital for Sick Children, University of Toronto, Ontario, Canada
* Corresponding author. Developmental Neurosciences, UCL Great Ormond Street Institute of Child Health, University College London, 30 Guilford Street, London WC1N 1EH, UK.
E-mail address: Rory.Piper.20@ucl.ac.uk

Neurosurg Clin N Am 35 (2024) 17–25
https://doi.org/10.1016/j.nec.2023.09.002
1042-3680/24/© 2023 Elsevier Inc. All rights reserved.

the propagation of seizure activity.[5] Two intracranial neuromodulation approaches exist within current epilepsy practice: (1) *deep brain stimulation* (DBS), which is the particular focus of this review and (2) *responsive neurostimulation* (RNS). Anterior nucleus of thalamus (ANT) DBS is available in the United States and some health care systems in Europe for the treatment of adults with focal-onset seizures. In the UK National Health Service, ANT DBS is approved with specific conditions but not commissioned,[6] whereas there is no approval for DBS using other intracranial targets for treating either adults or children with generalized-onset seizures. Other forms of intracranial neuromodulation, such as other forms of cortical stimulation, and extracranial neuromodulation, such as vagus nerve stimulation and transcranial neuromodulation, must be noted but are not covered in detail here.

This literature review and commentary addresses the use of *DBS to treat children with drug-resistant generalized epilepsy*. This review discusses the rationale and postulated therapeutic mechanisms for DBS in these children and current evidence to support its clinical efficacy. Furthermore, the authors discuss this therapy in terms of its current availability across health care systems, barriers to adoption, particular considerations and user needs for treating children, and recommendations for future research.

RATIONALE FOR USING DEEP BRAIN STIMULATION TO TREAT CHILDREN WITH GENERALIZED EPILEPSY

Epilepsy affects approximately 5/1000 children in the United States.[7] Although pediatric epilepsy is a heterogeneous condition in several respects, incidence studies suggest that a large proportion of children presenting with epilepsy have some form of generalized-onset seizure disorder.[8] The International League Against Epilepsy includes four distinct syndromes within the category of "idiopathic generalized epilepsies" (IGE): juvenile myoclonic epilepsy, childhood absence epilepsy, juvenile absence epilepsy, and epilepsy with generalized tonic–clonic seizures alone.[9] Other generalized epilepsies include developmental encephalopathic epilepsies, including Lennox–Gastaut syndrome (LGS),[10,11] Dravet syndrome,[12] and epilepsy with myotonic-atonic seizures.

ASM remains the primary treatment for children with generalized-onset seizures, but some children continue to have seizures despite adequate trials of ASM. The number of children who have drug-resistance varies across the different forms of generalized epilepsies. DRE is present in 10%

to 15% of children with IGE[13] but is much higher in and forms part of the defining features of other generalized epilepsies such as LGS and Dravet syndrome.[12] Potential alternative therapies include ketogenic diet and vagus nerve stimulation. Despite the existence of a relatively sizable subcohort of patients with DRE and generalized-onset seizures, a relatively small number of trials sparsely distributed over time have investigated DBS as a form of therapy for generalized epilepsy; the authors discuss these in a later section.

Mechanisms of action of DBS to reduce seizure frequency in generalized epilepsy are not well understood. Epilepsy is increasingly being considered a disorder of brain networks,[14–16] and the treatments of epilepsy are now being approached in this light, particularly within the field of epilepsy surgery including neuromodulation.[5,17,18] Given historical academic focus on refining epilepsy surgery for patients with focal-onset seizures, we know comparatively less about the network implications of treating generalized-onset seizures with neurostimulation. The therapeutic mechanism of DBS to treat generalized-onset seizures is debated and may involve one or a combination of the following mechanisms: (1) limiting the propagation of seizure activity in the brain by gating key propagation points (eg, the thalamus); (2) inducing a plastic functional reorganization of the epileptogenic network; or (3) modulating the epileptogenic brain toward normal physiologic activity.[5]

The centromedian nucleus of the thalamus (CMT) has become the most common brain target in reported cases of DBS for patients with generalized-onset seizures. The CMT is an intralaminar nucleus in the thalamus with diffuse cortical and subcortical connections, including the brainstem (reticular formation, nucleus solitarius, and nucleus ambiguus) and basal ganglia structures.[5,19,20] Bilateral CMT DBS, therefore, is intended to modulate a widespread brain network implicated in generalized-onset epilepsy. An interesting fMRI study by Torres Diaz and colleagues describes a diffuse cortical connectivity pattern linked to the CMT, with the strongest connections to the anterior cingulate cortex, supplementary motor area, central lobe, and insula.[21] Scalp electroencephalography data recording CMT stimulation have shown cortical activation particularly within the cingulate and frontotemporal regions.[22] The CMT is implicated in the seizure network in generalized epilepsy, with intracranial EEG studies showing simultaneous seizure activity within the CMT and cortex,[23] and debate continues as to whether the cortex or thalamus initiates generalized-onset seizures.[23,24] In addition, the CMT is considered to be a key node in the epileptic network of LGS, which is suggested to be a cortically driven network that later involves the thalamus and brainstem.[24,25]

As the authors detail in the next section and demonstrate in **Fig. 1**, the CMT dominates the reported intracranial neuromodulation targets for treating generalized-onset seizures and only a small number of studies or case reports have explored other targets. For example, ANT DBS has been shown to reduce electrographic and clinical seizure counts target for a 17-year-old girl with absence seizures.[26] Extrapolating evidence from RNS data, a recent case series detailed three adults with genetic generalized epilepsy who were treated with ANT RNS and two of the three were determined to be significant clinical responders, whereas the third patient needed device explanation due to infection.[27] Another report of ANT RNS for genetic generalized epilepsy demonstrated efficacy also.[28] It may be that there are other thalamic nuclei that are more suitable for treating generalized-onset seizures but remain yet to be discovered. For example, a recent intracranial EEG study by Wu and colleagues showed that it was the pulvinar rather than the ANT that was first region to be involved in temporal lobe seizures,[29] but there have been no similar intracranial studies to prompt other thalamic targets for patients with generalized epilepsy. Extra-thalamic targets reported in cases of DBS for children with generalized-onset seizures include the posterior hypothalamus, hippocampus, and caudal zona incerta,[30] but further research is required to bring confidence to these approaches.

To summarize this section, using DBS for treating children with generalized-onset DRE is supported by a cohort in need for novel therapies to achieve seizure burden reduction, a plausible network theory to explain its therapeutic action and the availability of a rationalised neuromodulation target. Further evidence is required to support this therapy option for specific subgroups of children with generalized epilepsy, including those with childhood absence epilepsy.[31]

CLINICAL EFFICACY OF DEEP BRAIN STIMULATION FOR TREATING CHILDREN WITH GENERALIZED-ONSET SEIZURES/DRUG-RESISTANT EPILEPSY

DBS was first established as an effective therapy for adult patients with DRE and supported by Level 1 evidence from the *SANTE (Stimulation of the Anterior Nucleus of the Thalamus for Epilepsy) trial*.[32] The authors discuss further data from the most recent systematic reviews of the outcomes of DBS to treat children with DRE[30,33] but highlight the persisting lack of similarly high quality of evidence to encourage its adoption.

Similar to studies of DBS for treating focal-onset epilepsy, the vast majority of available data for DBS for generalized epilepsy are from adult patients. Early data from Velasco and colleagues in the 1980s demonstrated that CMT

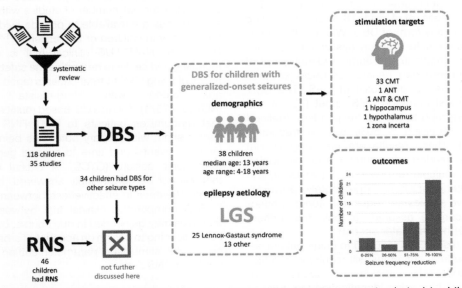

Fig. 1. Intracranial neuromodulation (deep brain stimulation and responsive neurostimulation) in children with drug-resistant epilepsy: a systematic review. ANT, anterior nucleus of thalamus; CMT, centromedian nucleus of thalamus; DBS, deep brain stimulation; RNS, responsive neurostimulation. (*Adapted from* supplementary data provided by Khan et al, 2021.[30])

DBS is able to deliver favorable results for patients with IGE,[34] supported by data from Valentín and colleagues,[35] but otherwise supported sparsely over time and inconsistently by other studies. A recent and arguably the most robust trial of CMT DBS was the *Electrical Stimulation of Thalamus for Epilepsy of Lennox–Gastaut phenotype (ESTEL) trial* by Dalic and colleagues. The ESTEL study was a randomized controlled clinical trial investigating relative seizure frequency reduction after 3 months in patients with LGS treated with CMT DBS.[36] The ESTEL trial recruited 20 young adults (aged 17–37 years) and showed that 50% in the stimulation group were responders (≥50% seizure reduction measured on patient diaries) compared with 22% of patients in the sham group, although this did not reach statistical significance. Analysis of the scalp EEG, however, demonstrated a statistically significant relative reduction in seizures compared with baseline in the stimulation group. No such study providing Level 1 evidence for CMT DBS has been performed in the treatment of children with LGS. Although retrospective and only including adult patients with generalized-onset DRE, other studies have shown encouraging results, for example, a retrospective cohort study by Yang and colleagues had 10/12 patients considered responders.[37]

The most recent systematic review investigating the clinical effectiveness of intracranial neurostimulation to treat children with DRE was by Khan and colleagues.[30] This review identified 35 studies that included data from 72 children between the ages of 4 and 18 years who were treated with any form of DBS. When further interrogating the results (publicly available in the supplementary material), the authors identified 38 of the 72 children had generalized-onset seizures and 25/38 had a diagnosis of LGS. The CMT was the most common DBS target (33/38) and 31/38 were reported to be 'responders' (defined as those receiving > 50% seizure frequency reduction). These results are encouraging, but caution is needed when interpreting the pooled data from multiple retrospective, open-label, and small volume studies. Appropriately powered, prospective studies are required before the effectiveness can be assured—a topic the authors discuss further in a later section.

Further research is required to guide patient selection. Optimal outcomes will require a multifactorial approach, including nuances of preoperative biomarker identification (eg, EEG or MRI features), individualized lead targeting,[38] refinement and personalization of stimulation parameters, and potentially closed-loop solutions.

BEYOND SEIZURE FREEDOM: WHAT ABOUT QUALITY OF LIFE, CARER BURDEN, AND COGNITION?

Primary outcomes in trials of DBS for DRE have thus far focused on seizure reduction, either relative seizure frequency reduction or rate of responders (>50% seizure frequency reduction). However, epilepsy is associated with other comorbidities and we require data to inform us about other important factors that could be improved by DBS in children with DRE (generalized or focal onset). For example, we need to understand the efficacy of DBS in terms of cognition, quality of life, carer burden, and socioeconomic gain. The ESTEL trial investigated cognition outcomes in young adults with LGS receiving CMT DBS, but findings were confounded by the "floor effect" due to low baseline scores.[39] The question remains, therefore, whether initiating DBS therapy earlier (ie, in childhood) will deliver a better chance of cognitive improvement.

RESPONSIVE NEUROSTIMULATION

Although this review focuses on DBS, it is important to acknowledge responsive neurostimulation (RNS), by *NeuroPace*: an alternative intracranial neurostimulation that remains similarly unvalidated in the treatment of children with DRE and generalized-onset seizures. Similar to the SANTE trial in DBS, the pivotal trial of RNS did not include children and the US FDA-approval does not extend to children or patients with generalized-onset seizures. Only a small number of studies with modest sample sizes are available to provide evidence for this therapy in children or adolescents.[31,40–44] The NeuroPace NAUTILUS clinical trial is currently recruiting and seeks to determine the safety and efficacy of using RNS to treat patients (aged 12 years and older) with drug-resistant IGE[45] (NCT05147571). This is a US-based multicenter trial that randomizes patients to CMT RNS therapy versus sham with primary outcomes being safety (adverse events) and time to second generalized tonic-clonic seizure (GTCS). A critical question that will not be convincingly answered, however, is the difference in effectiveness between DBS or RNS A comparative clinical trial between these therapies may be needed in due course, but would be challenging to design on account of arbitrary decisions for stimulation parameter setting in both DBS and RNS arms.

AVAILABILITY AND BARRIERS TO ADOPTION

Currently, DBS for epilepsy is a therapy that is unavailable in routine clinical practice in most health care settings. In the United States, where ANT DBS is FDA-approved and available to adults with focal-onset seizures, DBS can only be used off-label for children or adults with DRE and generalized-onset seizures.[46] A similar scenario exists in most European countries. In the United Kingdom, the National Institute for Health and Care Excellence (NICE) has approved DBS only for adults with focal DRE, but the service has not been formally commissioned.

DBS for children with both generalized and focal epilepsy is hampered by the same barriers that affect the adoption of most device-based therapies in pediatrics: small market/population, particular design considerations (discussed next), low return on investment, and complex regulatory processes.[47] A key consideration for the translation of this therapy is its economic viability and ignoring this will hamper adoption, particularly in public health care systems.[48] Only a handful of studies have investigated the cost-effectiveness of DBS for adults with DRE in terms of quality-adjusted life years,[49] but none to our knowledge have included children.

PATIENT AND CARER PERCEPTIONS: NUANCES OF DEEP BRAIN STIMULATION FOR EPILEPSY IN CHILDREN

To reiterate a key message of this review, the translation of DBS for the treatment of children with DRE has lagged behind adult practice. Part of this delay is explained by the hesitation to apply results from the adult population to children with potentially different disease profiles. Children are not small adults,[50,51] and as per any therapy, device-based therapies such as DBS proven out in adult sectors should not be directly translated to pediatric practice without consideration for additional factors.[47] The authors recently wrote a commentary to this point that integrated clinical, engineering, and children's perspective of DBS device design for children and identified the following areas of consideration[52] (**Fig. 2**):

- Device (including battery) longevity
- Rechargeable mechanisms that are noninvasive, acceptable, and sustainable
- Resistance or dynamic ability to endure the growth of the child
- Minimized risk of infection
- Personalized, adaptive neuromodulation to maximize clinical effect
- Remote programming abilities
- Device trust and acceptance to the child and to their family/carers

Understanding the needs of children and their carers and designing intentional, child-focused devices and practices will be critical in the translation of DBS as a therapy for children with epilepsy.[53,54]

RECOMMENDATIONS FOR FURTHER RESEARCH

Robust evidence to support the clinical effectiveness of DBS to treat children with generalized-onset seizures is still required. The gold standard of evidence in this field would be large-scale and multicenter clinical trials, similar to the design of

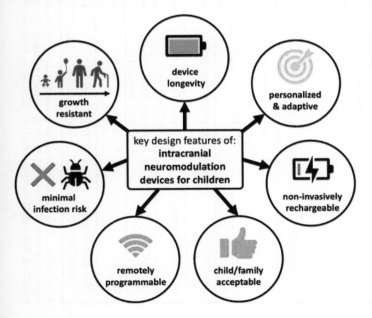

Fig. 2. Key design features of DBS devices for treating children with DRE. (*Adapted from* our commentary published in the Lancet Child and Adolescent Health.[52])

Table 1
Summary of ongoing clinical trials investigating the utility of intracranial neuromodulation for treating children with drug-resistant generalized epilepsy

	DBSpostVNS	CADET Pilot	CADET Trial	NAUTILUS
Primary objective(s)	• Efficacy	• Safety • Trial feasibility (of subsequent CADET trial)	• Efficacy	• Safety and efficacy
Trial design	• Prospective • Single center (Canada) • Patient-preference randomization: DBS vs continued VNS	• Prospective • Multicenter (UK) • Open-label	• Prospective • Multicenter (UK) • Randomized: ON vs OFF phase followed by open-label phase	• Prospective • Multicenter (USA) • Randomized: ON vs OFF phase followed by open-label phase
Primary outcome measure(s)	• Seizure reduction (Engel Epilepsy Surgery Outcome Scale)	• Adverse events • Participant willingness for recruitment • Participant completion of study • Device and re-charge and maintenance	• Seizure frequency reduction at 6 months following initiation of active stimulation	• 12-wk postoperative serious device-related adverse event rate • Time to second GTCS during the 9-mo effectiveness evaluation period
Key eligibility criteria (not exhaustive)	• Age 8–18 y • Diagnosis of DRE • Failure to respond to at least 12-mo of VNS therapy	• Age 5–14 y • Diagnosis of LGS • At least 10 seizures per month	• Age 5–14 y • Diagnosis of LGS • At least 10 seizures per month	• Age 12 y and older • Diagnosis of DRE • EEG with features consistent with IGE • At least two GTCS at baseline
Recruitment target	• 50	• 4	• 22	• 80–100
Device	• Percept (Medtronic)	• Picostim DyNeuMo (Bioinduction Ltd)	• Picostim DyNeuMo (Bioinduction Ltd)	• RNS system
Intracranial target	• Centromedian nucleus of the thalamus	• Centromedian nucleus of the thalamus	• Centromedian nucleus of the thalamus	• Centromedian nucleus of the thalamus
Sponsor	• Academic (Sick Kid's Hospital, Toronto)	• Academic (University College London, UK)	• Academic (University College London, UK)	• Commercial (NeuroPace, USA)
Status	• Recruiting	• Recruiting	• Recruitment pending results of CADET pilot	• Recruiting
ClinicalTrials.gov identifier	• NCT04181229	• NCT05437393	• Pending	• NCT05147571

Abbreviations: CADET, the children's adaptive deep brain stimulation for epilepsy trial[57]; CMT, centromedian nucleus of the thalamus; DBSpostVNS, deep brain stimulation post-vagus nerve stimulation trial[56]; DRE, drug-resistant epilepsy; DyNeuMo, dynamic neuromodulator Mk-1[58]; GTCS, generalized tonic-clonic seizure; LGS, Lennox–Gastaut syndrome; NAUTILUS, RNS system responsive thalamic stimulation for primary generalized seizures study.[45]

the SANTE[32] of ANT DBS or the NeuroPace trial of RNS.[55] As previously discussed, however, the existing published literature for DBS therapy for children with generalized-onset seizures is temporally sparse, limited to small samples, and either retrospective or uncontrolled studies. Given the relatively limited numbers in pediatrics and referral hesitancy, this would require a high-cost, multi-center, and multinational effort, which has inherent challenges.

Before large-scale studies can be conducted, provisional clinical efficacy and safety data are required to generate confidence in the pediatric community. Here, the authors highlight two ongoing studies that seek to provide this (summarized in **Table 1**). First, the *"Deep Brain Stimulation Post Failed Vagal Nerve Stimulation (DBSpostVNS)"*[56] is a prospective clinical trial that uses a patient-preference model to dichotomize children into a DBS therapy cohort or a continuing VNS therapy cohort. This trial will recruit 50 children (age 8–18 years) with DRE to receive CMT DBS, and the primary outcome is relative seizure frequency reduction at 12 month, measured using the Engel Epilepsy Surgery Outcome Scale. This trial does not specifically address generalized epilepsies but is expected to provide an understanding of the utility of DBS in children who have failed VNS therapy. A question remains, however, as to whether DBS will be additionally beneficial before treating with VNS therapy. Second, the *Children's Adaptive Deep brain stimulation for Epilepsy Trial (CADET)* is being prepared as a prospective, multicenter trial of CMT DBS for children (5–14 years) with LGS.[57] The primary outcome of the trial is relative seizure frequency reduction measured using carer-recorded diaries after 6 months of active stimulation. CADET is using a novel Picostim device (Bioinduction Ltd) that is a cranially mounted system with adaptive capabilities for future studies.[58]

While waiting for the results of large-scale RCTs, a pragmatic approach for advancing this field is to collaboratively and propsectively collate the results from multiple institutions to assess real-world application and effectiveness of DBS for children with epilepsy. A successful application of this approach is exemplified by the European MORE trial—a prospective assessment of 170 adults with focal-onset seizures implanted with DBS as part of routine clinical practice.[59]

A collaborative, multicenter effort to collate prospective evidence of outcomes for this therapy must pay attention to common data elements. To this end, the *Child & Youth CompreHenslve Longitudinal Database for Deep Brain Stimulation* (CHILD-DBS) project led by the University of Toronto[60] is a collaborative, multi-institution longitudinal data registry designed to collect longitudinal data from children receiving DBS therapy for all indications. CHILD-DBS collects standardized clinician-reported data (including clinical history, DBS programming settings, and complications), patient-/carer-reported data (including quality of life), neuroimaging data (including structural, diffusion, and functional MRI) and electrophysiological data (including intraoperative microelectrode recordings).

SUMMARY

In summary, DBS and other intracranial neuromodulation approaches have the potential to translate as valuable therapeutic options for children with drug-resistant generalized-onset seizures. The authors anticipate that the ongoing clinical trials will be beneficial in determining the effectiveness of DBS in this context, but a great deal of research and translational support is still required to ensure that treatment becomes attainable to those children who would benefit from it.

CLINICS CARE POINTS

- Based on current evidence, the CMT is a rational DBS target for patients with generalized-onset and drug-resistant seizures.

- The evidence base for CMT DBS in children with generalized-onset seizures is limited and further high-quality studies are required to guide our clinical practice in this field.

- DBS device design and treatment in pediatrics should pay attention to the needs of the children and their carers.

- We do not yet understand if CMT DBS has benefits for children with generalized-epilepsy beyond seizure frequency reduction.

DISCLOSURE

R.J. Piper has nothing to disclose. G.M. Ibrahim has received research funding as well as consulting and advisory fees from LivaNova, United Kingdom. M.M. Tisdall has received honoraria from Medtronic, sponsorship from Renishaw, and research funding from the Oakgrove Foundation.

REFERENCES

1. Devinsky O, Vezzani A, O'Brien TJ, et al. Epilepsy. Nat Rev Dis Prim 2018;4(1):18024.

2. Fisher RS, Acevedo C, Arzimanoglou A, et al. ILAE official report: a practical clinical definition of epilepsy. Epilepsia 2014;55(4):475–82.

3. Cross JH, Reilly C, Gutierrez Delicado E, et al. Epilepsy surgery for children and adolescents: evidence-based but underused. Lancet Child Adolesc Heal 2022;6(7):484–94.

4. Fisher RS, Velasco AL. Electrical brain stimulation for epilepsy. Nat Rev Neurol 2014;10(5):261–70.

5. Piper RJ, Richardson RM, Worrell G, et al. Towards network-guided neuromodulation for epilepsy. Brain 2022;145(10):3347–62.

6. National Institute of Clinical Excellence N. Deep Brain Stimulation for Refractory Epilepsy in Adults.; 2020. https://www.nice.org.uk/guidance/ipg678.

7. Cowan LD, Bodensteiner JB, Leviton A, et al. Prevalence of the epilepsies in children and adolescents. Epilepsia 1989;30(1):94–106.

8. Camfield P, Camfield C. Incidence, prevalence and aetiology of seizures and epilepsy in children. Epileptic Disord 2015;17(2):117–23.

9. Hirsch E, French J, Scheffer IE, et al. ILAE definition of the Idiopathic Generalized Epilepsy Syndromes: Position statement by the ILAE Task Force on Nosology and Definitions. Epilepsia 2022;63(6):1475–99.

10. Cross JH, Auvin S, Falip M, et al. Expert opinion on the management of lennox–gastaut syndrome: treatment algorithms and practical considerations. Front Neurol 2017;8:505.

11. Arzimanoglou A, French J, Blume WT, et al. Lennox-Gastaut syndrome: a consensus approach on diagnosis, assessment, management, and trial methodology. Lancet Neurol 2009;8(1):82–93.

12. Wirrell EC, Hood V, Knupp KG, et al. International consensus on diagnosis and management of Dravet syndrome. Epilepsia 2022;63(7):1761–77.

13. Gesche J, Beier CP. Drug resistance in idiopathic generalized epilepsies: Evidence and concepts. Epilepsia 2022;63(12):3007–19.

14. Fisher RS, Cross JH, French JA, et al. Operational classification of seizure types by the International League Against Epilepsy: Position Paper of the ILAE Commission for Classification and Terminology. Epilepsia 2017;58(4):522–30.

15. Royer J, Bernhardt BC, Larivière S, et al. Epilepsy and brain network hubs. Epilepsia 2022;63(3):537–50.

16. Richardson MP. Large scale brain models of epilepsy: dynamics meets connectomics. J Neurol Neurosurg Psychiatry 2012;83(12):1238–48.

17. Chari A, Seunarine KK, He X, et al. Drug-resistant focal epilepsy in children is associated with increased modal controllability of the whole brain and epileptogenic regions. Commun Biol 2022;5(1):394.

18. Richardson RM. Closed-loop brain stimulation and paradigm shifts in epilepsy surgery. Neurol Clin 2022;40(2):355–73.

19. Vetkas A, Germann J, Elias G, et al. Identifying the neural network for neuromodulation in epilepsy through connectomics and graphs. Brain Commun 2022; 4(3). https://doi.org/10.1093/braincomms/fcac092.

20. Warsi NM, Yan H, Suresh H, et al. The anterior and centromedian thalamus: Anatomy, function, and dysfunction in epilepsy. Epilepsy Res 2022;182:106913.

21. Torres Diaz CV, González-Escamilla G, Ciolac D, et al. Network substrates of centromedian nucleus deep brain stimulation in generalized pharmacoresistant epilepsy. Neurotherapeutics 2021;18(3):1665–77.

22. Kim SH, Lim SC, Yang DW, et al. Thalamo-cortical network underlying deep brain stimulation of centromedian thalamic nuclei in intractable epilepsy: a multimodal imaging analysis. Neuropsychiatr Dis Treat 2017;13:2607–19.

23. Martín-López D, Jiménez-Jiménez D, Cabañés-Martínez L, et al. The role of thalamus versus cortex in epilepsy: evidence from human ictal centromedian recordings in patients assessed for deep brain stimulation. Int J Neural Syst 2017;27(7):1750010.

24. Dalic LJ, Warren AEL, Young JC, et al. Cortex leads the thalamic centromedian nucleus in generalized epileptic discharges in Lennox-Gastaut syndrome. Epilepsia 2020;61(10):2214–23.

25. Warren AEL, Harvey AS, Vogrin SJ, et al. The epileptic network of Lennox-Gastaut syndrome. Neurology 2019;93(3):e215–26.

26. Lee C-Y, Lim S-N, Wu T, et al. Successful Treatment of Refractory Status Epilepticus Using Anterior Thalamic Nuclei Deep Brain Stimulation. World Neurosurg 2017;99:14–8.

27. O'Donnell CM, Swanson SJ, Carlson CE, et al. Responsive neurostimulation of the anterior thalamic nuclei in refractory genetic generalized epilepsy: a case series. Brain Sci 2023;13(2):324.

28. Herlopian A, Cash SS, Eskandar EM, et al. Responsive neurostimulation targeting anterior thalamic nucleus in generalized epilepsy. Ann Clin Transl Neurol 2019;6(10):2104–9.

29. Wu TQ, Kaboodvand N, McGinn RJ, et al. Multisite thalamic recordings to characterize seizure propagation in the human brain. Brain 2023;4. https://doi.org/10.1093/brain/awad121.

30. Khan M, Paktiawal J, Piper RJ, et al. Intracranial neuromodulation with deep brain stimulation and responsive neurostimulation in children with drug-resistant epilepsy: a systematic review. J Neurosurg Pediatr 2022;29(2):208–17.

31. Welch WP, Hect JL, Abel TJ. Case Report: responsive neurostimulation of the centromedian thalamic nucleus for the detection and treatment of seizures in pediatric primary generalized epilepsy. Front Neurol 2021;12:656585.

32. Fisher R, Salanova V, Witt T, et al. Electrical stimulation of the anterior nucleus of thalamus for treatment of refractory epilepsy. Epilepsia 2010;51(5):899–908.

33. Yan H, Toyota E, Anderson M, et al. A systematic review of deep brain stimulation for the treatment of drug-resistant epilepsy in childhood. J Neurosurg Pediatr 2018;23(3):274–84.

34. Velasco F, Velasco M, Ogarrio C, et al. Electrical stimulation of the centromedian thalamic nucleus in the treatment of convulsive seizures: a preliminary report. Epilepsia 1987;28(4):421–30.

35. Valentín A, García Navarrete E, Chelvarajah R, et al. Deep brain stimulation of the centromedian thalamic nucleus for the treatment of generalized and frontal epilepsies. Epilepsia 2013;54(10):1823–33.

36. Dalic LJ, Warren AEL, Bulluss KJ, et al. DBS of thalamic centromedian nucleus for lennox–gastaut syndrome (ESTEL Trial). Ann Neurol 2022;91(2): 253–67.

37. Yang JC, Bullinger KL, Isbaine F, et al. Centromedian thalamic deep brain stimulation for drug-resistant epilepsy: single-center experience. J Neurosurg 2022;137(6):1591–600.

38. Warren AEL, Dalic LJ, Bulluss KJ, et al. The optimal target and connectivity for DBS in Lennox-Gastaut syndrome. Ann Neurol 2022. https://doi.org/10. 1002/ana.26368.

39. Dalic LJ, Warren AEL, Malpas CB, et al. Cognition, adaptive skills and epilepsy disability/severity in patients with Lennox–Gastaut syndrome undergoing deep brain stimulation for epilepsy in the ESTEL trial. Seizure 2022;101(July):67–74.

40. Nagahama Y, Zervos TM, Murata KK, et al. Real-world preliminary experience with responsive neurostimulation in pediatric epilepsy: a multicenter retrospective observational study. Neurosurgery 2021;0(0):1–8.

41. Singhal NS, Numis AL, Lee MB, et al. Responsive neurostimulation for treatment of pediatric drug-resistant epilepsy. Epilepsy Behav case reports 2018;10:21–4.

42. Panov F, Ganaha S, Haskell J, et al. Safety of responsive neurostimulation in pediatric patients with medically refractory epilepsy. J Neurosurg Pediatr 2020;26(5):525–32.

43. Sisterson ND, Kokkinos V, Urban A, et al. Responsive neurostimulation of the thalamus improves seizure control in idiopathic generalised epilepsy: initial case series. J Neurol Neurosurg Psychiatry 2022;93(5):491–8.

44. Kwon C-S, Schupper AJ, Fields MC, et al. Centromedian thalamic responsive neurostimulation for Lennox-Gastaut epilepsy and autism. Ann Clin Transl Neurol 2020;7(10):2035–40.

45. Morrell MJ. RNS System NAUTILUS Study (NAUTILUS). ClinicalTrials.gov. https://clinicaltrials.gov/ct2/show/NCT05147571.

46. Haneef Z, Skrehot HC. Neurostimulation in generalized epilepsy: a systematic review and meta-analysis. Epilepsia 2023;16. https://doi.org/10.1111/epi.17524.

47. Espinoza J, Cooper K, Afari N, et al. Innovation in pediatric medical devices: proceedings from the west coast consortium for technology & innovation in pediatrics 2019 annual stakeholder summit. JMIR Biomed Eng 2020;5(1):e17467.

48. Borton DA, Dawes HE, Worrell GA, et al. Developing collaborative platforms to advance neurotechnology and its translation. Neuron 2020;108(2):286–301.

49. Chan HY, Wijnen BFM, Majoie MHJM, et al. Economic evaluation of deep brain stimulation compared with vagus nerve stimulation and usual care for patients with refractory epilepsy: A lifetime decision analytic model. Epilepsia 2022;63(3):641–51.

50. The Lancet. Time to be serious about children's health care. Lancet 2001;358(9280):431.

51. Gillis J, Loughlan P. Not just small adults: the metaphors of paediatrics. Arch Dis Child 2007;92(11): 946–7.

52. Piper RJ, Fleming J, Valentín A, et al. Neurostimulation devices for children: lessons learned. Lancet Child Adolesc Heal 2022;6(6):359–61.

53. Elkaim LM, Niazi F, Levett JJ, et al. Deep brain stimulation in children and youth: perspectives of patients and caregivers gleaned through Twitter. Neurosurg Focus 2022;53(4):E11.

54. Bergeron D, Iorio-Morin C, Bonizzato M, et al. Use of invasive brain-computer interfaces in pediatric neurosurgery: technical and ethical considerations. J Child Neurol 2023. https://doi.org/10.1177/08830738231167736. 8830738231167736.

55. Morrell MJ, RNS System in Epilepsy Study Group. Responsive cortical stimulation for the treatment of medically intractable partial epilepsy. Neurology 2011;77(13):1295–304.

56. Siegel L, Ibrahim G. Deep brain stimulation post failed vagal nerve stimulation (DBSpostVNS). ClinicalTrials.gov; 2023. https://clinicaltrials.gov/ct2/show/NCT04181229?term=ibrahim&cond=Epilepsy&draw=2&rank=1.

57. Piper RJ, Tisdall MM. Children's adaptive deep brain stimulation for epilepsy trial (CADET): pilot (CADET pilot). ClinicalTrials.gov; 2023. https://clinicaltrials.gov/ct2/show/NCT05437393.

58. Zamora M, Toth R, Morgante F, et al. DyNeuMo Mk-1: Design and pilot validation of an investigational motion-adaptive neurostimulator with integrated chronotherapy. Exp Neurol 2022;351:113977.

59. Peltola J, Colon AJ, Pimentel J, et al. Deep brain stimulation of the anterior nucleus of the thalamus in drug-resistant epilepsy in the more multicenter patient registry. Neurology 2023;100(18):e1852–65.

60. Yan H, Siegel L, Breitbart S, et al. The child & youth comprehensive longitudinal database for deep brain stimulation (CHILD-DBS). Childs Nerv Syst 2021; 37(2):607–15.

Neurostimulation for Generalized Epilepsy
Should Therapy be Syndrome-specific?

Aaron E.L. Warren, PhD[a],*, Steven Tobochnik, MD[b],
Melissa M.J. Chua, MD[a], Hargunbir Singh, MBBS[a], Michaela A. Stamm, MS[a],
John D. Rolston, MD, PhD[a]

KEYWORDS

- Epilepsy • Generalized seizures • Lennox-Gastaut syndrome • Idiopathic generalized epilepsy
- Thalamus • Deep brain stimulation • Responsive neurostimulation • Neuromodulation

KEY POINTS

- Lennox-Gastaut syndrome (LGS) and Idiopathic Generalized Epilepsy (IGE) show electroclinical differences, including distinct interictal epileptiform discharges and predominant seizure types.
- Neurostimulation devices, including deep brain stimulation and responsive neurostimulation, aim to therapeutically modulate epileptic brain networks.
- Recent neuroimaging studies suggest that the brain networks underlying LGS and IGE are syndrome-specific.
- These findings may have important implications for syndrome-specific optimization of stimulation targeting and programming.

INTRODUCTION

One-third of people with epilepsy have *generalized onset seizures*,[1,2] which appear to begin in both hemispheres simultaneously on scalp electroencephalography (EEG). This contrasts with *focal onset seizures*, which originate in one hemisphere and have a unilateral EEG appearance.[2] Although the borders between these seizure types are not always clear, the distinction between focal and generalized epilepsy has strong implications for diagnosis and treatment.

The clinical manifestations of a generalized seizure vary widely, from motor (eg, tonic stiffening, atonia, clonic or myoclonic jerking) to nonmotor symptoms (eg, impaired awareness), either alone or in combination. The EEG appearance can also show various seizure onset patterns, including repetitive spike-wave discharges, paroxysmal fast activity, rhythmic activity, and diffuse electrodecrement, each suggestive of a unique neuronal firing pattern (**Fig. 1**).

Combined with other electroclinical features, patients with generalized seizures may be categorized into distinct *epilepsy syndromes*,[3] each having a unique profile with respect to typical onset age, etiology, comorbidities, quality of life, and impact on families and caregivers, all of which are important to consider when designing treatments and predicting outcomes.

Neurostimulation is rapidly changing the treatment landscape for generalized epilepsy. Clinically available options include continuous and duty-cycling deep brain stimulation (DBS), responsive neurostimulation (RNS), and vagus nerve stimulation.[4] However, current applications are largely agnostic to the syndrome and seizure type or types being treated, and only carry Food and Drug Administration approvals in the United States for focal epilepsy, despite increasing off-label use.

[a] Department of Neurosurgery, Brigham and Women's Hospital, Harvard Medical School, Boston, MA, USA;
[b] Department of Neurology, Brigham and Women's Hospital, Harvard Medical School, Boston, MA, USA
* Corresponding author. Hale Building for Transformative Medicine, Brigham and Women's Hospital, 60 Fenwood Road, Boston, MA 02115.
E-mail address: awarren15@bwh.harvard.edu

Neurosurg Clin N Am 35 (2024) 27–48
https://doi.org/10.1016/j.nec.2023.08.001
1042-3680/24/© 2023 Elsevier Inc. All rights reserved.

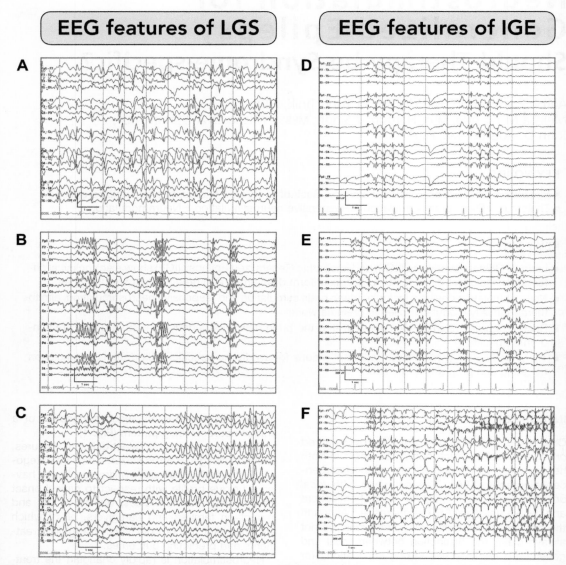

Fig. 1. Characteristic EEG features of LGS versus IGE. LGS and IGE are associated with different generalized IEDs and ictal patterns on scalp EEG. (*A*) Interictally, LGS is characterized by generalized SSW discharges occurring at a frequency of ≤2.5 Hz, typically on an abnormal background of diffuse theta-delta slowing. (*B*) Bursts of interictal >10 Hz GPFA are also seen, particularly during sleep. (*C*) Ictally, tonic seizures of LGS consist of a burst of bilateral >10 Hz fast activity (resembling GPFA) followed by diffuse decrement evolving to higher-amplitude spike and slow-wave discharges. (*D*) Interictally, patients with IGE show a well-organized background with superimposed "faster" ~3 to 6 Hz GSW and/or (*E*) generalized polyspike-wave (GPSW) activity. (*F*) Ictally, generalized tonic-clonic seizures of IGE typically demonstrate an onset of bilateral polyspikes and/or evolving spike/polyspike-wave discharges.

A salient example is DBS, where the same anatomic site, the thalamic centromedian nucleus, has been targeted for Lennox-Gastaut syndrome (LGS)[5–9] and idiopathic (genetic) generalized epilepsies (IGE),[7,9–11] among others (eg, patients with focal, multifocal, and combined generalized and focal epilepsy).[8,9,12–17] Many retrospective DBS studies have used broad inclusion criteria, with outcomes collapsed across syndromes and seizure types. This likely reflects the still-emerging state of the field and the small number of prospective and controlled studies performed relative to other DBS indications, such as movement disorders.

Applications of neurostimulation have progressed in parallel with—but, we would argue, often independent of—a growing understanding of the syndrome- and seizure-specific brain networks underlying generalized epilepsy[18–20] and its associated cognitive and behavioral comorbidities.[21] The concept of generalized epilepsy networks has been advanced through neuroimaging studies using anatomic[22–27] and diffusion-weighted MRI,[28–32] simultaneous EEG with functional MRI (EEG-fMRI),[33–44] resting-state fMRI,[45–51] PET,[52–56] single-photon emission computed tomography (SPECT),[57–60] and magnetoencephalography (MEG),[61–65] among others.

A commonly stated goal of neurostimulation is to reduce seizures by modulating the specific brain area or areas thought to generate them or their pathways of propagation. For example, in patients with focal seizures who are not candidates for resective neurosurgery, RNS can be delivered directly to one or more cortical seizure foci.[66,67] However, this goal is more difficult to define in the context of generalized epilepsy, for several reasons. Generalized seizures are seemingly expressed synchronously across widespread brain regions,[2] which impedes defining a discrete seizure focus and, consequently, stimulation target. Patients with generalized epilepsy also commonly experience multiple seizure types, which, as reviewed in later discussion, engage different brain networks. In addition, generalized epilepsy can occur in patients with focal lesions,[33,68,69] complicating the treatment target: is it the generalized seizure network, the lesion, or both?

SCOPE OF THIS REVIEW

Recent reviews of neurostimulation for generalized epilepsy have focused on clinical efficacy,[4,70–73] targets,[18,74,75] and surgical techniques.[76] The present review compares the 2 main syndromic "archetypes" of generalized epilepsy—LGS and IGE—and focuses on the 2 neurostimulation approaches most actively being studied in recent and ongoing clinical trials: DBS and RNS.

First, evidence from neuroimaging studies is reviewed describing differences in the brain networks underlying LGS and IGE. Second, potential mechanisms mediating neurostimulation efficacy, how they may differ by syndrome and seizure type, and how these differences may inform selection of appropriate targets and paradigms for DBS/RNS are discussed. Third, how LGS and IGE evolve over short (eg, between wakefulness and sleep) and long (eg, childhood to adulthood) timescales and how stimulation programming may be dynamically adjusted to respond to these changes are considered.

We structure the review as a series of 5 clinical questions that are encountered when assessing a patient with generalized epilepsy for neurostimulation therapy.

WHAT EPILEPSY SYNDROME DOES THE PATIENT HAVE?

Differentiation of LGS and IGE can be traced as far back as the first EEG studies of epilepsy performed by Gibbs, Gibbs, and Lennox in the 1930s[77–79] and 1940s.[80,81] Although the syndromes were not known as such at that time, Gibbs and colleagues described EEG differences in patients with generalized epilepsy, which were later elaborated upon by Gastaut and colleagues[82,83] and Dravet.[84] They described a "fast" ($\geq$3 Hz) generalized spike-wave (GSW) pattern and a "slow" ($\leq$2.5 Hz) spike-wave (SSW) pattern (see **Fig. 1**) and found that the 2 tended to be associated with different clinical profiles.[81] Patients with SSW often had severe cognitive impairment, greater treatment resistance, tonic seizures, and other EEG patterns, including >10 Hz generalized paroxysmal fast activity (GPFA). In contrast, patients with GSW tended to show more preserved cognitive function, usually responded better to antiseizure medications, and did not have tonic seizures.

These 2 phenotypes are similar to what are now recognized as LGS and IGE (**Table 1**). The 2022 International League Against Epilepsy classification[85] defines LGS by the following 3 key features: (i) multiple drug-resistant seizure types with onset <18 years, including tonic seizures; (ii) cognitive and/or behavioral impairments (typically mild to profound intellectual disability); and (iii) SSW and GPFA (see **Fig. 1**). Although often considered "rare" (0.24–0.28 per 1000 births),[86–88] the intractability of seizures in LGS leads to a disproportionately high prevalence, with the syndrome accounting for ~4% of children with epilepsy[89] and up to 17% of epilepsy patients with intellectual disability.[90]

IGE is one of the most common forms of epilepsy, accounting for 15% to 20% of all epilepsy diagnoses.[91] IGE comprises 4 subsyndromes (see **Table 1**) associated with different onset ages and predominant seizure types[92] but sharing similar EEG findings, including normal background activity, ~3- to 6-Hz GSW and/or generalized polyspike-wave discharges (see **Fig. 1**). Tonic seizures, SSW, GPFA, and intellectual disability are not typically seen; however, some patients with IGE can develop GPFA, which may be associated with greater treatment resistance.[93,94]

LGS and IGE are etiologically divergent. Genomic studies show that IGE has a genetic,

Table 1
Typical electroclinical characteristics of Lennox-Gastaut syndrome and idiopathic generalized epilepsy

	Lennox-Gastaut Syndrome (LGS)	Idiopathic Generalized Epilepsy Subsyndromes			
		Childhood Absence Epilepsy (CAE)	Juvenile Absence Epilepsy	Juvenile Myoclonic Epilepsy	Epilepsy with Generalized Tonic-Clonic Seizures Alone
EEG background	Diffuse theta-delta slowing and disorganization	Occipital intermittent rhythmic delta activity in 21%–30%	Normal	Normal	Normal
Interictal EEG patterns	Awake: Generalized slow ≤2.5 Hz spike-wave; Asleep: Generalized paroxysmal fast ≥10 Hz activity	Awake: 2.5–4 Hz generalized spike-wave; Asleep: polyspike-wave primarily in drowsiness/sleep	Awake: 3–5.5 Hz generalized spike-wave; Asleep: polyspike-wave primarily in drowsiness/sleep	Generalized 3–5.5 Hz spike-wave and polyspike-wave	Generalized 3–5.5 Hz spike-wave and polyspike-wave
Ictal EEG patterns	Tonic seizures: bilateral ≥10 Hz bursts of fast activity with recruiting rhythm	Regular 2.5–4 Hz generalized spike-wave, infrequent disorganized discharges	Regular 3–5.5 Hz generalized spike-wave; 8× more frequent disorganized discharges than CAE	Absences: 3.5–6 Hz generalized spike-wave/polyspike-wave (more disorganized discharges than CAE); Myoclonic jerks: generalized polyspike-wave; GTCs: generalized spikes (tonic phase), spike-wave (clonic phase)	Generalized spikes (tonic phase), spike-wave (clonic phase)
Seizure type or types	Tonic seizures + at least one additional seizure type (eg, atypical absence, atonic, myoclonic, focal impaired awareness, GTC, epileptic spasms)	Daily to multiple daily 3- to 20-s typical absence seizures	Less than daily 5- to 30-s typical absence seizures; commonly have GTCs during periods of frequent absence seizures	Myoclonic (mostly upon awakening); GTCs common, preceded by myoclonic jerks; 1/3 have brief 3- to 8-s typical absence seizures (infrequent)	Infrequent GTCs (usually within 2 h of awakening; occurs yearly or less)

Cognitive profile	Mild to severe intellectual disability that often worsens over time	Typically, normal development; ADHD, mood disorders, or learning disabilities can occur	Typically, normal development; ADHD, mood disorders, or learning disabilities can occur	Typically, normal development; ADHD, mood disorders, or learning disabilities can occur	Typically, normal development; ADHD, mood disorders, or learning disabilities can occur
Typical seizure onset age	18 mo to 8 y (rarely 8–18 y)	4–10 y	9–13 y	10–24 y	10–25 y
Presumed/known causes	Structural (most common), genetic (usually de novo), infectious, metabolic, and/or immune causes	Genetic susceptibility (polygenic > monogenic)	Genetic susceptibility (polygenic > monogenic)	Genetic susceptibility (polygenic > monogenic)	Genetic susceptibility (polygenic > monogenic)

LGS and IGE (and it subsyndromes) differ with respect to their interictal and ictal EEG features, predominant seizure type or types, cognitive profiles, onset ages, and causes. There is often electroclinical overlap between the IGE subsyndromes, and one subsyndrome can evolve to another as patients age.

Abbreviations: ADHD, attention-deficit/hyperactivity disorder; GTC, generalized tonic-clonic.

Example structural MRI findings in LGS

Examples in IGE

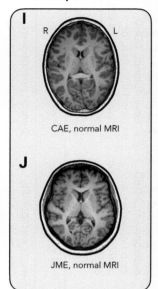

A Focal cortical dysplasia

B Rasmussen's encephalitis

C Bilateral polymicrogyria

D Perinatal ischemic injury

E Band heterotopia, *DCX* mutation

F DNET + partial monosomy 18p

G Schizencephaly, PVNH

H Normal MRI, unknown cause

I CAE, normal MRI

J JME, normal MRI

Fig. 2. Radiological MRI findings in LGS versus IGE. T1-weighted MRI scans in patients with LGS (*A–H*) and IGE (*I–J*). (*A*) Adult with LGS aged in their 20s with a left frontal lobe focal cortical dysplasia (histopathology: balloon cells). (*B*) Adult with LGS aged in their 20s with diffuse right frontal atrophy and ventricular dilation owing to Rasmussen's encephalitis. (*C*) Adult with LGS aged in their 30s with bilateral perisylvian polymicrogyria. (*D*) Adult with LGS aged in their 30s with right temporal atrophy and gliosis owing to a perinatal infarction. (*E*) Adolescent with LGS and bilateral band heterotopia (double cortex syndrome) and a *DCX* gene mutation. (*F*) Child with LGS and a right medial temporal lobe dysembryoplastic neuroepithelial tumor (DNET) on the background of a chromosomal abnormality (partial monosomy 18p). (*G*) Adult with LGS aged in their 20s with a complex malformation of cortical development involving bilateral periventricular nodular heterotopia (PVNH) and left posterior schizencephaly. (*H*) Adolescent with LGS with normal MRI and unknown cause of epilepsy. (*I*) Child with IGE (childhood absence epilepsy [CAE]) with normal MRI. (*J*) Adolescent with IGE (juvenile myoclonic epilepsy [JME]) with normal MRI. *Interpretation:* LGS develops secondarily to diverse etiologies, with structural causes accounting for 30% to 50% of patients.[98–100] In contrast, structural abnormalities are not typically seen in IGE, although subtle alterations are described in quantitative analyses.

typically polygenic, basis.[92,95] Monogenic cases are also reported.[92] On structural MRI, patients with IGE show visually normal anatomy (**Fig. 2**), although altered cortical thickness and regional brain volumes have been described in quantitative analyses.[96]

In contrast, the etiologic profile of LGS is heterogeneous, with a variety of structural, genetic, infectious, immune, and metabolic factors.[97] Thirty percent to 50%[98–100] have abnormal structural MRI findings, ranging from malformations of cortical development to acquired brain lesions (see **Fig. 2**). The shared phenotype of LGS is thought to reflect a common "reaction" of the brain to these causes—that is, LGS develops secondarily,[83,97] potentially via convergent neurodevelopmental alterations caused by seizures and other risk factors in early life.[34]

In summary, LGS and IGE differ with respect to their predominant seizure types (and thus also the target seizure types for treatments including neurostimulation), EEG signatures, cognitive comorbidities, and etiologic profiles. In the next section, neuroimaging evidence is reviewed showing that these syndromic differences may be underpinned by distinct patterns of brain network pathology condition.

WHAT BRAIN NETWORKS ARE INVOLVED?

Generalized epilepsy is a disorder of bilateral brain networks,[2,101] that is, spatially distributed regions connected structurally and/or functionally, within which seizures begin and manifest clinically. These networks can be defined and studied at multiple scales, from synaptic connectivity between neurons to large-scale neuronal ensembles spanning lobes and hemispheres. The latter is the level where neuroimaging techniques operate, to which our attention now turns.

We first consider the similarities bewteen LGS and IGE. First, although the diffuse EEG appearance of LGS and IGE might suggest equal participation of all brain areas during seizures and interictal epileptiform discharges (IEDs), functional neuroimaging studies indicate otherwise. Combined EEG-fMRI, which measures blood-oxygen-level-dependent (BOLD) responses time-locked to EEG events, reveals that generalized IEDs of LGS[34,38] and IGE[41,42] engage bilateral but select brain regions (**Figs. 3** and **4**). Furthermore, the response patterns of involved regions vary, with some showing BOLD increases and others showing BOLD decreases,[33,41,42] likely indicating distinct neuronal responses between different areas during the same IEDs.

However, beyond these superficial similarities, important brain network differences can be observed between LGS and IGE, and between different epileptiform event types in the same syndrome. During GPFA, which is characteristic of LGS and shows EEG similarities to tonic seizures (see **Fig. 1**), BOLD signal increases occur in diffuse frontal and parietal "association" (ie, nonprimary) cortices together with the thalamus, basal ganglia (caudate and putamen), cerebellum, and pontomedullary reticular formation (see **Fig. 3**).[33,34] This pattern is similar between children and adults[34] and between individual patients with various causes of LGS,[33,34] suggesting it reflects a "secondary network" response to the specific epileptogenic insult.[97] It is also similar to the cerebral perfusion changes seen during the early phase of tonic seizures, as revealed by SPECT.[58]

In patients with LGS secondary to a focal cortical lesion, EEG-fMRI involvement of the anatomic lesion can be seen together with the recognized group-level functional patterns

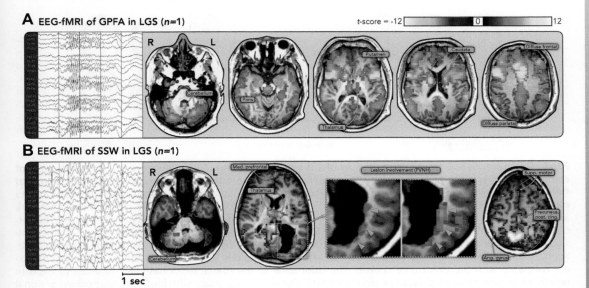

Fig. 3. Simultaneous EEG-fMRI findings in GPFA versus SSW of LGS and involvement of patient-specific lesions. Representative individual-level event-related statistical parametric mapping (SPM) of BOLD signal changes associated with scalp EEG-recorded discharges in 2 patients with LGS. (*A*) EEG-fMRI acquired during natural sleep in a patient aged in their 20s with LGS on a background of tuberous sclerosis complex. Bursts of GPFA were manually marked on the in-scanner EEG. GPFA onsets and durations were convolved with the canonical hemodynamic response function (HRF) in SPM software (http://www.fil.ion.ucl.ac.uk/spm). One-sample *t* tests were used to obtain a spatial map of significant GPFA-related BOLD changes (thresholded using a cluster-level, false discovery rate-corrected threshold of *P*<.05 with a cluster-defining threshold of *P*<.001, uncorrected). Orange/yellow colors indicate regions showing BOLD increases and blue/light blue colors indicate BOLD decreases. Results are overlaid upon the patient's T1-weighted MRI scan. (*B*) EEG-fMRI acquired during natural sleep in a patient aged in their 20s with LGS on the background of a complex malformation of cortical development (including bilateral PVNH and a left posterior schizencephaly). Bursts of SSW were manually marked on the in-scanner EEG. Zoomed-in views show BOLD activation in the patient's lesions (periventricular nodules; *arrowheads*) that are seen together with the more distributed cortical and subcortical SSW-related pattern. *Interpretation:* GPFA and SSW of LGS show distinct patterns of brain network involvement. In patients with lesions, EEG-fMRI involvement of the lesion can occur together with the more distributed patterns seen in patients with or without lesions,[33,34,105] suggesting that epileptiform activity of LGS is expressed via a shared "secondary network."[97] Ang, angular; med, medial; post. cing., posterior cingulate.

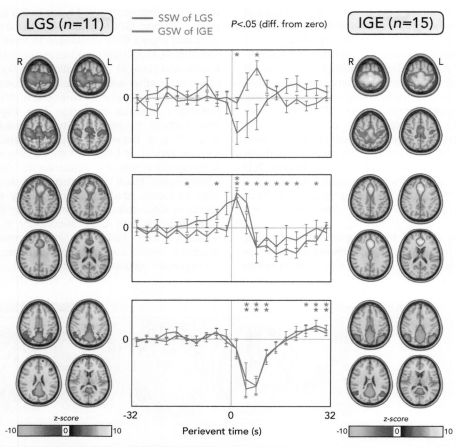

Fig. 4. Simultaneous EEG-fMRI findings in SSW of LGS versus GSW of IGE. Group-level event-related independent component analysis,[108] which uses a flexible modeling approach to estimate time courses and spatial sources of fMRI activity associated with EEG events, was performed in 11 patients with LGS (mean age = 34 years) and 15 patients with IGE/childhood absence epilepsy (mean age = 10 years). Each row shows a different brain network and its associated fMRI time course, over the period −32 to +32 seconds relative to SSW or GSW onset. The vertical line in each plot indicates the time of GSW or SSW onset, and the horizontal line indicates the baseline fMRI signal level. Asterisks indicate where the fMRI signal is significantly different from baseline ($P<.05$, uncorrected). Spatial maps (left and right columns) are z-statistic images, thresholded to show significant ($P<.05$) clusters of voxels associated with the event time courses. The color scale of the spatial maps has been adjusted to indicate whether the brain network shows a predominant fMRI signal decrease (maps with blue/light blue colors) or signal increase (maps with orange/yellow colors) in response to SSW or GSW. *Interpretation:* Sensorimotor cortex (*first row*) shows decreased fMRI signal in response to SSW of LGS, whereas it shows increased fMRI signal in response to GSW of IGE. However, both SSW and GSW involve increased fMRI signal in supplementary motor cortex/anterior cingulate (*second row*) and decreased fMRI signal in regions of the "default-mode network" (*third row*). Figure created using findings from Warren and colleagues.[107] Diff, difference.

shared by patients with or without lesions (see **Fig. 3**).[33,102] Prompt lesion removal can sometimes have significant benefits,[33,102,103] including seizure control, developmental improvement, and abolition of generalized EEG abnormalities. In such patients, lesionectomy may be the preferred first-line surgical treatment over neurostimulation,[104] particularly when the lesion is identified early after epilepsy onset. These considerations do not occur in the context of IGE, where focal cortical lesions are not seen (see **Fig. 2**).[92]

The pattern of epileptic involvement during GPFA differs from that seen during SSW of LGS. EEG-fMRI of SSW shows a distinct pattern of cortical changes, with BOLD *decreases* being more prominent than increases (see **Fig. 3**).[105] The distribution of BOLD decreases resembles the "default-mode network" in healthy subjects (including posterior cingulate, precuneus, angular gyrus, and medial prefrontal cortex), which is thought to support self-oriented cognitive processes, including awareness and autobiographical memory, among other functions.[106] SSW-related inhibition of this network is hypothesized to contribute to the clinical manifestation of blank staring and impaired awareness during prolonged runs of SSW and atypical absence seizures.[33,97] SSW-related BOLD increases are also reported in supplementary motor cortex, anterior cingulate, thalamus, and cerebellum (see **Fig. 3**), although these appear to be more variable than the default-mode network inhibition.[105] The shape and timing of the BOLD response to SSW can deviate from typical hemodynamic assumptions used in EEG-fMRI analysis,[33] which may contribute to some of this variability.

The brain networks underlying GSW of IGE show similarities and differences to SSW of LGS (see **Fig. 4**). Like SSW, EEG-fMRI studies of GSW have detected BOLD decreases in the default-mode network,[41,42,44] and this is similarly linked to impaired awareness during typical absence seizures of IGE.[44] BOLD increases are also reported in supplementary motor cortex, anterior cingulate, thalamus, and cerebellum, but again, these changes are thought to be more variable,[44] possibly owing to hemodynamic response variability.

However, when this variability is accounted for, differences emerge between SSW and GSW. One EEG-fMRI study[107] used a flexible analysis approach that made fewer assumptions about the shape and timing of hemodynamic responses to IEDs[108] and found that SSW of LGS showed BOLD *decreases* in sensorimotor cortex, whereas the same areas showed BOLD *increases* during GSW of IGE (see **Fig. 4**). Sensorimotor activation during GSW may contribute to myoclonic jerking seen during seizures of some IGE variants[109] or may reflect the evolving nature of IGE subsyndromes across age (eg, from absence seizure-predominant childhood absence epilepsy to myoclonic seizure-predominant juvenile myoclonic epilepsy).[92] It is also consistent with early sensorimotor activation seen during GSW in rodent models,[110,111] and with findings from MEG studies.[65] Hence, although SSW and GSW both involve inhibition of the default-mode network, sensorimotor differences may be one factor contributing to their distinct EEG appearances and clinical correlates.

In addition to these functional changes, there are potential differences in brain network structural alterations between LGS and IGE, although direct comparisons are lacking. In one study of 10 adults with LGS, there was widespread gray- and white-matter atrophy relative to controls, notably in medial frontal cortex and the pons,[26] as measured by voxel-based morphometry of T1-weighted MRI. In contrast, a study of 289 adults with mixed forms of IGE found maximal gray-matter atrophy in precentral/paracentral cortex and the thalamus,[25] echoing the pattern of GSW-related sensorimotor activation described above.[107]

There is emerging evidence of brain network differences between IGE subsyndromes. For example, differences in dopamine uptake are seen in PET scans of juvenile myoclonic epilepsy versus epilepsy with generalized tonic-clonic seizures alone, the former showing reduced tracer binding in the midbrain and the latter showing reductions in the putamen.[54] Similarly, differences in diffusion MRI white-matter architecture[28] and fMRI connectivity[50] are found between refractory and nonrefractory forms of IGE, and between IGE subsyndromes,[112] suggesting unique patterns of seizure engagement and their related network alterations.

WHAT IS THE OPTIMAL STIMULATION TARGET?

If LGS and IGE are expressed via different brain networks, the optimal stimulation targets may also differ—if neurostimulation exerts therapeutic effects by acting on the specific neural generators of seizures and not a more seizure type-agnostic mechanism,[113] such as modulating overall cortical arousal.

The thalamic centromedian nucleus is the most widely explored stimulation target for LGS and IGE, or at least the most widely *intended* target, as different neurosurgical targeting and postimplantation programming strategies likely have differing accuracies[114] with respect to electrode trajectories and stimulation field effects on the centromedian nucleus versus surrounding structures.

Evidence for efficacy of centromedian stimulation, specifically duty-cycling or continuous DBS, is more mature for LGS than it is for IGE. Centromedian DBS has been studied in LGS for more than 30 years, starting with the pioneering work of Velasco and colleagues[6,115–118] and Fisher and colleagues.[15] Benefits have also been described in several unblinded studies.[8,9,13,14] Most recently, the efficacy of duty-cycling bilateral centromedian DBS was evaluated in a randomized, double-blind, placebo-controlled trial (*Electrical Stimulation of Thalamus for Epilepsy of Lennox-Gastaut phenotype* [ESTEL]), showing a significantly greater reduction in EEG-recorded—but not diary-recorded—seizures after 3 months in the treatment versus control groups, with outcomes measured as the sum of multiple seizure types.[5] There have been no such randomized controlled trials of centromedian DBS for IGE, but a small number of case studies give reason to be optimistic, with seizure reductions of 75% to 97% reported.[9,11] One single-blind trial including 4 patients with IGE found a 50% to 100% reduction in absence and generalized tonic-clonic seizures after 3 months of DBS.[7] Additional evidence comes from unblinded case reports of centromedian RNS for IGE.[10,119–121]

The rationale for centromedian stimulation in generalized epilepsy stems from a long-held view implicating this nucleus in modulating diffuse cortical excitability, as supported by the observation of generalized cortical potentials evoked by stimulating it,[74,122] and by a somewhat contentious notion of the centromedian nucleus being a "nonspecific" thalamic region with "widespread" cortical and subcortical connections.[123] However, more recent work suggests a greater degree of specificity in the functions and connectivity of this nucleus than perhaps previously thought.[124,125] Axonal tracing studies in nonhuman primates show it is a major source of excitatory input to the striatum (particularly sensorimotor striatal territories, including caudal putamen and caudate), whereas its projections to the cortex (which are mostly to central and precentral regions of sensorimotor cortex) and extrastriatal basal ganglia are comparatively sparse.[126–128] The centromedian nucleus also receives brainstem inputs from the reticular formation, vestibular nucleus, and solitary nucleus.[125] Similar patterns are seen in human neuroimaging studies,[13,114,129] including an analysis of diffusion MRI data from the Human Connectome Project[130] performed as part of the current review (Fig. 5).

How might this connectivity pattern relate to efficacy of centromedian stimulation for LGS and IGE? One hypothesis is that overlaps exist between these connections and the epileptic networks underlying each syndrome. For example, both the centromedian nucleus and the network implicated in GPFA/tonic seizures of LGS connect to the brainstem, putamen, caudate, and cerebellum (see Figs. 3 and 5). Similarly, regarding GSW of IGE, a key overlap may be sensorimotor cortex (see Figs. 4 and 5). Supporting this hypothesis is the recent finding from the ESTEL trial that DBS efficacy for LGS is positively correlated with structural connectivity between thalamic stimulation sites and areas of GPFA-related BOLD activation.[131]

However, there are also areas of nonoverlap, which may be relevant to understanding the seizure types for which centromedian stimulation is most efficacious or may speak to therapeutic mechanisms other than direct connections with the specific brain regions driving seizures. For example, connections between the centromedian nucleus and areas of the default-mode network (which shows prominent inhibition during SSW and GSW) are less apparent, for example, with the precuneus and posterior cingulate (see Fig. 5). This contrasts with the reported efficacy, at least in some individuals, of centromedian DBS for absence seizures,[6–8] the ictal correlate of GSW. One interpretation is that therapeutic effects are instead mediated via less direct means, such as shifting the brain to a state where absence seizures are less likely to occur.[132] For example, absence seizures show an inverse correlation with vigilance, being less frequent during periods of high arousal, including cognitive or physical tasks.[133,134] Such states are known to disengage the default-mode network,[106] and there is some evidence that centromedian DBS alters cortical arousal levels.[135]

Another possibility is that stimulation targets other than—or additional to—the centromedian nucleus may be more effective for specific syndromes or seizure types, owing to differences in the brain networks involved. For example, Valentín and colleagues[7] found that centromedian DBS was significantly more effective for 6 patients with mixed forms of generalized epilepsy (4 with IGE) compared with 5 with frontal lobe epilepsy, potentially reflecting preferential seizure networks modulated by centromedian stimulation. The optimal stimulation site in the ESTEL trial included the anterior and inferolateral "parvocellular" subregion of the centromedian nucleus, but also extended into the adjacent ventral lateral nucleus,[131] raising the potential strategy of stimulating other and/or multiple thalamic targets for LGS (as may be possible with, for example, current steering[136] or dual thalamic implant[137] approaches). Within the centromedian nucleus, Son and colleagues[14] found that DBS was more effective in different nuclear subregions for LGS (optimal in anterior and inferolateral subregion, like in ESTEL[131]) versus multilobar epilepsy (optimal in dorsal subregion). The pulvinar[138] and central lateral[139] thalamic nuclei show connectivity with cortical regions of the default-mode network, this being potentially relevant to the inhibition patterns seen during SSW and GSW (see Figs. 3 and 4); these nuclei are being targeted in ongoing trials.[140,141] Other studied targets for generalized epilepsy include the caudate[142] and cerebellum,[142–144] both of which appear involved in the epileptic networks of LGS and IGE.

To date, most neurostimulation studies for generalized epilepsy have focused on the subcortex, predominantly the thalamus. However, the affected regions are more widespread, and there

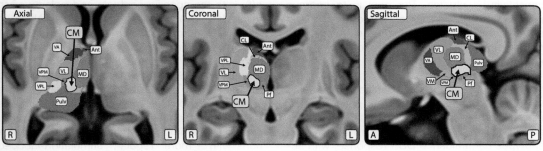

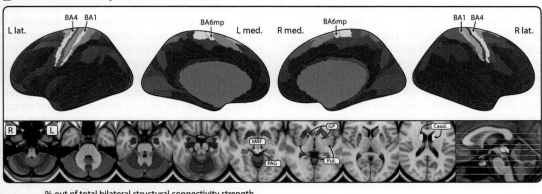

Fig. 5. Thalamic anatomy and structural connectivity of the centromedian nucleus. (*A*) Thalamic anatomy defined by the Krauth/Morel atlas,[186] including the centromedian nucleus (*yellow*). (*B*) Results of a structural connectivity analysis performed using diffusion MRI scans in the "100 unrelated subjects" dataset of healthy young adults (mean age = 29 years) from the Human Connectome Project.[130] Analysis followed our previously described pipe-line,[131] using MRtrix3 software (https://www.mrtrix.org). Briefly, whole-brain probabilistic tractography (20 million streamlines) and spherically informed filtering of tractograms (SIFT2) were performed per HCP subject. The resulting SIFT2-weighted tractograms were used to calculate structural connectivity strength between left and right masks of the thalamic centromedian nucleus[186] and a whole-brain parcellation of gray matter (https://identifiers.org/neurovault.collection:11930).[131] Left and right connectivity values were summed together and then results were averaged across all 100 HCP subjects. For display, these subject-averaged values were converted to percentages (out of the total bilateral connectivity strength across all parcels). Cortical hemisphere views were generated using *ggsegGlasser* software (https://github.com/ggseg/ggsegGlasser).[187] Positions of subcortical axial views are indicated by the dotted white lines on the sagittal view. *Interpretation:* Cortically, the centromedian nucleus shows strongest connectivity with primary motor (Brodmann area 4), primary somato-sensory (Brodmann area 1), and medial posterior supplementary motor cortex (Brodmann area 6mp). Subcorti-cally, there is strongest connectivity with posterior caudate, posterior putamen, globus pallidus, midbrain reticular formation, and peri-aqueductal gray area. A, anterior; Ant, anterior nuclear group; BA1, Brodmann area 1; BA4, Brodmann area 4; BA6mp, Brodmann area 6 medial posterior; Caud, caudate; CL, central lateral nu-cleus; CM, centromedian nucleus; GP, globus pallidus; L, left; Lat, lateral; MD, mediodorsal nucleus; Med, medial; MRF, midbrain reticular formation; P, posterior; PAG, peri-aqueductal gray area; Pulv, pulvinar nucleus; Put, pu-tamen; VA, ventral anterior nucleus; VL, ventral lateral nucleus; VM, ventral medial nucleus; VPL, ventral posterior lateral nucleus; VPM, ventral posterior medial nucleus.

is evidence that the cortex may participate earlier than the thalamus during some epileptiform event types in LGS[34,145] and IGE,[110,146,147] at least with respect to EEG onset times. These observations have led to the concept of dual thalamic *and* cortical neurostimulation,[17,148] including an ongoing single-blind clinical trial of RNS in LGS.[149] In this trial, bilateral neurostimulators are implanted, each with a depth lead targeting the centromedian nucleus and a cortical strip lead targeting a "hotspot" in LGS—premotor frontal cortex—recently identified from a multimodal synthesis of EEG-fMRI,[34] PET,[56] and structural connectivity[131] studies. The goal is to improve the speed and precision of seizure detection (and thus responsive stimulations) and to provide broader modulation of the epileptic network underlying LGS.

There are myriad other factors that likely influence a stimulation target's efficacy, including those that occur at the individual patient (rather than syndrome) level. In other conditions, such as Parkinson disease, there is evidence that individual genotypes can influence DBS response, with superior outcomes for patients carrying certain mutations (eg, *LRRK2*) compared with others (eg, *GBA*).[150] Similar findings occur in the pharmacologic treatment of generalized epilepsy, where outcomes are dependent on the genetic cause.[151,152] Genetic factors also influence many properties that govern how brain tissue responds to stimulation, including variability in glutamate signaling,[153] which can affect clinical response.[154,155] We envision that personalized treatment approaches based on individual causes or genotypes will soon be adopted in epilepsy neurostimulation to enable targeted selection of patients most likely to benefit.

WHAT IS THE OPTIMAL STIMULATION PARADIGM?

Beyond the targets, neurostimulation involves decisions regarding parameters including stimulation frequency, amplitude, pulse width, constant voltage or current, bipolar or referential polarity, unilateral or bilateral, and continuous or duty-cycling (on/off) or closed-loop detection thresholds.

This vast parameter space remains largely unexplored in generalized epilepsy. Most DBS and RNS studies employ stimulation settings used in previous trials, likely owing to regulatory and safety considerations, as well as extending generalizability by using settings already known to "work," at the expense of investigating novel ones that may yield superior outcomes. Practical constraints also limit the number of settings that can feasibly be explored, given that outcomes typically take several months to assess; multiple paradigms would require lengthy trial durations. Anecdotally, more exploration happens outside the trial context, with device adjustments occurring in the course of ongoing clinical management, but the insights gained tend to be specific to individual patients.

In centromedian DBS, typical choices[5,8,9] include bilateral, high-frequency (eg, 130–145 Hz) stimulation, delivered either continuously or in a duty-cycling fashion (eg, 1 minute on/5 minutes off), with the specific contacts and polarity often tailored to avoid patient side effects. Although the exact neurophysiologic effects are unknown, and likely differ between patients and anatomic targets, it is commonly thought that high-frequency DBS mimics "lesioning" by inhibiting neuronal firing,[156,157] which theoretically reduces excitability. However, more recent hypotheses suggest the mechanism may be more complex, such as "overriding" pathologic neuronal oscillations with a more "regular," stimulation-induced pattern,[158] modulating wider dysfunctional circuits connected to the target,[159] or inducing long-term neuroplastic changes[160] (which may contribute to the progressive seizure improvements seen over months and years of DBS).[161]

One strategy that may facilitate faster and more systematic identification of optimal paradigms is to develop disease biomarkers against which stimulation can be rapidly titrated. In other indications, such as Parkinson's disease, there are established electrophysiologic biomarkers that are measurable intraoperatively or postoperatively and correlate with disease symptoms and DBS response, including beta-band (∼ 11–30 Hz) frequency power of local field potentials[162] and evoked resonant neural activity ("ERNA").[163] These can inform stimulation adjustments, like selecting paradigms that suppress beta-band power.[164]

At present, no such biomarkers are clinically used for neurostimulation in generalized epilepsy, although some are proposed.[165–168] For example, the burden of scalp EEG-recorded GPFA discharges correlates with seizure outcomes in DBS for LGS.[169] Other measures may be imported from the broader domain of epilepsy neurosurgery, where several electrophysiologic biomarkers have been identified[170] to tailor resections (eg, high-frequency oscillations); these may hold similar value in optimizing stimulation targeting and paradigms.

In addition, the choice of stimulation paradigm may depend on the therapeutic goal. Is it to "chase and abort" seizures while having minimal impact on normal brain function to avoid potential stimulation side effects (as may be more effectively achieved by the intermittent stimulations given in closed-loop approaches)? Or is to create a lasting neuroplastic change from a state of abnormal brain organization, of which seizures are a symptom (as may be more effectively achieved by delivering more frequent stimulation, or stimulating during periods when the brain is most capable of such "reorganization")? Supporting the latter goal is the recent—and somewhat counterintuitive—observation that closed-loop stimulation for focal epilepsy leads to better outcomes when stimulation is provided during periods of *less* epileptiform activity and *lower* seizure susceptibility,[171] suggesting the interictal period may be when the brain is more amenable to the neuroplastic changes required for prolonged seizure reduction. Whether the same holds true in generalized epilepsy, and whether this differs between LGS and IGE, will be important to confirm in ongoing RNS trials.[149,172]

WHAT IS THE PLAN FOR ADJUSTING STIMULATION OVER TIME?

Stimulation programming is typically static in the short term (hours and days), but often adjusted in the long term (months and years). However, generalized epilepsy is dynamic and presents differently over time, suggesting stimulation paradigms may also need to flexibly adapt to these changes.

Regarding short-term changes, epileptiform activity of LGS and IGE shows circadian variation. In LGS, seizures and IEDs occur most frequently during non–rapid eye movement (NREM) sleep and are comparatively less frequent during wakefulness and rapid eye movement (REM) sleep.[173,174] A similar pattern is seen in IGE.[175] Sleep is not typically factored into stimulation programming for generalized epilepsy, despite evidence that DBS can alter sleep architecture, including by changing the timing and duration of REM and NREM sleep stages in subthalamic DBS for Parkinson disease,[176] or by increasing the number of nighttime arousals in anterior thalamic DBS for focal epilepsy.[177] Hence, stimulation programming for LGS and IGE may benefit from considering impacts on sleep cycles, given their close association with seizure susceptibility.

Seizure occurrence also varies over multiday cycles (eg, weekly to monthly),[178] with the exact timing seemingly patient-specific and associated with endogenous cycles in heart rate,[179] body temperature,[180] electrodermal activity,[180] and other physiologic systems. There is also evidence that seizure occurrence may even be influenced by environmental factors, including elevated carbon monoxide concentrations owing to ambient air pollution.[181] These multiday cycles have mostly been investigated in the context of focal epilepsy, and it will be important to confirm whether similar patterns are also observed in LGS and IGE. However, they raise the potential of dynamically adjusting stimulation using information from long-term physiologic or environmental recording devices, which are already being used to, for example, forecast risk states associated with sudden unexpected death in epilepsy via subcutaneous cardiac monitors.[182]

In the longer term, LGS and IGE show significant evolution over the course of a patient's life. At onset of LGS (peak age 3–5 years), not all electroclinical features may be present in combination,[85] and some seizure types can wax and wane over time. For example, tonic and atypical absence seizures tend to persist into adulthood, whereas atonic seizures can sometimes diminish.[100] In addition, the nature of caregiver burden in LGS can change over time, with cognitive, behavioral, and physical impairments (eg, sleep disturbances) often becoming equally or even more challenging to manage than seizures as patients become older.[183,184] Whether neurostimulation therapies can play a role in managing these nonseizure consequences remains largely unstudied in epilepsy.[185]

A similar evolution occurs in IGE, where there is often an age-related shift from one subsyndrome to another (eg, from childhood absence epilepsy to juvenile myoclonic epilepsy; see **Table 1**). Given emerging evidence of variability in the brain network substrates of different IGE sub-syndromes,[28,50,54,112] stimulation programming may need to be adjusted to respond to the evolving nature of IGE.

SUMMARY

We are early in the journey toward optimizing neurostimulation therapy for generalized epilepsy. There is accumulating evidence of efficacy for select targets and paradigms, including DBS of the thalamic centromedian nucleus. However, generalized epilepsy is not a uniform disease, suggesting that the optimal forms of neurostimulation may lie beyond the prevailing "one-target-fits-all" approach.

LGS and IGE differ with respect to their EEG signatures, predominant seizure types, cognitive comorbidities, etiologic profiles, and prognosis. Recent neuroimaging studies demonstrate that these differences may be underpinned by syndrome-specific patterns of brain network pathology condition. Hence, therapeutic efficacy of neurostimulation may be enhanced by applying knowledge of the underlying brain networks and how they evolve over short and long timescales.

CLINICS CARE POINTS

- Lennox-Gastaut syndrome and idiopathic generalized epilepsy are distinct generalized epilepsy syndromes.

- Different brain networks underlie Lennox-Gastaut syndrome and idiopathic generalized epilepsy.
- Neurostimulation is not currently tailored to each syndrome.
- Optimal stimulation targets and programming may be syndrome specific.

FUNDING

S. Tobochnik is supported in part by a VA Career Development Award (V1CDA2022–68) and has received research support from Eisai. J.D. Rolston is supported in part by an NIH/NINDS career development award (K23 NS114178). The EEG-fMRI data acquired and analyzed in this article were supported by NHMRC project grants #628725 and #1108881 (PI: A/Prof John Archer, University of Melbourne).

DISCLOSURE

A.E.L. Warren, Steven Tobochnik, Melissa M.J. Chua, Hargunbir Singh, and Michaela A. Stamm have no disclosures to report. John D. Rolston has received consulting payments from Medtronic, Corlieve, and NeuroPace.

REFERENCES

1. Camfield CS, Camfield PR, Gordon K, et al. Incidence of epilepsy in childhood and adolescence: a population-based study in Nova Scotia from 1977 to 1985. Epilepsia 1996;37(1):19–23. https://doi.org/10.1111/j.1528-1157.1996.tb00506.x.
2. Berg AT, Berkovic SF, Brodie MJ, et al. Revised terminology and concepts for organization of seizures and epilepsies: report of the ILAE Commission on Classification and Terminology, 2005–2009. Epilepsia 2010;51(4):676–85. https://doi.org/10.1111/j.1528-1167.2010.02522.x.
3. Wirrell EC, Nabbout R, Scheffer IE, et al. Methodology for classification and definition of epilepsy syndromes with list of syndromes: Report of the ILAE Task Force on Nosology and Definitions. Epilepsia 2022;63(6):1333–48. https://doi.org/10.1111/epi.17237.
4. Touma L, Dansereau B, Chan AY, et al. Neurostimulation in people with drug-resistant epilepsy: Systematic review and meta-analysis from the ILAE Surgical Therapies Commission. Epilepsia 2022;63(6):1314–29. https://doi.org/10.1111/epi.17243.
5. Dalic LJ, Warren AEL, Bulluss KJ, et al. DBS of Thalamic Centromedian Nucleus for Lennox-Gastaut Syndrome (ESTEL Trial). Ann Neurol 2022;91(2):253–67. https://doi.org/10.1002/ana.26280.
6. Velasco AL, Velasco F, Jiménez F, et al. Neuromodulation of the centromedian thalamic nuclei in the treatment of generalized seizures and the improvement of the quality of life in patients with Lennox–Gastaut syndrome. Epilepsia 2006;47(7):1203–12. https://doi.org/10.1111/j.1528-1167.2006.00593.x.
7. Valentín A, García Navarrete E, Chelvarajah R, et al. Deep brain stimulation of the centromedian thalamic nucleus for the treatment of generalized and frontal epilepsies. Epilepsia 2013;54(10):1823–33. https://doi.org/10.1111/epi.12352.
8. Cukiert A, Cukiert CM, Burattini JA, et al. Seizure outcome during bilateral, continuous, thalamic centromedian nuclei deep brain stimulation in patients with generalized epilepsy: a prospective, open-label study. Seizure 2020;81:304–9. https://doi.org/10.1016/j.seizure.2020.08.028.
9. Yang JC, Bullinger KL, Isbaine F, et al. Centromedian thalamic deep brain stimulation for drug-resistant epilepsy: single-center experience. J Neurosurg 2022;137(6):1591–600. https://doi.org/10.3171/2022.2.JNS212237.
10. Welch WP, Hect JL, Abel TJ. Case Report: Responsive Neurostimulation of the Centromedian Thalamic Nucleus for the Detection and Treatment of Seizures in Pediatric Primary Generalized Epilepsy. Front Neurol 2021;12:656585. https://doi.org/10.3389/fneur.2021.656585.
11. Agashe S, Burkholder D, Starnes K, et al. Centromedian Nucleus of the Thalamus Deep Brain Stimulation for Genetic Generalized Epilepsy: A Case Report and Review of Literature. Front Hum Neurosci 2022;16:858413. https://doi.org/10.3389/fnhum.2022.858413.
12. Alcala-Zermeno JL, Gregg NM, Wirrell EC, et al. Centromedian thalamic nucleus with or without anterior thalamic nucleus deep brain stimulation for epilepsy in children and adults: A retrospective case series. Seizure 2021;84:101–7. https://doi.org/10.1016/j.seizure.2020.11.012.
13. Kim SH, Lim SC, Yang DW, et al. Thalamo–cortical network underlying deep brain stimulation of centromedian thalamic nuclei in intractable epilepsy: a multimodal imaging analysis. Neuropsychiatr Dis Treat 2017;13:2607. https://doi.org/10.2147/NDT.S148617.
14. Son B-c, Shon YM, Choi J-g, et al. Clinical Outcome of Patients with Deep Brain Stimulation of the Centromedian Thalamic Nucleus for Refractory Epilepsy and Location of the Active Contacts. Stereotact Funct Neurosurg 2016;94(3):187–97. https://doi.org/10.1159/000446611.
15. Fisher RS, Uematsu S, Krauss GL, et al. Placebo-Controlled Pilot Study of Centromedian Thalamic

Stimulation in Treatment of Intractable Seizures. Epilepsia 1992;33(5):841–51. https://doi.org/10.1111/j.1528-1157.1992.tb02192.x.

16. Torres Diaz CV, Gonzalez-Escamilla G, Ciolac D, et al. Network Substrates of Centromedian Nucleus Deep Brain Stimulation in Generalized Pharmacoresistant Epilepsy. Neurotherapeutics 2021; 18(3):1665–77. https://doi.org/10.1007/s13311-021-01057-y.

17. Burdette DE, Haykal MA, Jarosiewicz B, et al. Brain-responsive corticothalamic stimulation in the centromedian nucleus for the treatment of regional neocortical epilepsy. Epilepsy Behav 2020;112:107354. https://doi.org/10.1016/j.yebeh.2020.107354.

18. Piper RJ, Richardson RM, Worrell G, et al. Towards network-guided neuromodulation for epilepsy. Brain 2022;145(10):3347–62. https://doi.org/10.1093/brain/awac234.

19. Pittau F, Vulliemoz S. Functional brain networks in epilepsy: recent advances in noninvasive mapping. Curr Opin Neurol 2015;28(4):338–43. https://doi.org/10.1097/WCO.0000000000000221.

20. Richardson M. Current themes in neuroimaging of epilepsy: brain networks, dynamic phenomena, and clinical relevance. Clin Neurophysiol 2010;121(8):1153–75. https://doi.org/10.1016/j.clinph.2010.01.004.

21. Hermann BP, Struck AF, Busch RM, et al. Neurobehavioural comorbidities of epilepsy: towards a network-based precision taxonomy. Nat Rev Neurol 2021;17(12):731–46. https://doi.org/10.1038/s41582-021-00555-z.

22. Betting LE, Mory SB, Lopes-Cendes I, et al. MRI reveals structural abnormalities in patients with idiopathic generalized epilepsy. Neurology 2006; 67(5):848–52. https://doi.org/10.1212/01.wnl.0000233886.55203.bd.

23. Kim EH, Shim WH, Lee JS, et al. Altered Structural Network in Newly Onset Childhood Absence Epilepsy. J Clin Neurol 2020;16(4):573–80. https://doi.org/10.3988/jcn.2020.16.4.573.

24. Lariviere S, Royer J, Rodriguez-Cruces R, et al. Structural network alterations in focal and generalized epilepsy assessed in a worldwide ENIGMA study follow axes of epilepsy risk gene expression. Nat Commun 2022;13(1):4320. https://doi.org/10.1038/s41467-022-31730-5.

25. Lariviere S, Rodriguez-Cruces R, Royer J, et al. Network-based atrophy modeling in the common epilepsies: A worldwide ENIGMA study. Sci Adv 2020;6(47). https://doi.org/10.1126/sciadv.abc6457.

26. Newham BJ, Curwood EK, Jackson GD, et al. Pontine and cerebral atrophy in Lennox-Gastaut syndrome. Epilepsy Res 2016;120:98–103. https://doi.org/10.1016/j.eplepsyres.2015.12.005.

27. Woermann FG, Free SL, Koepp MJ, et al. Abnormal cerebral structure in juvenile myoclonic epilepsy demonstrated with voxel-based analysis of MRI. Brain 1999;122(Pt 11):2101–8. https://doi.org/10.1093/brain/122.11.2101.

28. McKavanagh A, Kreilkamp BAK, Chen Y, et al. Altered Structural Brain Networks in Refractory and Nonrefractory Idiopathic Generalized Epilepsy. Brain Connect 2022;12(6):549–60. https://doi.org/10.1089/brain.2021.0035.

29. Hatton SN, Huynh KH, Bonilha L, et al. White matter abnormalities across different epilepsy syndromes in adults: an ENIGMA-Epilepsy study. Brain 2020; 143(8):2454–73. https://doi.org/10.1093/brain/awaa200.

30. Caeyenberghs K, Powell HW, Thomas RH, et al. Hyperconnectivity in juvenile myoclonic epilepsy: a network analysis. Neuroimage Clin 2015;7:98–104. https://doi.org/10.1016/j.nicl.2014.11.018.

31. Vulliemoz S, Vollmar C, Koepp MJ, et al. Connectivity of the supplementary motor area in juvenile myoclonic epilepsy and frontal lobe epilepsy. Epilepsia 2011;52(3):507–14. https://doi.org/10.1111/j.1528-1167.2010.02770.x.

32. O'Muircheartaigh J, Vollmar C, Barker GJ, et al. Abnormal thalamocortical structural and functional connectivity in juvenile myoclonic epilepsy. Brain 2012;135(12):3635–44. https://doi.org/10.1093/brain/aws296.

33. Archer JS, Warren AEL, Stagnitti MR, et al. Lennox-Gastaut Syndrome and Phenotype: secondary network epilepsies. Epilepsia 2014;55(8):1245–54. https://doi.org/10.1111/epi.12682.

34. Warren AEL, Harvey AS, Vogrin SJ, et al. The epileptic network of Lennox-Gastaut syndrome: Cortically driven and reproducible across age. Neurology 2019;93(3):e215–26. https://doi.org/10.1212/WNL.0000000000007775.

35. Tyvaert L, Chassagnon S, Sadikot A, et al. Thalamic nuclei activity in idiopathic generalized epilepsy: an EEG-fMRI study. Neurology 2009; 73(23):2018–22. https://doi.org/10.1212/WNL.0b013e3181c55d02.

36. Siniatchkin M, Van Baalen A, Jacobs J, et al. Different neuronal networks are associated with spikes and slow activity in hypsarrhythmia. Epilepsia 2007;48(12):2312–21. https://doi.org/10.1111/j.1528-1167.2007.01195.x.

37. Moeller F, Groening K, Moehring J, et al. EEG-fMRI in myoclonic astatic epilepsy (Doose syndrome). Neurology 2014. https://doi.org/10.1212/WNL.0000000000000359.

38. Siniatchkin M, Coropceanu D, Moeller F, et al. EEG-fMRI reveals activation of brainstem and thalamus in patients with Lennox-Gastaut syndrome. Epilepsia 2011;52(4):766–74. https://doi.org/10.1111/j.1528-1167.2010.02948.x.

39. Siniatchkin M, Groening K, Moehring J, et al. Neuronal networks in children with continuous

spikes and waves during slow sleep. Brain 2010; 133(9):2798–813. https://doi.org/10.1093/brain/awq183.

40. Archer JS, Abbott DF, Waites AB, et al. fMRI "deactivation" of the posterior cingulate during generalized spike and wave. Neuroimage 2003;20(4):1915–22. https://doi.org/10.1016/s1053-8119(03)00294-5.

41. Aghakhani Y, Bagshaw A, Benar C, et al. fMRI activation during spike and wave discharges in idiopathic generalized epilepsy. Brain 2004;127(5):1127–44. https://doi.org/10.1093/brain/awh136.

42. Gotman J, Grova C, Bagshaw A, et al. Generalized epileptic discharges show thalamocortical activation and suspension of the default state of the brain. Proc Natl Acad Sci U S A 2005;102(42):15236–40. https://doi.org/10.1073/pnas.0504935102.

43. Maki Y, Natsume J, Ito Y, et al. Involvement of the Thalamus, Hippocampus, and Brainstem in Hypsarrhythmia of West Syndrome: Simultaneous Recordings of Electroencephalography and fMRI Study. AJNR Am J Neuroradiol 2022;43(10):1502–7. https://doi.org/10.3174/ajnr.A7646.

44. Carney P, Masterton R, Harvey A, et al. The core network in absence epilepsy Differences in cortical and thalamic BOLD response. Neurology 2010;75(10):904–11. https://doi.org/10.1212/WNL.0b013e3181f11c06.

45. Warren AEL, Abbott DF, Vaughan DN, et al. Abnormal cognitive network interactions in Lennox-Gastaut Syndrome: A potential mechanism of epileptic encephalopathy. Epilepsia 2016;57(5):812–22. https://doi.org/10.1111/epi.13342.

46. Warren AEL, Abbott DF, Jackson GD, et al. Thalamocortical functional connectivity in Lennox–Gastaut syndrome is abnormally enhanced in executive-control and default-mode networks. Epilepsia 2017;58(12):2085–97. https://doi.org/10.1111/epi.13932.

47. Luo C, Li Q, Lai Y, et al. Altered functional connectivity in default mode network in absence epilepsy: a resting-state fMRI study. Hum Brain Mapp 2011;32(3):438–49. https://doi.org/10.1002/hbm.21034.

48. Ji G-J, Zhang Z, Xu Q, et al. Identifying corticothalamic network epicenters in patients with idiopathic generalized epilepsy. AJNR Am J Neuroradiol 2015;36(8):1494–500. https://doi.org/10.3174/ajnr.A4308.

49. Wang Z, Lariviere S, Xu Q, et al. Community-informed connectomics of the thalamocortical system in generalized epilepsy. Neurology 2019;93(11):e1112–22. https://doi.org/10.1212/WNL.0000000000008096.

50. Pegg EJ, McKavanagh A, Bracewell RM, et al. Functional network topology in drug resistant and well-controlled idiopathic generalized epilepsy: a resting state functional MRI study. Brain Commun 2021;3(3):fcab196. https://doi.org/10.1093/braincomms/fcab196.

51. Tangwiriyasakul C, Perani S, Abela E, et al. Sensorimotor network hypersynchrony as an endophenotype in families with genetic generalized epilepsy: A resting-state functional magnetic resonance imaging study. Epilepsia 2019;60(3):e14–9. https://doi.org/10.1111/epi.14663.

52. Chugani HT, Mazziotta JC, Engel J, et al. The Lennox-Gastaut syndrome: Metabolic subtypes determined by 2-deoxy-2 [18F] fluoro-d-glucose positron emission tomography. Ann Neurol 1987;21(1):4–13. https://doi.org/10.1002/ana.410210104.

53. Prevett MC, Duncan JS, Jones T, et al. Demonstration of thalamic activation during typical absence seizures using H2(15)O and PET. Neurology 1995;45(7):1396–402. https://doi.org/10.1212/wnl.45.7.1396.

54. Ciumas C, Wahlin TB, Espino C, et al. The dopamine system in idiopathic generalized epilepsies: identification of syndrome-related changes. Neuroimage 2010;51(2):606–15. https://doi.org/10.1016/j.neuroimage.2010.02.051.

55. Ligot N, Archambaud F, Trotta N, et al. Default mode network hypometabolism in epileptic encephalopathies with CSWS. Epilepsy Res 2014;108(5):861–71. https://doi.org/10.1016/j.eplepsyres.2014.03.014.

56. Balfroid T, Warren AEL, Dalic LJ, et al. Frontoparietal 18F-FDG-PET hypo-metabolism in Lennox-Gastaut syndrome: further evidence highlighting the key network. Epilepsy Res 2023;192:107131. https://doi.org/10.1016/j.eplepsyres.2023.107131.

57. Blumenfeld H, Westerveld M, Ostroff RB, et al. Selective frontal, parietal, and temporal networks in generalized seizures. Neuroimage 2003;19(4):1556–66. https://doi.org/10.1016/s1053-8119(03)00204-0.

58. Intusoma U, Abbott DF, Masterton RA, et al. Tonic seizures of Lennox-Gastaut syndrome: Periictal single-photon emission computed tomography suggests a corticopontine network. Epilepsia 2013;54(12):2151–7. https://doi.org/10.1111/epi.12398.

59. Yeni SN, Kabasakal L, Yalcinkaya C, et al. Ictal and interictal SPECT findings in childhood absence epilepsy. Seizure 2000;9(4):265–9. https://doi.org/10.1053/seiz.2000.0400.

60. Gaggero R, Caputo M, Fiorio P, et al. SPECT and epilepsy with continuous spike waves during slow-wave sleep. Childs Nerv Syst 1995;11(3):154–60. https://doi.org/10.1007/BF00570256.

61. Stefan H, Paulini-Ruf A, Hopfengartner R, et al. Network characteristics of idiopathic generalized epilepsies in combined MEG/EEG. Epilepsy Res 2009;85(2–3):187–98. https://doi.org/10.1016/j.eplepsyres.2009.03.015.

62. Stier C, Loose M, Kotikalapudi R, et al. Combined electrophysiological and morphological phenotypes in patients with genetic generalized epilepsy and their healthy siblings. Epilepsia 2022;63(7):1643–57. https://doi.org/10.1111/epi.17258.

63. Tenney JR, Williamson BJ, Kadis DS. Cross-Frequency Coupling in Childhood Absence Epilepsy. Brain Connect 2022;12(5):489–96. https://doi.org/10.1089/brain.2021.0119.

64. Gadad V, Sinha S, Mariyappa N, et al. Source analysis of epileptiform discharges in absence epilepsy using Magnetoencephalography (MEG). Epilepsy Res 2018;140:46–52. https://doi.org/10.1016/j.eplepsyres.2017.12.003.

65. Aung T, Tenney JR, Bagic AI. Contributions of Magnetoencephalography to Understanding Mechanisms of Generalized Epilepsies: Blurring the Boundary Between Focal and Generalized Epilepsies? Front Neurol 2022;13:831546. https://doi.org/10.3389/fneur.2022.831546.

66. Morrell MJ, Group, RNSSiES. Responsive cortical stimulation for the treatment of medically intractable partial epilepsy. Neurology 2011;77(13):1295–304. https://doi.org/10.1212/WNL.0b013e3182302056.

67. Nair DR, Laxer KD, Weber PB, et al. Nine-year prospective efficacy and safety of brain-responsive neurostimulation for focal epilepsy. Neurology 2020;95(9):e1244–56. https://doi.org/10.1212/WNL.0000000000010154.

68. Wyllie E, Lachhwani D, Gupta A, et al. Successful surgery for epilepsy due to early brain lesions despite generalized EEG findings. Neurology 2007;69(4):389–97. https://doi.org/10.1212/01.wnl.0000266386.55715.3f.

69. Freeman J, Harvey A, Rosenfeld J, et al. Generalized epilepsy in hypothalamic hamartoma Evolution and postoperative resolution. Neurology 2003;60(5):762–7. https://doi.org/10.1212/01.wnl.0000049457.05670.7d.

70. Haneef Z, Skrehot HC. Neurostimulation in generalized epilepsy: A systematic review and meta-analysis. Epilepsia 2023;64(4):811–20. https://doi.org/10.1111/epi.17524.

71. Vetkas A, Fomenko A, Germann J, et al. Deep brain stimulation targets in epilepsy: Systematic review and meta-analysis of anterior and centromedian thalamic nuclei and hippocampus. Epilepsia 2022;63(3):513–24. https://doi.org/10.1111/epi.17157.

72. Yan H, Toyota E, Anderson M, et al. A systematic review of deep brain stimulation for the treatment of drug-resistant epilepsy in childhood. J Neurosurg Pediatr 2018;23(3):274–84. https://doi.org/10.3171/2018.9.PEDS18417.

73. Khan M, Paktiawal J, Piper RJ, et al. Intracranial neuromodulation with deep brain stimulation and responsive neurostimulation in children with drug-resistant epilepsy: a systematic review. J Neurosurg Pediatr 2021;1–10. https://doi.org/10.3171/2021.8.PEDS21201.

74. Velasco F, Saucedo-Alvarado PE, Reichrath A, et al. Centromedian Nucleus and Epilepsy. J Clin Neurophysiol 2021;38(6):485–93. https://doi.org/10.1097/WNP.0000000000000735.

75. Remore LG, Omidbeigi M, Tsolaki E, et al. Deep brain stimulation of thalamic nuclei for the treatment of drug-resistant epilepsy: Are we confident with the precise surgical target? Seizure 2023;105:22–8. https://doi.org/10.1016/j.seizure.2023.01.009.

76. Bullinger KL, Alwaki A, Gross. RE. Surgical Treatment of Drug-Resistant Generalized Epilepsy. Curr Neurol Neurosci Rep 2022;22(8):459–65. https://doi.org/10.1007/s11910-022-01210-w.

77. Gibbs FA, Gibbs E, Lennox WG. Influence of the blood sugar level on the wave and spike formation in petit mal epilepsy. Arch NeurPsych 1939;41(6):1111–6. https://doi.org/10.1001/archneurpsyc.1939.02270180039002.

78. Gibbs F, Davis H, Lennox W. The electroencephalogram in epilepsy and in conditions of impaired consciousness. Arch NeurPsych 1935;34(6):1133–48. https://doi.org/10.1001/archneurpsyc.1935.02250240002001.

79. Gibbs F, Lennox W, Gibbs EL. The electroencephalogram in diagnosis and in localization of epileptic seizures. Arch NeurPsych 1936;36(6):1225–35. https://doi.org/10.1001/archneurpsyc.1936.02260120072005.

80. Gibbs FA, Gibbs EL, Lennox WG. Electroencephalographic classification of epileptic patients and control subjects. Arch NeurPsych 1943;50(2):111–28. https://doi.org/10.1001/archneurpsyc.1943.02290200011001.

81. Lennox WG, Davis JP. Clinical correlates of the fast and the slow spike-wave electroencephalogram. Pediatrics 1950;5(4):626–44. https://doi.org/10.1542/peds.5.4.626.

82. Gastaut H, Roger J, Ocjahchi S, et al. An electroclinical study of generalized epileptic seizures of tonic expression. Epilepsia 1963;4(1-4):15–44. https://doi.org/10.1111/j.1528-1157.1963.tb05206.x.

83. Gastaut H, Roger J, Soulayrol R, et al. Childhood Epileptic Encephalopathy with Diffuse Slow Spike-Waves (otherwise known as "Petit Mal Variant") or Lennox Syndrome. Epilepsia 1966;7(2):139–79. https://doi.org/10.1111/j.1528-1167.1966.tb06263.x.

84. Dravet C. Encéphalopathie épileptique de l'enfant avec pointe-onde lente diffuse (petit mal variant). Marseilles, France: University of Marseilles; 1965.

85. Specchio N, Wirrell EC, Scheffer IE, et al. International League Against Epilepsy classification and definition of epilepsy syndromes with onset in childhood: Position paper by the ILAE Task Force

on Nosology and Definitions. Epilepsia 2022;63(6): 1398–442. https://doi.org/10.1111/epi.17241.

86. Beaumanoir A. The Lennox-Gastaut syndrome: a personal study. Electroencephalogr Clin Neurophysiol Suppl 1982;(35):85–99.

87. Heiskala H. Community-Based Study of Lennox-Gastaut Syndrome. Epilepsia 1997;38(5): 526–31. https://doi.org/10.1111/j.1528-1157.1997.tb01136.x.

88. Rantala H, Putkonen T. Occurrence, Outcome, and Prognostic Factors of Infantile Spasms and Lennox-Gastaut Syndrome. Epilepsia 1999;40(3): 286–9. https://doi.org/10.1111/j.1528-1157.1999.tb00705.x.

89. Trevathan E, Murphy CC, Yeargin-Allsopp M. Prevalence and descriptive epidemiology of Lennox-Gastaut syndrome among Atlanta children. Epilepsia 1997;38(12):1283–8. https://doi.org/10.1111/j.1528-1157.1997.tb00065.x.

90. Millichap J. Prevalence of Lennox-Gastaut Syndrome in Atlanta. Pediatr Neurol Briefs 1998; 12(1). https://doi.org/10.15844/pedneurbriefs-12-1-11.

91. Jallon P, Latour P. Epidemiology of idiopathic generalized epilepsies. Epilepsia 2005;46(Suppl 9):10–4. https://doi.org/10.1111/j.1528-1167.2005.00309.x.

92. Hirsch E, French J, Scheffer IE, et al. ILAE definition of the Idiopathic Generalized Epilepsy Syndromes: Position statement by the ILAE Task Force on Nosology and Definitions. Epilepsia 2022;63(6):1475–99. https://doi.org/10.1111/epi.17236.

93. Bansal L, Vargas Collado L, Pawar K, et al. Electroclinical Features of Generalized Paroxysmal Fast Activity in Typical Absence Seizures. J Clin Neurophysiol 2019;36(1):36–44. https://doi.org/10.1097/WNP.0000000000000535.

94. Gesche J, Beier CP. Drug resistance in idiopathic generalized epilepsies: Evidence and concepts. Epilepsia 2022;63(12):3007–19. https://doi.org/10.1111/epi.17410.

95. International League Against Epilepsy Consortium on Complex E. Genome-wide mega-analysis identifies 16 loci and highlights diverse biological mechanisms in the common epilepsies. Nat Commun 2018;9(1):5269. https://doi.org/10.1038/s41467-018-07524-z.

96. Whelan CD, Altmann A, Botia JA, et al. Structural brain abnormalities in the common epilepsies assessed in a worldwide ENIGMA study. Brain 2018;141(2):391–408. https://doi.org/10.1093/brain/awx341.

97. Archer JS, Warren AEL, Jackson GD, et al. Conceptualising Lennox-Gastaut Syndrome as a secondary network epilepsy. Front Neurol 2014;5(225):11. https://doi.org/10.3389/fneur.2014.00225.

98. Goldsmith IL, Zupanc ML, Buchhalter JR. Long-Term Seizure Outcome in 74 Patients with Lennox–Gastaut Syndrome: Effects of Incorporating MRI Head Imaging in Defining the Cryptogenic Subgroup. Epilepsia 2000;41(4):395–9. https://doi.org/10.1111/j.1528-1157.2000.tb00179.x.

99. Kim HJ, Kim HD, Lee JS, et al. Long-term prognosis of patients with Lennox–Gastaut syndrome in recent decades. Epilepsy Res 2015;110:10–9. https://doi.org/10.1016/j.eplepsyres.2014.11.004.

100. Vignoli A, Oggioni G, De Maria G, et al. Lennox–Gastaut syndrome in adulthood: Long-term clinical follow-up of 38 patients and analysis of their recorded seizures. Epilepsy Behav 2017;77:73–8. https://doi.org/10.1016/j.yebeh.2017.09.006.

101. Spencer SS. Neural networks in human epilepsy: evidence of and implications for treatment. Epilepsia 2002;43(3):219–27. https://doi.org/10.1046/j.1528-1157.2002.26901.x.

102. Warren AE, Harvey AS, Abbott DF, et al. Cognitive network reorganization following surgical control of seizures in Lennox-Gastaut syndrome. Epilepsia 2017;58(5):e75–81. https://doi.org/10.1111/epi.13720.

103. Kang JW, Eom S, Hong W, et al. Long-term Outcome of Resective Epilepsy Surgery in Patients With Lennox-Gastaut Syndrome. Pediatrics 2018; 142(4). https://doi.org/10.1542/peds.2018-0449.

104. Thirunavu V, Du R, Wu JY, et al. The role of surgery in the management of Lennox-Gastaut syndrome: A systematic review and meta-analysis of the clinical evidence. Epilepsia 2021;62(4):888–907. https://doi.org/10.1111/epi.16851.

105. Pillay N, Archer JS, Badawy RA, et al. Networks underlying paroxysmal fast activity and slow spike and wave in Lennox-Gastaut syndrome. Neurology 2013;81(7):665–73. https://doi.org/10.1212/WNL.0b013e3182a08f6a.

106. Raichle ME, MacLeod AM, Snyder AZ, et al. A default mode of brain function. Proc Natl Acad Sci U S A 2001;98(2):676–82. https://doi.org/10.1073/pnas.98.2.676.

107. Warren AEL, Abbott DF, Carney P, et al. EEG-fMRI event-related ICA of spike-wave in genetic generalised epilepsy compared to Lennox-Gastaut syndrome. Victoria, Australia: *Epilepsy Melbourne @ MBC*. Parkville; 2014.

108. Masterton RA, Jackson GD, Abbott DF. Mapping brain activity using event-related independent components analysis (eICA): specific advantages for EEG-fMRI. Neuroimage 2013;70:164–74. https://doi.org/10.1016/j.neuroimage.2012.12.025.

109. Nasser H, Lopez-Hernandez E, Ilea A, et al. Myoclonic jerks are commonly associated with absence seizures in early-onset absence epilepsy. Epileptic Disord 2017;19(2):137–46. https://doi.org/10.1684/epd.2017.0905.

110. Meeren HK, Pijn JPM, Van Luijtelaar EL, et al. Cortical focus drives widespread corticothalamic networks during spontaneous absence seizures in rats. J Neurosci 2002;22(4):1480–95. https://doi.org/10.1523/JNEUROSCI.22-04-01480.2002.

111. Polack PO, Guillemain I, Hu E, et al. Deep layer somatosensory cortical neurons initiate spike-and-wave discharges in a genetic model of absence seizures. J Neurosci 2007;27(24):6590–9. https://doi.org/10.1523/JNEUROSCI.0753-07.2007.

112. Liu M, Concha L, Beaulieu C, et al. Distinct white matter abnormalities in different idiopathic generalized epilepsy syndromes. Epilepsia 2011;52(12):2267–75. https://doi.org/10.1111/j.1528-1167.2011.03313.x.

113. McIntyre CC, Hahn PJ. Network perspectives on the mechanisms of deep brain stimulation. Neurobiol Dis 2010;38(3):329–37. https://doi.org/10.1016/j.nbd.2009.09.022.

114. Warren AEL, Dalic LJ, Thevathasan W, et al. Targeting the centromedian thalamic nucleus for deep brain stimulation. J Neurol Neurosurg Psychiatry 2020;91(4):339–49. https://doi.org/10.1136/jnnp-2019-322030.

115. Velasco F, Velasco M, Ogarrio C, et al. Electrical stimulation of the centromedian thalamic nucleus in the treatment of convulsive seizures: a preliminary report. Epilepsia 1987;28(4):421–30. https://doi.org/10.1111/j.1528-1157.1987.tb03668.x.

116. Velasco M, Velasco F, Alcalá H, et al. Epileptiform EEG Activity of the Centromedian Thalamic Nuclei in Children with Intractable Generalized Seizures of the Lennox-Gastaut Syndrome. Epilepsia 1991;32(3):310–21. https://doi.org/10.1111/j.1528-1157.1991.tb04657.x.

117. Velasco M, Velasco F, Velasco AL, et al. Effect of chronic electrical stimulation of the centromedian thalamic nuclei on various intractable seizure patterns: II. Psychological performance and background EEG activity. Epilepsia 1993;34(6):1065–74. https://doi.org/10.1111/j.1528-1157.1993.tb02135.x.

118. Velasco F, Velasco M, Velasco AL, et al. Effect of chronic electrical stimulation of the centromedian thalamic nuclei on various intractable seizure patterns: I. Clinical seizures and paroxysmal EEG activity. Epilepsia 1993;34(6):1052–64. https://doi.org/10.1111/j.1528-1157.1993.tb02134.x.

119. Sisterson ND, Kokkinos V, Urban A, et al. Responsive neurostimulation of the thalamus improves seizure control in idiopathic generalised epilepsy: initial case series. J Neurol Neurosurg Psychiatry 2022;93(5):491–8. https://doi.org/10.1136/jnnp-2021-327512.

120. Kokkinos V, Urban A, Sisterson ND, et al. Responsive Neurostimulation of the Thalamus Improves Seizure Control in Idiopathic Generalized Epilepsy: A Case Report. Neurosurgery 2020;87(5):E578–83. https://doi.org/10.1093/neuros/nyaa001.

121. Zillgitt AJ, Haykal MA, Chehab A, et al. Centromedian thalamic neuromodulation for the treatment of idiopathic generalized epilepsy. Front Hum Neurosci 2022;16:907716. https://doi.org/10.3389/fnhum.2022.907716.

122. Dempsey EW, Morison RS. The production of rhythmically recurrent cortical potentials after local thalamic stimulation. Am J Physiol 1941;135(2):293–300. https://doi.org/10.1152/AJPLEGACY.1941.135.2.293.

123. McLardy T. Diffuse thalamic projection to cortex: an anatomical critique. Electroencephalogr Clin Neurophysiol 1951;3(2):183–8. https://doi.org/10.1016/0013-4694(51)90009-0.

124. Groenewegen HJ, Berendse HW. The specificity of the 'nonspecific' midline and intralaminar thalamic nuclei. Trends Neurosci 1994;17(2):52–7. https://doi.org/10.1016/0166-2236(94)90074-4.

125. Ilyas A, Pizarro D, Romeo AK, et al. The centromedian nucleus: Anatomy, physiology, and clinical implications. J Clin Neurosci 2019;63:1–7. https://doi.org/10.1016/j.jocn.2019.01.050.

126. Sadikot AF, Rymar VV. The primate centromedian–parafascicular complex: anatomical organization with a note on neuromodulation. Brain Res Bull 2009;78(2):122–30. https://doi.org/10.1016/j.brainresbull.2008.09.016.

127. Sadikot AF, Parent A, Francois C. Efferent connections of the centromedian and parafascicular thalamic nuclei in the squirrel monkey: a PHA-L study of subcortical projections. J Comp Neurol 1992;315(2):137–59. https://doi.org/10.1002/cne.903150203.

128. Sadikot AF, Parent A, Francois C. The centre median and parafascicular thalamic nuclei project respectively to the sensorimotor and associative-limbic striatal territories in the squirrel monkey. Brain Res 1990;510(1):161–5. https://doi.org/10.1016/0006-8993(90)90746-x.

129. Eckert U, Metzger CD, Buchmann JE, et al. Preferential networks of the mediodorsal nucleus and centromedian-parafascicular complex of the thalamus—a DTI tractography study. Hum Brain Mapp 2012;33(11):2627–37. https://doi.org/10.1002/hbm.21389.

130. Glasser MF, Sotiropoulos SN, Wilson JA, et al. The minimal preprocessing pipelines for the Human Connectome Project. Neuroimage 2013;80:105–24. https://doi.org/10.1016/j.neuroimage.2013.04.127.

131. Warren AEL, Dalic LJ, Bulluss KJ, et al. The Optimal Target and Connectivity for Deep Brain Stimulation in Lennox-Gastaut Syndrome. Ann Neurol 2022;92(1):61–74. https://doi.org/10.1002/ana.26368.

132. Danielson NB, Guo JN, Blumenfeld H. The default mode network and altered consciousness in epilepsy. Behav Neurol 2011;24(1):55–65. https://doi.org/10.3233/BEN-2011-0310.

133. Van Luijtelaar EL, Van der Werf SJ, Vossen JM, et al. Arousal, performance and absence seizures in rats. Electroencephalogr Clin Neurophysiol 1991;79(5):430–4. https://doi.org/10.1016/0013-4694(91)90208-I.

134. Matsuoka H, Nakamura M, Ohno T, et al. The role of cognitive-motor function in precipitation and inhibition of epileptic seizures. Epilepsia 2005;46(Suppl 1):17–20. https://doi.org/10.1111/j.0013-9580.2005.461006.x.

135. Martin RA, Cukiert A, Blumenfeld H. Short-term changes in cortical physiological arousal measured by electroencephalography during thalamic centromedian deep brain stimulation. Epilepsia 2021;62(11):2604–14. https://doi.org/10.1111/epi.17042.

136. Butson CR, McIntyre CC. Current steering to control the volume of tissue activated during deep brain stimulation. Brain Stimul 2008;1(1):7–15. https://doi.org/10.1016/j.brs.2007.08.004.

137. Kundu B, Arain A, Davis T, et al. Using chronic recordings from a closed-loop neurostimulation system to capture seizures across multiple thalamic nuclei. Ann Clin Transl Neurol 2023;10(1):136–43. https://doi.org/10.1002/acn3.51701.

138. Cunningham SI, Tomasi D, Volkow ND. Structural and functional connectivity of the precuneus and thalamus to the default mode network. Hum Brain Mapp 2017;38(2):938–56. https://doi.org/10.1002/hbm.23429.

139. Li J, Curley WH, Guerin B, et al. Mapping the subcortical connectivity of the human default mode network. Neuroimage 2021;245:118758. https://doi.org/10.1016/j.neuroimage.2021.118758.

140. Blumenfeld, H. Stimulation of the Thalamus for Arousal Restoral in Temporal Lobe Epilepsy (START); 2023. https://clinicaltrials.gov/ct2/show/NCT04897776. Accessed April 25, 2023.

141. Marseille, APHD. Pulvinar Stimulation in Epilepsy: a Pilot Study (PULSE); 2023. https://clinicaltrials.gov/ct2/show/NCT04692701. Accessed April 25, 2023.

142. Chkhenkeli SA, Sramka M, Lortkipanidze GS, et al. Electrophysiological effects and clinical results of direct brain stimulation for intractable epilepsy. Clin Neurol Neurosurg 2004;106(4):318–29. https://doi.org/10.1016/j.clineuro.2004.01.009.

143. Cooper IS, Amin I, Riklan M, et al. Chronic cerebellar stimulation in epilepsy. Clinical and anatomical studies. Arch Neurol 1976;33(8):559–70. https://doi.org/10.1001/archneur.1976.00500080037006.

144. Wright G, McLellan D, Brice J. A double-blind trial of chronic cerebellar stimulation in twelve patients with severe epilepsy. J Neurol Neurosurg Psychiatry 1984;47(8):769–74. https://doi.org/10.1136/jnnp.47.8.769.

145. Dalic LJ, Warren AEL, Young JC, et al. Cortex leads the thalamic centromedian nucleus in generalized epileptic discharges in Lennox-Gastaut syndrome. Epilepsia 2020;61(10):2214–23. https://doi.org/10.1111/epi.16657.

146. Vaudano AE, Laufs H, Kiebel SJ, et al. Causal hierarchy within the thalamo-cortical network in spike and wave discharges. PLoS One 2009;4(8):e6475. https://doi.org/10.1371/journal.pone.0006475.

147. Szaflarski JP, DiFrancesco M, Hirschauer T, et al. Cortical and subcortical contributions to absence seizure onset examined with EEG/fMRI. Epilepsy Behav 2010;18(4):404–13. https://doi.org/10.1016/j.yebeh.2010.05.009.

148. Elder C, Friedman D, Devinsky O, et al. Responsive neurostimulation targeting the anterior nucleus of the thalamus in 3 patients with treatment-resistant multifocal epilepsy. Epilepsia Open 2019;4(1):187–92. https://doi.org/10.1002/epi4.12300.

149. NeuroPace. RNS System LGS Feasibility Study; 2023. https://clinicaltrials.gov/ct2/show/NCT05339126. Accessed April 25, 2023.

150. Ligaard J, Sannaes J, Pihlstrom L. Deep brain stimulation and genetic variability in Parkinson's disease: a review of the literature. NPJ Parkinsons Dis 2019;5:18.

151. Arsov T, Mullen SA, Damiano JA, et al. Early onset absence epilepsy: 1 in 10 cases is caused by GLUT1 deficiency. Epilepsia 2012;53(12):e204–7. https://doi.org/10.1111/epi.12007.

152. Ceulemans B, Boel M, Leyssens K, et al. Successful use of fenfluramine as an add-on treatment for Dravet syndrome. Epilepsia 2012;53(7):1131–9. https://doi.org/10.1111/j.1528-1167.2012.03495.x.

153. Baranzini SE, Srinivasan R, Khankhanian P, et al. Genetic variation influences glutamate concentrations in brains of patients with multiple sclerosis. Brain 2010;133(9):2603–11. https://doi.org/10.1093/brain/awq192.

154. Tawfik VL, Chang SY, Hitti FL, et al. Deep brain stimulation results in local glutamate and adenosine release: investigation into the role of astrocytes. Neurosurgery 2010;67(2):367–75. https://doi.org/10.1227/01.NEU.0000371988.73620.4C.

155. Minelli A, Congiu C, Ventriglia M, et al. Influence of GRIK4 genetic variants on the electroconvulsive therapy response. Neurosci Lett 2016;626:94–8. https://doi.org/10.1016/j.neulet.2016.05.030.

156. Benazzouz A, Gao DM, Ni ZG, et al. Effect of high-frequency stimulation of the subthalamic nucleus on the neuronal activities of the substantia nigra pars reticulata and ventrolateral nucleus of the thalamus in the rat. Neuroscience 2000;99(2):289–95. https://doi.org/10.1016/s0306-4522(00)00199-8.

157. Filali M, Hutchison WD, Palter VN, et al. Stimulation-induced inhibition of neuronal firing in human subthalamic nucleus. Exp Brain Res 2004;156(3): 274–81. https://doi.org/10.1007/s00221-003-1784-y.

158. Zhuang QX, Li GY, Li B, et al. Regularizing firing patterns of rat subthalamic neurons ameliorates parkinsonian motor deficits. J Clin Invest 2018;128(12): 5413–27. https://doi.org/10.1172/JCI99986.

159. Lozano AM, Lipsman N. Probing and regulating dysfunctional circuits using deep brain stimulation. Neuron 2013;77(3):406–24. https://doi.org/10.1016/j.neuron.2013.01.020.

160. Bambico FR, Bregman T, Diwan M, et al. Neuroplasticity-dependent and -independent mechanisms of chronic deep brain stimulation in stressed rats. Transl Psychiatry 2015;5(11):e674. https://doi.org/10.1038/tp.2015.166.

161. Salanova V, Witt T, Worth R, et al. Long-term efficacy and safety of thalamic stimulation for drug-resistant partial epilepsy. Neurology 2015;84(10): 1017–25. https://doi.org/10.1212/WNL.0000000000001334.

162. Eusebio A, Thevathasan W, Doyle Gaynor L, et al. Deep brain stimulation can suppress pathological synchronisation in parkinsonian patients. J Neurol Neurosurg Psychiatry 2011;82(5):569–73. https://doi.org/10.1136/jnnp.2010.217489.

163. Sinclair NC, McDermott HJ, Bulluss KJ, et al. Subthalamic nucleus deep brain stimulation evokes resonant neural activity. Ann Neurol 2018;83(5): 1027–31. https://doi.org/10.1002/ana.25234.

164. Feldmann LK, Lofredi R, Neumann WJ, et al. Toward therapeutic electrophysiology: beta-band suppression as a biomarker in chronic local field potential recordings. NPJ Parkinsons Dis 2022;8(1):44. https://doi.org/10.1038/s41531-022-00301-2.

165. Maturana MI, Meisel C, Dell K, et al. Critical slowing down as a biomarker for seizure susceptibility. Nat Commun 2020;11(1):2172. https://doi.org/10.1038/s41467-020-15908-3.

166. Deutschova B, Klimes P, Jordan Z, et al. Thalamic oscillatory activity may predict response to deep brain stimulation of the anterior nuclei of the thalamus. Epilepsia 2021;62(5):e70–5. https://doi.org/10.1111/epi.16883.

167. Tong X, Wang J, Qin L, et al. Analysis of power spectrum and phase lag index changes following deep brain stimulation of the anterior nucleus of the thalamus in patients with drug-resistant epilepsy: A retrospective study. Seizure 2022;96:6–12. https://doi.org/10.1016/j.seizure.2022.01.004.

168. Dell KL, Cook MJ, Maturana MI. Deep Brain Stimulation for Epilepsy: Biomarkers for Optimization. Curr Treat Options Neurol 2019;21(10):47. https://doi.org/10.1007/s11940-019-0590-1.

169. Dalic LJ, Warren AEL, Spiegel C, et al. Paroxysmal fast activity is a biomarker of treatment response in deep brain stimulation for Lennox-Gastaut syndrome. Epilepsia 2022;63(12):3134–47. https://doi.org/10.1111/epi.17414.

170. Bernabei JM, Li A, Revell AY, et al. Quantitative approaches to guide epilepsy surgery from intracranial EEG. Brain 2023. https://doi.org/10.1093/brain/awad007. Online ahead of print.

171. Anderson DN, Charlebois CM, Smith EH, et al. Closed-loop neurostimulation for epilepsy leads to improved outcomes when stimulation episodes are delivered during periods with less epileptiform activity. medRxiv 2022. https://doi.org/10.1101/2022.11.28.22282784.

172. NeuroPace. RNS System NAUTILUS Study (NAUTILUS); 2023. https://clinicaltrials.gov/ct2/show/NCT05147571. Accessed April 25, 2023 2023.

173. Sforza E, Mahdi R, Roche F, et al. Nocturnal interictal epileptic discharges in adult Lennox-Gastaut syndrome: the effect of sleep stage and time of night. Epileptic Disord 2016;18(1):44–50. https://doi.org/10.1684/epd.2016.0793.

174. Eisensehr I, Parrino L, Noachtar S, et al. Sleep in Lennox–Gastaut syndrome: the role of the cyclic alternating pattern (CAP) in the gate control of clinical seizures and generalized polyspikes. Epilepsy Res 2001;46(3):241–50. https://doi.org/10.1016/s0920-1211(01)00280-7.

175. Martins da Silva A, Aarts JH, Binnie CD, et al. The circadian distribution of interictal epileptiform EEG activity. Electroencephalogr Clin Neurophysiol 1984;58(1):1–13. https://doi.org/10.1016/0013-4694(84)90195-0.

176. Sharma VD, Sengupta S, Chitnis S, et al. Deep Brain Stimulation and Sleep-Wake Disturbances in Parkinson Disease: A Review. Front Neurol 2018; 9:697. https://doi.org/10.3389/fneur.2018.00697.

177. Voges BR, Schmitt FC, Hamel W, et al. Deep brain stimulation of anterior nucleus thalami disrupts sleep in epilepsy patients. Epilepsia 2015;56(8): e99–103. https://doi.org/10.1111/epi.13045.

178. Karoly PJ, Rao VR, Gregg NM, et al. Cycles in epilepsy. Nat Rev Neurol 2021;17(5):267–84. https://doi.org/10.1038/s41582-021-00464-1.

179. Karoly PJ, Stirling RE, Freestone DR, et al. Multiday cycles of heart rate are associated with seizure likelihood: An observational cohort study. EBioMedicine 2021;72:103619. https://doi.org/10.1016/j.ebiom.2021.103619.

180. Gregg NM, Pal Attia T, Nasseri M, et al. Seizure occurrence is linked to multiday cycles in diverse physiological signals. Epilepsia 2023. https://doi.org/10.1111/epi.17607. Online ahead of print.

181. Chen Z, Yu W, Xu R, et al. Ambient air pollution and epileptic seizures: A panel study in Australia. Epilepsia 2022;63(7):1682–92. https://doi.org/10.1111/epi.17253.

182. Sivathamboo S, Liu Z, Sutherland F, et al. Serious Cardiac Arrhythmias Detected by Subcutaneous Long-

term Cardiac Monitors in Patients With Drug-Resistant Epilepsy. Neurology 2022;98(19):e1923–32. https://doi.org/10.1212/WNL.0000000000200173.

183. Camfield PR, Gibson PA, Douglass LM. Strategies for transitioning to adult care for youth with Lennox-Gastaut syndrome and related disorders. Epilepsia 2011;52(s5):21–7. https://doi.org/10.1111/j.1528-1167.2011.03179.x.

184. Gibson PA. Lennox-Gastaut syndrome: impact on the caregivers and families of patients. J Multidiscip Healthc 2014;7:441–8. https://doi.org/10.2147/JMDH.S69300.

185. Berg AT, Gaebler-Spira D, Wilkening G, et al. Non-seizure consequences of Dravet syndrome, KCNQ2-DEE, KCNB1-DEE, Lennox-Gastaut syndrome, ESES: A functional framework. Epilepsy Behav 2020;111:107287. https://doi.org/10.1016/j.yebeh.2020.107287.

186. Krauth A, Blanc R, Poveda A, et al. A mean three-dimensional atlas of the human thalamus: generation from multiple histological data. Neuroimage 2010;49(3):2053–62. https://doi.org/10.1016/j.neuroimage.2009.10.042.

187. Mowinckel AM, Vidal-Piñeiro D. Visualization of Brain Statistics With R Packages ggseg and ggseg3d. Advances in Methods and Practices in Psychological Science 2020;3(4):466–83. https://doi.org/10.1177/2515245920928009.

Epilepsy Surgery for Cognitive Improvement in Epileptic Encephalopathy

John R. McLaren, MD[a,b,1], Kristopher T. Kahle, MD, PhD[b,c],
R. Mark Richardson, MD, PhD[b,d], Catherine J. Chu, MD, MA, MMSc[a,b],*

KEYWORDS

- Neurodevelopment • Outcome • Pediatric epilepsy surgery • Interictal localization
- Developmental epileptic encephalopathy • ESES • CSWS • Case report

KEY POINTS

- In patients with epileptic encephalopathy, continued abundant epileptiform activity and continued antiseizure medications can both contribute negatively to cognitive and behavioral outcomes in children.
- Epilepsy surgery can often cure or reduce the pathologic epileptic activity contributing to cognitive dysfunction in epileptic encephalopathy.
- Modern surgical diagnostic and treatment approaches can be used to evaluate and treat children with epileptic encephalopathies.
- Improved outcome measures that can detect changes in developmental trajectory across multiple domains in children with epileptic encephalopathies are required.
- Patients expected to have cognitive and/or behavioral benefit from epilepsy surgery should be offered this treatment option.

INTRODUCTION

Epilepsy surgery is an effective, but underutilized, evidence-based treatment of drug-resistant epilepsy.[1] Although most reported outcomes focus on seizure control, cognitive dysfunction due to epilepsy negatively impacts quality of life (QOL) to the same degree as drug-resistant seizures.[2] Further, larger, positive influences on developmental outcome are seen with surgical interventions.[3] Yet less than 3% of eligible patients receive epilepsy surgery in the United States, only after an average of 22 years from diagnosis.[4] Ambivalence in current guidelines about the role of epilepsy surgery to improve neurodevelopmental outcomes contributes to this devastating treatment gap.

One in 540 children has a developmental or epileptic encephalopathy, defined by the presence of frequent epileptiform activity that causes neurodevelopmental slowing or regression.[5] Such abnormal neurophysiology can often be surgically cured following similar localization procedures used to address drug refractory seizures. However, current consensus-based indications for epilepsy surgery require the presence of drug refractory seizures.[6,7] Further, current metrics for surgical success focus on seizure control. Despite the evidence that epilepsy surgery can reverse or ameliorate cognitive and behavioral decline in epileptic encephalopathies, only rare case series report offering surgery for patients in the absence of drug refractory seizures.[8–10] Expert consensus

a Department of Neurology, Massachusetts General Hospital, Boston, MA 02114, USA; b Harvard Medical School; c Department of Neurosurgery, Massachusetts General Hospital, 55 Fruit Street, Wang Building Room 333, Boston, MA 02114, USA; d Department of Neurosurgery, Massachusetts General Hospital, 55 Fruit Street, Their Building, 4th Floor, Boston, MA 02114, USA
1 Present address: 100 Cambridge Street, 20th floor, Boston, MA 02140.
* Corresponding author. 100 Cambridge Street, Office 2036, Boston, MA 02140.
E-mail address: cjchu@mgh.harvard.edu

recognizes that epilepsy surgery should be considered in lesional patients even if they are seizure free[6] but this position results in the exclusion of nonlesional or lesional but seizure-free patients with epileptic encephalopathy who stand to benefit cognitively and behaviorally from epilepsy surgery. Here, we review the evidence for epilepsy surgery to improve neurodevelopment in children with drug refractory epilepsy and in children with epileptic encephalopathies. We also share one case of epilepsy surgery from our institution in a child with epileptic encephalopathy without drug refractory seizures to highlight adjustments to the surgical evaluation that can be taken to assess and address the pathologic interictal activity in epileptic encephalopathy. In patients with epileptic encephalopathy, we propose that cognitive improvement alone is a sufficient indication to recommend surgical intervention in experienced centers.

COGNITIVE IMPACT OF EPILEPSY SURGERY VERSUS CONTINUED MEDICATION

The only available randomized prospective clinical trial in children with drug refractory epilepsy found that among 63 children randomized to either epilepsy surgery (n = 30) or continued medication treatment (n = 33), those that received surgery trended to have improved intelligence quotient (IQ) compared with those who did not ($P = .06$).[1] Those that received continued medication showed a decrease in IQ ($P < .001$) during the 12-month follow-up that was not observed in the surgery group ($P = .3$). A similar result was observed in a case-control study, which also found that discontinuing antiseizure medications in the setting of seizure control after surgery correlates with further improved cognitive scores.[11] These data highlight the known negative influence of antiseizure medications on cognitive function,[12,13] which should be considered when weighing the cognitive risks and benefits of epilepsy surgery.

PREDICTORS OF COGNITIVE IMPROVEMENT AFTER PEDIATRIC EPILEPSY SURGERY

Cognitive improvements after surgery have been linked to postoperative seizure-control[14,15] but this association has not born out in all studies.[16] Higher cognitive improvements after surgery have also been linked to younger age at surgery,[17] shorter duration of epilepsy,[14,16] lower premorbid IQ,[17,18] greater integrity of the residual brain,[11,19] and longer duration of follow-up.[11] However, many of these associations have not been consistently found.[19–21] Most studies do not control for the influence of continued or withdrawn antiseizure medication treatment after epilepsy surgery, which may explain some of the inconsistencies seen.

EPILEPSY SURGERY FOR DEVELOPMENTAL AND EPILEPTIC ENCEPHALOPATHIES

In developmental and epileptic encephalopathies, ongoing epileptic activity directly contributes to neurodevelopmental symptoms including neuropsychological deceleration, plateau, or regression.[22–25] The mechanisms through which epileptic activity impair cognitive function is poorly understood but emerging evidence suggests that epileptiform activity can interfere with memory encoding[26–28] and memory consolidation.[29–32] In this way, reduction or resolution of the epileptic activity is expected to mitigate or resolve the cerebral dysfunction caused by the epileptic activity.

At present, 11 specific developmental and epileptic encephalopathies are recognized by the International League Against Epilepsy, including 4 with onset in infancy,[22] 5 with onset in childhood,[23] and 2 with onset at variable ages.[24] Surgical options are available for each, including destructive procedures or neuromodulation. Because disconnection surgeries are the only definitive treatments available for Rasmussen syndrome, a syndrome characterized by progressive hemispheric cerebral atrophy, progressive focal seizures, and progressive cognitive impairment,[24] we do not include this syndrome in our review. A scoping review of the literature detailing cognitive outcomes following epilepsy surgery in each of the remaining epileptic encephalopathy syndromes is provided below.

Early Infantile Developmental and Epileptic Encephalopathy

Early infantile developmental and epileptic encephalopathy (EIDEE) is a syndrome characterized by early onset of frequent, drug-resistant tonic and/or myoclonic seizures and/or epileptic spasms and an EEG showing diffuse slowing with either burst suppression or multifocal discharges. Children typically present within the first few months of life with an abnormal neurologic examination and develop moderate to profound developmental impairment.[22] Both pathologic gene variants and structural brain abnormalities are common in children with EIDEE. When the latter are identified, children may benefit from resective epilepsy surgery. In one case series, 2 of 2 infants were reported to wean off of antiseizure medication and make developmental progress following surgery.[33] The authors describe 9 further children with similar positive outcomes from the literature. A second case series included 12 infants with EIDEE due to hemimegalencephaly treated with hemispherotomy. Although 8 children (67%) were seizure free postoperatively, only the 4 children (33%) who were weaned off antiseizure medications experienced gains in their postoperative developmental quotient, whereas 6 of 8 who maintained (n = 1) or increased (n = 5) antiseizure medications postoperatively were found to have decreased postoperative developmental quotient (DQ).[34]

Early Infantile Migrating Focal Seizures

Epilepsy of infancy with migrating focal features (EIMFS) is characterized by focal motor clonic or tonic seizures in which the seizures migrate from one cortical region to another on EEG.[22] Genetic causes can be identified in up to half of cases and neuroimaging is normal. Because resective targets are difficult to identify in this developmental epileptic encephalopathies (DEE), neuromodulation may be considered. One case series describes 3 patients with EIMFS treated with a vagal nerve stimulator between 0.7 and 1.4 years of life.[35] A 40% to 60% seizure reduction was reported in 2 patients (66%) and improvement in psychomotor function was reported in one child (33%). All children continued antiseizure medication polytherapy.

Infantile Epileptic Spasms Syndrome

Infantile epileptic spasms syndrome (IESS) is characterized by the onset of clusters of epileptic spasms and either interictal hypsarrhythmia or focal or multifocal epileptiform discharges on EEG in the first 2 years of life.[22] Children often have developmental slowing concordant with the onset of spasms that is expected to worsen without effective treatment. Neuroimaging is abnormal in one-half to two-thirds of children, and an early surgical assessment is recommended.[22] Using modern neurosurgical techniques, including magnetoencephalogram (MEG), fluoro-deoxyglucose-positron emission tomography (FDG-PET), and invasive recordings when required, postoperative seizure freedom in IESS has been reported in 61% to 83% of lesional cases (n = 225)[36] and 9/18 (50%) nonlesional cases,[37] comparable to outcomes reported for other drug refractory lesional epilepsies. Several case series report children with accelerated development after epilepsy surgery, as measured by formal neuropsychological testing, often concordant with antiseizure medication taper.[17,38,39]

Dravet Syndrome

Dravet syndrome (DS) is characterized by prolonged febrile and afebrile focal and/or generalized clonic seizures in the first year of life followed by cognitive and behavioral impairments that are evident by the second year.[22] Brain imaging does not reveal a structural brain lesion and a pathogenic mutation in SCN1A is present in more than 80% to 85% of patients. The EEG shows focal, multifocal, or generalized discharges. Given the challenges in identifying a resective target, neuromodulation may be offered to children with DS. A recent systemic review of 15 published studies describing 107 patients treated with open loop vagal nerve stimulation (VNS) found that 56% of patients had a 50% or greater reduction in seizures and 7.5% were seizure free.[40] Those authors reviewed one study describing 2 patients with DS who underwent open-loop deep brain thalamic stimulation (DBS) of the anterior nucleus of the thalamus. Both patients had seizure reduction over the subsequent decade of 67% to 93% although medications were also adjusted in the interim. Among patients with VNS, using subjective measures, 2 case series report improved alertness in 2 out of 8 children (25%),[41] and 4 out of 12 children (33%).[42] In studies that evaluated preoperative and postoperative neuropsychological testing, 9 out of 9 children (100%) had improved alertness and communication skills[43,44] and 1 of these children (12.5%) also showed improvements in adaptive behavior.[43]

Epilepsy with Myoclonic Atonic Seizures

Epilepsy with myoclonic atonic seizures (EMAts) is clinically characterized by the onset of mixed generalized seizures during childhood, including myotonic-atonic seizures concordant with developmental slowing and generalized discharges on EEG. Seizures spontaneously remit in up to a quarter of patients with EMAts.[23] Brain imaging does not show a structural lesion and surgical options focus on neuromodulation. One case series reported that of 5 patients with EMAts and drug refractory seizures who underwent VNS implantation, 3 (60%) had greater than 50% reduction in seizures.[45] Three separate case reports report 3 out of 3 children had dramatic seizure reduction (2 became seizure free), each with subjective cognitive improvement after VNS surgery at the age of 4 years,[46] 5 years,[47] and 9 years.[48] The 5-year-old patient developed symptomatic bradycardia at age 13 years requiring the VNS to be turned off and epileptic seizures did not recur.

Lennox-Gastaut Syndrome

Lennox-Gastaut syndrome (LGS) is characterized by the development of tonic seizures alongside other seizure types during childhood, cognitive and behavioral delay, alongside EEG findings of diffuse slow spike-and-wave and generalized paroxysmal fast activity.[23] A recent large meta-analysis evaluated the influence of VNS, corpus callosotomy (CC), DBS, and resective surgery on seizure control, medication usage, QOL, and neurodevelopmental outcomes in 892 patients with LGS.[49] Reduction in seizures was 54.6% for VNS (17 studies, n = 370 patients), 74.1% for CC (19 studies, n = 337 patients), 88.9% for resective surgery (4 studies, n = 138 patients), 100% for DBS (1 study, n = 13 patients), 88% for combined CC and DBS (2 studies, n = 25 patients), and 56% for combined CC and VNS (1 study, n = 9 patients). Among studies that reported cognitive and/or behavioral outcomes after VNS surgery, 69 out of 103 children (67%) were reported to have subjective improvements in alertness and/or attention,[43,50–54] 6 out of 24 children (25%) were reported to have subjective improvement in verbal skills,[50] 4 out of 24 children (17%) had subjective improvement in memory,[50] 13 out of 30 children (43%) had subjective improvements in school performance and/or learning,[50,54] 5 out of 6 children (83%) had subjective improvements in independence,[54] and 2 out of 4 children (50%) had subjective improvement in behavior.[43] Using formal neuropsychological testing, one study reported no cognitive change following VNS surgery in 4 out of 4 children (100%). In the studies that commented on behavior and/or cognitive change after CC alone, 20 out of 24 children (85%) were noted to have subjective improvements in attention,[51] 4 out of 5 children (80%) had improvement in behavior,[55] and 10 out of 23 children (43%) had improved IQ on formal neuropsychological testing.[56] Two studies that included a total of 21 children reported no change IQ or cognition based on preoperative and postoperative neuropsychological testing.[57,58] In the 3 studies that commented on behavior and/or cognitive changes after resective surgery, one reported improved IQ in 60% (n = 20) and improved memory in 40% (n = 20),[59] one reported improved behavioral functioning in 90% (n = 21),[60] and one reported no difference in preoperative and postoperative social functioning.[61]

Developmental/Epileptic Encephalopathy with Spike Wave Activation in Sleep

Developmental epileptic encephalopathies with spike wave activation during sleep (DEE-SWAS) and epileptic encephalopathy with spike wave activation during sleep (EE-SWAS) are characterized by deceleration or regression in neurodevelopment alongside EEG recordings that show marked increases in interictal epileptiform activity during non-rapid eye movement sleep in children with either a preexisting neurodevelopmental disorder (DEE-SWAS) or previously normal development (EE-SWAS).[23] In a large, pooled analyses of 575 patients with epileptic encephalopathy related to SWAS from 112 articles, cognitive improvement was reported in 80% of patients after surgery.[62] This rate was higher than reported for treatment with traditional antiseizure medications (40%) or treatment with benzodiazepines (50%) and comparable to that reported after treatment with steroids (78%). Qualitatively similar results were reported in subgroup analysis including only studies that enrolled patients consecutively. In subsequent case series, subjective cognitive and behavioral improvements were observed in 6 of 9 (66%),[63] 8 of 11 (73%),[64] and 2 of 2 (100%) children[65] after disconnection procedures, and 5 of 5 (100%) after varying resective procedures[66] for EE-SWAS. Notable, pathologic evaluation of tissue resected following intracranial investigation identified focal cortical dysplasia that had not been evident on preoperative MRIs in 3 cases in the latter series. In contrast, improvements were only reported in 3 of 14 children (21%) with EE-SWAS treated with multiple subpial transections.[67] In studies evaluating preoperative and postoperative function using formal neuropsychological testing, 9 of 14 patients (64%) displayed arrest of decline, gains in performance or stability of presurgical function following disconnection or resective surgeries,[9] whereas only 1 of 3 (33%) children had improved DQ or IQ after CC.[8] A separate study found that 6 of 11 patients (55%) with EE-SWAS treated with hemispherotomy had a greater than 10 point gain in language skills assessed using the Wechsler Intelligence Scale for Children (WISC) language subtests, 4 had stable findings (36%), and 1 had a greater than 10 point loss in language skills (9%) after surgery.[68] Cognitive improvement correlated with discontinuing antiseizure medication even when comparing only children who were seizure free (P = .011).

Hemiconvulsion-hemiplegic Syndrome

Hemiconvulsion-hemiplegic syndrome is characterized by initial focal motor status epilepticus in infancy or early childhood followed by drug refractory focal seizures and motor and/or language deficits.[23] Successful seizure outcomes have been reported after epilepsy surgery but cognitive outcomes were not included.[69,70] In a separate case series, 1 of 3 cases (33%) was noted to have improved cognitive dysfunction after functional hemispherotomy.[71]

Febrile Infection-related Epilepsy Syndrome

Febrile infection-related epilepsy syndrome (FIRES) is characterized by new onset super-refractory status epilepticus following febrile illness followed by variable intellectual disabilities after resolution of the status epilepticus. MRI does not reveal a structural lesion in FIRES and EEG typically shows multifocal abnormalities.[24] One of 3 (33%) children with FIRES treated surgically with open-loop DBS of the bilateral centromedian nucleus of the thalamus was reported to have cognitive improvement.[72,73] One child with FIRES treated with cortical closed-loop RNS was reported to have reduced seizures and improvement across most cognitive domains on neuropsychological testing 6 to 8 months after RNS, although the patient was also noted to have been started on stimulant medications over this time.[74]

Progressive Myoclonic Epilepsy

The progressive myoclonic epilepsies (PMEs) include Unverricht-Lundborg disease, Lafora disease, neuronal ceroid lipofuscinosis, mitochondrial disorders, and sialidosis. These diseases are electroclinically related by the shared features of myoclonus; progressive cerebral dysfunction including cognitive, motor, sensory, and cerebellar impairments; and abnormal slowing on EEG.[24] Given the diffuse nature of this disease, surgical interventions have focused on neuromodulation. The case reports to date have focused on stimulation targets used in movement disorders, including the subthalamic nucleus (STN) and substantia nigra (SNr). In 7 adult patients with PME treated with open-loop bilateral DBS targeting the STN and SNr, a qualitative improvement in cognitive functioning was reported on average in a cohort of 5 patients,[75] in 1 of 1 patient,[76] and was not commented on for 1 of 1 patient.[77] Improvements in seizure control and motor symptoms were observed in all 7 patients.[76]

CONSIDERATIONS IN EPILEPSY SURGERY EVALUATION FOR EPILEPTIC ENCEPHALOPATHY

The first consideration when assessing the risk–benefits of epilepsy surgery for a child with suspected epileptic encephalopathy is to determine to what degree the epileptic encephalopathy is contributing to cerebral dysfunction. This requires a sufficient longitudinal assessment to identify developmental slowing, plateau, or regression. In addition to standard electroclinical evaluations, we consider high-dose diazepam trials in those with suspected epileptic encephalopathies. Although not all children respond positively to high-dose diazepam, a positive cognitive response concurrent with suppression of epileptiform activity confirms the reversibility of cerebral dysfunction due to epileptic encephalopathy. Alternative medical treatments for this trial include high-dose steroids or intravenous immunoglobulin (IVIG), although they may be less effective.[62] In the absence of a positive response to high-dose diazepam, children may still be candidates for epilepsy surgery based on the overall risk–benefit ratio assessment made by the multidisciplinary epilepsy surgery team.

During the presurgical workup, similar to surgical evaluations in children with drug refractory seizures, evaluation of children with epileptic encephalopathy requires high-resolution MRI to evaluate for a structural lesion and video EEG to lateralize or localize the abnormal neurophysiology, focusing on the abundant, interictal epileptiform activity. Different interictal epileptiform populations may be present during different sleep stages, requiring capture of all stages of consciousness on the video EEG. The abundant interictal epileptiform activity can be focal, diffuse, generalized, or falsely generalized and careful attention needs to be paid to interictal propagation patterns during visual analysis. Interictal MEG studies can further help localize interictal epileptiform discharges and evaluate their propagation patterns. As abundant interictal activity increases local glucose metabolism, PET studies obtained during sleep or sedation can highlight the volume of the irritative zone as a hypermetabolic region. Intracranial EEG can further localize the region of interest, separating the initiating cortex from propagated activity. When interictal activity is abundant during sleep, as in EE-SWAS, intraoperative electrocorticography can be used to guide the extent and confirm the completion of a resection. In the case of resective treatments, postoperatively, EEGs are required to assess for the resolution of interictal activity. Resolution of interictal epileptiform activity may not be seen in disconnection procedures or palliative neuromodulatory treatments. Postoperatively, benefits of earlier antiseizure medication taper for cognitive benefits should be weighed against the risks of earlier detection of incomplete seizure control,[78] where successful tapering of antiseizure medications alone can accelerate cognitive gains.[1] An example surgical evaluation pathway for epileptic encephalopathies is provided in **Fig. 1**.

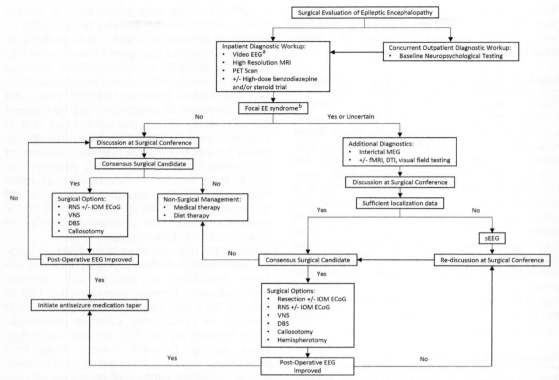

Fig. 1. An example epileptic encephalopathy surgical planning pathway. [a]All stages of sleep should be captured to fully characterize populations/burden. [b]Based on clinical and imaging features.

CASE EXAMPLE

Case 1: The child is an ex-31 week right-handed female with a history of in utero bilateral intraventricular hemorrhage (grade III on the left and grade IV on the right), expanding right frontoparietal porencephalic cyst status post fenestration, left hemiparesis, motor, and speech delay. At 20 months, she underwent an EEG to rule out seizures in the setting of staring spells and was found to have behavioral staring but also near-continuous bisynchronous and diffuse right hemispheric epileptiform spikes during sleep. She was started on clobazam with a modest reduction in epileptiform activity and was noted by parents to have concordant developmental leaps. She was subsequently referred for a surgical evaluation at age 34 months, at which time she was unable to walk independently and was speaking in 1 to 2 word sentences. As part of her treatment and presurgical evaluation, she underwent a high-dose diazepam trial (1 mg/kg) with a further modest reduction in amplitude and frequency of her epileptiform discharges during nonrapid eye movement sleep. Following high-dose diazepam, she was noted by her parents and teachers to have marked improvements

in language, attention, and gross motor skills. Most notably, she began to speak in 3 to 5 word sentences and began walking independently. Tapering of diazepam corresponded to worsened language but improved balance. Reintroducing diazepam again led to improvements in speech, attention, and confidence reported by parents, teachers, and therapists. On physical examination, she had evidence of some fractionated finger movements of the left hand. Ophthalmologic evaluation suggested possible left visual field cut but her efforts were inconsistent. Tractography revealed bilateral optic tracts and a foreshortened corticospinal tract in the right hemisphere. MEG study revealed interictal activity in the right temporal, parietal, and occipital lobes with a dense population in the right precuneus. PET study revealed an area of hypermetabolism in the right lateral parietal cortex and right precuneus. At discussion in the multidisciplinary epilepsy surgery conference, stereotactic intracranial EEG (sEEG) evaluation was recommended to guide a targeted resection of the irritative zone contributing to her encephalopathy. She subsequently underwent a 48-hour sEEG followed by topectomy of the lateral parietal region at 41 months. Pathology revealed a type 1a focal cortical dysplasia. EEG following resection showed persistent, abundant right temporal spikes. Postoperative MEG showed resolution of the temporal discharges but persistent spikes in the right parietal region, suggesting an incomplete resection. After rediscussion in surgical conference, the patient underwent a repeat 48-hour sEEG with denser sampling of the right precuneus in addition to lateral parietal and temporal coverage. sEEG revealed 2 spiking populations with near-continuous activity originating independently from the right inferior and superior medial precuneus regions and propagating to the temporal and occipital regions. She underwent resection including both of the precuneus targets at 47 months of age. Immediate postoperative EEG showed complete resolution of interictal spikes. Her repeated surgical procedures were complicated by a postoperative infection requiring a course of intravenous antibiotics. Despite the complexity of this child's course, her parents report notable gains in development postoperatively, including the use of more complex sentences, stronger memory of previous discussions, and the new use of "W" words (who, what, when, where, and why). She has successfully tapered off of several antiseizure medications with ongoing developmental gains. Example imaging results during the course of this patient's treatment is provided in **Fig. 2**.

MEASURES OF SUCCESS

Current measures of success after epilepsy surgery focus on seizure outcome.[79,80] A brief QOL survey has also been proposed to provide a more expansive assessment of meaningful improvements after epilepsy surgery[81,82] but this 10-item questionnaire includes only one question that addresses an aspect of cognitive and behavioral function. For epileptic encephalopathies, improved tools are required to capture the variable cognitive and behavioral changes that can be seen from epileptic activity impacting diverse cortical regions and networks. Even comprehensive formal neuropsychological assessments cannot capture some meaningful qualitative gains reported by parents.[83] For example, improvements in sleep-dependent memory consolidation cannot be detected in the memory assessments used in office visits because they are only performed during the wakeful state.[84] Several laboratories, including our own, are working to develop and validate neurophysiological measures of cognitive function to provide objective assessments of cognitive response.[29,85–87] Because quantitative neurophysiological or behavioral measures are not currently available, in our practice, we use subjective reports alongside formal preoperative and postoperative neuropsychological assessments, to assess outcomes. For these assessments, we

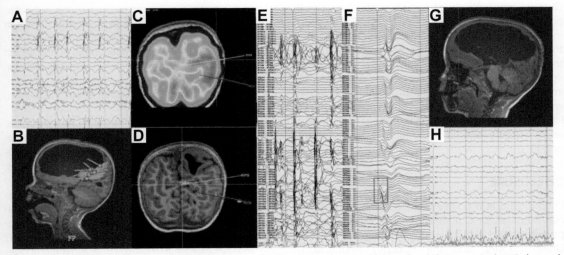

Fig. 2. Case example of surgical evaluation and course for epileptic encephalopathy. (*A*) Presurgical EEG showed near-continuous diffuse discharges during nonrapid eye movement sleep. (*B*) MEG localized the peak of the spikes primarily to the right precuneus region. (*C*) PET identified hypermetabolism in the right lateral parietal cortex. (*D*) Stereotactic intracranial EEG targeted several regions of interest. (*E*) Stereotactic intracranial EEG revealed diffuse, abundant epileptiform discharges involving multiple lobes. (*F*) Close inspection of discharges using a far-field noncephalic reference (here second cervical spinous process) revealed consistent propagation with spikes originating in the right precuneus region (*red box*) and secondarily propagating to other regions. (*G*) Postoperative MRI reveals resection of the right precuneus cortex. (*H*) Postoperative EEG reveals resolution of epileptiform spikes.

aim to gather longitudinal observations from multiple sources, including the child's caregivers at home, school, daycare, therapy sessions, and in the clinic. As the cognitive impact of epileptiform activity is increasingly understood, we hope that improved objective measures will be available for future application.

SUMMARY

In the United States alone, nearly US$700 million is spent annually on research to improve treatments for intellectual and developmental disabilities[88] and disability-associated expenditures account for more than one-third of health-care costs.[89] In patients with epileptic encephalopathy, surgical intervention is a unique, available treatment option that can often successfully cure or reduce the pathologic epileptic activity contributing to cognitive dysfunction. Modern surgical evaluations include advanced techniques to localize pathologic epileptic networks and modern surgical treatments include both destructive and neuromodulatory options.[90] Determining the risk and benefits of surgery for an individual patient requires careful evaluation and partnering with family to understand their personal determinants of health and well-being[91,92] so that decisions can be made together. Barriers due to knowledge gaps, socioeconomic bias, and misperceived goals imposed by medical providers are critical to overcome.[93] Current assessments of cognitive and behavioral outcomes after surgery include qualitative assessments by caregivers. Reliable outcome measures that can detect changes in developmental trajectory across multiple domains in children with epileptic encephalopathies are required to improve these assessments. Although much work remains to be done, patients expected to have cognitive and/or behavioral benefit from epilepsy surgery should be offered this treatment option.

DISCLOSURE

Dr C.J. Chu is a coinvestigator in the Neuropace Nautilus trial. Dr C.J. Chu receives research support from NIH NINDS, United States, NIH NIMH, United States, and the Epilepsy Foundation, United States New England and is a coinvestigator in the Neuropace Nautilus trial. Dr C.J. Chu has served as a consultant for Biogen Inc, Ionis Pharmaceuticals, Sun Pharmaceuticals, and Novartis within the last 2 years. Dr R.M. Richardson is PI in the Neuropace Nautilus trial and coinvestigator in the RNS System LGS Feasibility Study. Dr R.M. Richardson receives research support from NIH NINDS. Dr K.T. Kahle receives research support from NIH NINDS.

REFERENCES

1. Dwivedi R, Ramanujam B, Chandra PS, et al. Surgery for Drug-Resistant Epilepsy in Children. N Engl J Med 2017;377(17):1639–47.
2. Piazzini A, Beghi E, Turner K, et al. LICE Quality of Life Group. Health-related quality of life in epilepsy: findings obtained with a new Italian instrument. Epilepsy Behav EB 2008;13(1):119–26.
3. Shurtleff HA, Barry D, Firman T, et al. Impact of epilepsy surgery on development of preschool children: identification of a cohort likely to benefit from early intervention. J Neurosurg Pediatr 2015;16(4):383–92.
4. Samanta D, Ostendorf AP, Willis E, et al. Underutilization of epilepsy surgery: Part I: A scoping review of barriers. Epilepsy Behav EB 2021;117: 107837.
5. Poke G, Stanley J, Scheffer IE, et al. Epidemiology of Developmental and Epileptic Encephalopathy and of Intellectual Disability and Epilepsy in Children. Neurology 2023;100(13):e1363–75.
6. Jehi L, Jette N, Kwon CS, et al. Timing of referral to evaluate for epilepsy surgery: Expert Consensus Recommendations from the Surgical Therapies Commission of the International League Against Epilepsy. Epilepsia 2022;63(10):2491–506.
7. Cross JH, Jayakar P, Nordli D, et al. Proposed criteria for referral and evaluation of children for epilepsy surgery: recommendations of the Subcommission for Pediatric Epilepsy Surgery. Epilepsia 2006;47(6):952–9.
8. Yokosako S, Muraoka N, Watanabe S, et al. Corpus callosotomy in pediatric patients with non-lesional epileptic encephalopathy with electrical status epilepticus during sleep. Epilepsy Behav Rep 2021; 16:100463.
9. Marashly A, Koop J, Loman M, et al. Examining the Utility of Resective Epilepsy Surgery in Children With Electrical Status Epilepticus in Sleep: Long Term Clinical and Electrophysiological Outcomes. Front Neurol 2019;10:1397.
10. Peltola ME, Liukkonen E, Granström ML, et al. The effect of surgery in encephalopathy with electrical status epilepticus during sleep. Epilepsia 2011; 52(3):602–9.
11. Skirrow C, Cross JH, Harrison S, et al. Temporal lobe surgery in childhood and neuroanatomical predictors of long-term declarative memory outcome. Brain J Neurol 2015;138(Pt 1):80–93.
12. Strzelczyk A, Schubert-Bast S. Psychobehavioural and Cognitive Adverse Events of Anti-Seizure Medications for the Treatment of Developmental and Epileptic Encephalopathies. CNS Drugs 2022; 36(10):1079–111.

13. Glauser TA, Cnaan A, Shinnar S, et al. Ethosuximide, valproic acid, and lamotrigine in childhood absence epilepsy. N Engl J Med 2010;362(9):790–9.

14. Jonas R, Nguyen S, Hu B, et al. Cerebral hemispherectomy: hospital course, seizure, developmental, language, and motor outcomes. Neurology 2004; 62(10):1712–21.

15. Lee YJ, Kang HC, Lee JS, et al. Resective pediatric epilepsy surgery in Lennox-Gastaut syndrome. Pediatrics 2010;125(1):e58–66.

16. D'Argenzio L, Colonnelli MC, Harrison S, et al. Cognitive outcome after extratemporal epilepsy surgery in childhood. Epilepsia 2011;52(11):1966–72.

17. Loddenkemper T, Holland KD, Stanford LD, et al. Developmental outcome after epilepsy surgery in infancy. Pediatrics 2007;119(5):930–5.

18. Korkman M, Granström ML, Kantola-Sorsa E, et al. Two-year follow-up of intelligence after pediatric epilepsy surgery. Pediatr Neurol 2005;33(3):173–8.

19. Boshuisen K, van Schooneveld MMJ, Leijten FSS, et al. Contralateral MRI abnormalities affect seizure and cognitive outcome after hemispherectomy. Neurology 2010;75(18):1623–30.

20. Westerveld M, Sass KJ, Chelune GJ, et al. Temporal lobectomy in children: cognitive outcome. J Neurosurg 2000;92(1):24–30.

21. Miranda C, Smith ML. Predictors of Intelligence after Temporal Lobectomy in Children with Epilepsy. Epilepsy Behav EB 2001;2(1):13–9.

22. Zuberi SM, Wirrell E, Yozawitz E, et al. ILAE classification and definition of epilepsy syndromes with onset in neonates and infants: Position statement by the ILAE Task Force on Nosology and Definitions. Epilepsia 2022;63(6):1349–97.

23. Specchio N, Wirrell EC, Scheffer IE, et al. International League Against Epilepsy classification and definition of epilepsy syndromes with onset in childhood: Position paper by the ILAE Task Force on Nosology and Definitions. Epilepsia 2022;63(6):1398–442.

24. Riney K, Bogacz A, Somerville E, et al. International League Against Epilepsy classification and definition of epilepsy syndromes with onset at a variable age: position statement by the ILAE Task Force on Nosology and Definitions. Epilepsia 2022;63(6): 1443–74.

25. Berg AT, Berkovic SF, Brodie MJ, et al. Revised terminology and concepts for organization of seizures and epilepsies: report of the ILAE Commission on Classification and Terminology, 2005-2009. Epilepsia 2010;51(4):676–85.

26. Henin S, Shankar A, Borges H, et al. Spatiotemporal dynamics between interictal epileptiform discharges and ripples during associative memory processing. Brain J Neurol 2021;144(5):1590–602.

27. Horak PC, Meisenhelter S, Song Y, et al. Interictal epileptiform discharges impair word recall in multiple brain areas. Epilepsia 2017;58(3):373–80.

28. Ung H, Cazares C, Nanivadekar A, et al. Interictal epileptiform activity outside the seizure onset zone impacts cognition. Brain J Neurol 2017;140(8):2157–68.

29. Kramer MA, Stoyell SM, Chinappen D, et al. Focal Sleep Spindle Deficits Reveal Focal Thalamocortical Dysfunction and Predict Cognitive Deficits in Sleep Activated Developmental Epilepsy. J Neurosci Off J Soc Neurosci 2021;41(8):1816–29.

30. Spencer ER, Chinappen D, Emerton BC, et al. Source EEG reveals that Rolandic epilepsy is a regional epileptic encephalopathy. NeuroImage Clin 2022;33:102956.

31. Schiller K, Avigdor T, Abdallah C, et al. Focal epilepsy disrupts spindle structure and function. Sci Rep 2022;12(1):11137.

32. Wodeyar A, Chinappen D, Mylonas D, et al. Human Thalamic Recordings Reveal That Epileptic Spikes Block Sleep Spindle Production during Non-Rapid Eye Movement Sleep. Neuroscience 2023.

33. Malik SI, Galliani CA, Hernandez AW, et al. Epilepsy surgery for early infantile epileptic encephalopathy (ohtahara syndrome). J Child Neurol 2013;28(12): 1607–17.

34. Honda R, Kaido T, Sugai K, et al. Long-term developmental outcome after early hemispherotomy for hemimegalencephaly in infants with epileptic encephalopathy. Epilepsy Behav EB 2013;29(1):30–5.

35. Zamponi N, Rychlicki F, Corpaci L, et al. Vagus nerve stimulation (VNS) is effective in treating catastrophic 1 epilepsy in very young children. Neurosurg Rev 2008;31(3):291–7.

36. Abel TJ, Losito E, Ibrahim GM, et al. Multimodal localization and surgery for epileptic spasms of focal origin: a review. Neurosurg Focus 2018;45(3):E4.

37. Chugani HT, Ilyas M, Kumar A, et al. Surgical treatment for refractory epileptic spasms: The Detroit series. Epilepsia 2015;56(12):1941–9.

38. Iwatani Y, Kagitani-Shimono K, Tominaga K, et al. Long-term developmental outcome in patients with West syndrome after epilepsy surgery. Brain Dev 2012;34(9):731–8.

39. Caplan R, Guthrie D, Komo S, et al. Infantile spasms: the development of nonverbal communication after epilepsy surgery. Dev Neurosci 1999;21(3–5):165–73.

40. Ding J, Wang L, Li W, et al. Up to What Extent Does Dravet Syndrome Benefit From Neurostimulation Techniques? Front Neurol 2022;13:843975.

41. Sirsi D, Khan M, Arnold S. Vagal Nerve Stimulation: Is It Effective in Children with Dravet Syndrome? J Pediatr Epilepsy 2015;05(01):007–10.

42. Fulton SP, Van Poppel K, McGregor AL, et al. Vagus Nerve Stimulation in Intractable Epilepsy Associated With SCN1A Gene Abnormalities. J Child Neurol 2017;32(5):494–8.

43. Zamponi N, Passamonti C, Cappanera S, et al. Clinical course of young patients with Dravet syndrome

after vagal nerve stimulation. Eur J Paediatr Neurol EJPN Off J Eur Paediatr Neurol Soc 2011;15(1): 8–14.

44. Spatola M, Jeannet PY, Pollo C, et al. Effect of vagus nerve stimulation in an adult patient with Dravet syndrome: contribution to sudden unexpected death in epilepsy risk reduction? Eur Neurol 2013;69(2): 119–21.

45. Caraballo RH, Chamorro N, Darra F, et al. Epilepsy with myoclonic atonic seizures: an electroclinical study of 69 patients. Pediatr Neurol 2013;48(5): 355–62.

46. Fan PC, Peng SSF, Yen RF, et al. Neuroimaging and electroencephalographic changes after vagus nerve stimulation in a boy with medically intractable myoclonic astatic epilepsy. J Formos Med Assoc Taiwan Yi Zhi 2014;113(4):258–63.

47. Cantarín-Extremera V, Ruíz-Falcó-Rojas ML, Tamaríz-Martel-Moreno A, et al. Late-onset periodic bradycardia during vagus nerve stimulation in a pediatric patient. A new case and review of the literature. Eur J Paediatr Neurol EJPN Off J Eur Paediatr Neurol Soc 2016;20(4):678–83.

48. Kanai S, Okanishi T, Nishimura M, et al. Successful corpus callosotomy for Doose syndrome. Brain Dev 2017;39(10):882–5.

49. Thirunavu V, Du R, Wu JY, et al. The role of surgery in the management of Lennox-Gastaut syndrome: A systematic review and meta-analysis of the clinical evidence. Epilepsia 2021;62(4):888–907.

50. Frost M, Gates J, Helmers SL, et al. Vagus nerve stimulation in children with refractory seizures associated with Lennox-Gastaut syndrome. Epilepsia 2001;42(9):1148–52.

51. Cukiert A, Cukiert CM, Burattini JA, et al. Long-term outcome after callosotomy or vagus nerve stimulation in consecutive prospective cohorts of children with Lennox-Gastaut or Lennox-like syndrome and nonspecific MRI findings. Seizure 2013;22(5):396–400.

52. Kostov K, Kostov H, Taubøll E. Long-term vagus nerve stimulation in the treatment of Lennox-Gastaut syndrome. Epilepsy Behav EB 2009;16(2): 321–4.

53. Shahwan A, Bailey C, Maxiner W, et al. Vagus nerve stimulation for refractory epilepsy in children: More to VNS than seizure frequency reduction. Epilepsia 2009;50(5):1220–8.

54. Hornig GW, Murphy JV, Schallert G, et al. Left vagus nerve stimulation in children with refractory epilepsy: an update. South Med J 1997;90(5):484–8.

55. Provinciali L, Del Pesce M, Censori B, et al. Evolution of neuropsychological changes after partial callosotomy in intractable epilepsy. Epilepsy Res 1990;6(2): 155–65.

56. Liang S, Zhang S, Hu X, et al. Anterior corpus callosotomy in school-aged children with Lennox-Gastaut syndrome: a prospective study. Eur J Paediatr

Neurol EJPN Off J Eur Paediatr Neurol Soc 2014; 18(6):670–6.

57. Turanli G, Yalnizoğlu D, Genç-Açikgöz D, et al. Outcome and long term follow-up after corpus callosotomy in childhood onset intractable epilepsy. Childs Nerv Syst ChNS Off J Int Soc Pediatr Neurosurg 2006;22(10):1322–7.

58. Tanriverdi T, Olivier A, Poulin N, et al. Long-term seizure outcome after corpus callosotomy: a retrospective analysis of 95 patients. J Neurosurg 2009; 110(2):332–42.

59. Ding P, Liang S, Zhang S, et al. Resective surgery combined with corpus callosotomy for children with non-focal lesional Lennox-Gastaut syndrome. Acta Neurochir 2016;158(11):2177–84.

60. Pati S, Deep A, Troester MM, et al. Lennox-Gastaut syndrome symptomatic to hypothalamic hamartoma: evolution and long-term outcome following surgery. Pediatr Neurol 2013;49(1):25–30.

61. Kang JW, Eom S, Hong W, et al. Long-term Outcome of Resective Epilepsy Surgery in Patients With Lennox-Gastaut Syndrome. Pediatrics 2018;142(4). e20180449.

62. van den Munckhof B, van Dee V, Sagi L, et al. Treatment of electrical status epilepticus in sleep: A pooled analysis of 575 cases. Epilepsia 2015; 56(11):1738–46.

63. Jeong A, Strahle J, Vellimana AK, et al. Hemispherotomy in children with electrical status epilepticus of sleep. J Neurosurg Pediatr 2017;19(1):56–62.

64. Wang S, Weil AG, Ibrahim GM, et al. Surgical management of pediatric patients with encephalopathy due to electrical status epilepticus during sleep (ESES). Epileptic Disord Int Epilepsy J Videotape 2020;22(1):39–54.

65. Fournier-Del Castillo C, García-Fernández M, Pérez-Jiménez MÁ, et al. Encephalopathy with electrical status epilepticus during sleep: cognitive and executive improvement after epilepsy surgery. Seizure 2014;23(3):240–3.

66. Alawadhi A, Appendino JP, Hader W, et al. Surgically Remediable Secondary Network Epileptic Encephalopathies With Continuous Spike Wave in Sleep: Lesions May Not Be Visible on Brain Magnetic Resonance Imaging (MRI). J Child Neurol 2022;37(12–14):992–1002.

67. Downes M, Greenaway R, Clark M, et al. Outcome following multiple subpial transection in Landau-Kleffner syndrome and related regression. Epilepsia 2015;56(11):1760–6.

68. Gröppel G, Dorfer C, Dressler A, et al. Immediate termination of electrical status epilepticus in sleep after hemispherotomy is associated with significant progress in language development. Dev Med Child Neurol 2017;59(1):89–97.

69. Kim DW, Kim KK, Chu K, et al. Surgical treatment of delayed epilepsy in hemiconvulsion-hemiplegia-

epilepsy syndrome. Neurology 2008;70(22 Pt 2): 2116–22.

70. Kwan SY, Wong TT, Chang KP, et al. Seizure outcome after corpus callosotomy: the Taiwan experience. Childs Nerv Syst ChNS Off J Int Soc Pediatr Neurosurg 2000;16(2):87–92.

71. Itamura S, Okanishi T, Arai Y, et al. Three Cases of Hemiconvulsion-Hemiplegia-Epilepsy Syndrome With Focal Cortical Dysplasia Type IIId. Front Neurol 2019;10:1233.

72. Hect JL, Fernandez LD, Welch WP, et al. Deep brain stimulation of the centromedian thalamic nucleus for the treatment of FIRES. Epilepsia Open 2022;7(1): 187–93.

73. Sa M, Singh R, Pujar S, et al. Centromedian thalamic nuclei deep brain stimulation and Anakinra treatment for FIRES - Two different outcomes. Eur J Paediatr Neurol EJPN Off J Eur Paediatr Neurol Soc 2019;23(5):749–54.

74. Theroux L, Shah Y, Cukier Y, et al. Improved seizure burden and cognitive performance in a child treated with responsive neurostimulation (RNS) following febrile infection related epilepsy syndrome (FIRES). Epileptic Disord Int Epilepsy J Videotape 2020; 22(6):811–6.

75. Wille C, Steinhoff BJ, Altenmüller DM, et al. Chronic high-frequency deep-brain stimulation in progressive myoclonic epilepsy in adulthood–report of five cases. Epilepsia 2011;52(3):489–96.

76. Vesper J, Steinhoff B, Rona S, et al. Chronic high-frequency deep brain stimulation of the STN/SNr for progressive myoclonic epilepsy. Epilepsia 2007; 48(10):1984–9.

77. di Giacopo A, Baumann CR, Kurthen M, et al. Selective deep brain stimulation in the substantia nigra reduces myoclonus in progressive myoclonic epilepsy: a novel observation and short review of the literature. Epileptic Disord Int Epilepsy J Videotape 2019;21(3):283–8.

78. Rubboli G, Sabers A, Uldall P, et al. Management of Antiepileptic Treatment After Epilepsy Surgery - Practices and Problems. Curr Pharm Des 2017; 23(37):5749–59.

79. Engel J. Outcome with respect to epileptic seizures. Raven Press; 1993. p. 609–21.

80. Wieser HG, Blume WT, Fish D, et al. ILAE Commission Report. Proposal for a new classification of outcome with respect to epileptic seizures following epilepsy surgery. Epilepsia 2001;42(2):282–6.

81. Cramer JA, Perrine K, Devinsky O, et al. A brief questionnaire to screen for quality of life in epilepsy: the QOLIE-10. Epilepsia 1996;37(6):577–82.

82. Sheikh S, Thompson N, Bingaman W, et al. (Re) Defining success in epilepsy surgery: The importance of relative seizure reduction in patient-reported quality of life. Epilepsia 2019;60(10): 2078–85.

83. Pulsipher DT, Stanford LD. Serial neuropsychological testing before and after hemispherectomy in a child with electrical status epilepticus in slow wave sleep. Epilepsy Behav Rep 2022;18:100539.

84. Walker MP, Stickgold R. Sleep-dependent learning and memory consolidation. Neuron 2004;44(1): 121–33.

85. Paixao L, Sikka P, Sun H, et al. Excess brain age in the sleep electroencephalogram predicts reduced life expectancy. Neurobiol Aging 2020;88:150–5.

86. Ye E, Sun H, Leone MJ, et al. Association of Sleep Electroencephalography-Based Brain Age Index With Dementia. JAMA Netw Open 2020;3(9). e2017357.

87. McLaren JR, Luo Y, Kwon H, et al. Preliminary Evidence of a Relationship between Sleep Spindles and Treatment Response in Epileptic Encephalopathy. Ann Clin Transl Neurol 2023;10(9):1513–24.

88. Estimates of Funding for Various Research, Condition, and Disease Categories (RCDC). NIH Research Portfolio Online Reporting Tools. Published March 31, 2023. https://report.nih.gov/funding/categorical-spending#/Accessed May 5, 2023.

89. Shahat ARS, Greco G. The Economic Costs of Childhood Disability: A Literature Review. Int J Environ Res Public Health 2021;18(7):3531.

90. Richardson RM. Decision Making in Epilepsy Surgery. Neurosurg Clin N Am 2020;31(3):471–9.

91. Swarztrauber K, Dewar S, Engel J. Patient attitudes about treatments for intractable epilepsy. Epilepsy Behav EB 2003;4(1):19–25.

92. Baca CB, Cheng EM, Spencer SS, et al, Multicenter Study of Epilepsy Surgery. Racial differences in patient expectations prior to resective epilepsy surgery. Epilepsy Behav EB 2009;15(4):452–5.

93. Samanta D, Singh R, Gedela S, et al. Underutilization of epilepsy surgery: Part II: Strategies to overcome barriers. Epilepsy Behav 2021;117:107853.

Section II: Network Surgery and the Evolution of Stereoelectroencephalography (SEEG)

Imaging and Stereotactic Electroencephalography Functional Networks to Guide Epilepsy Surgery

Derek J. Doss, BE[a,b,c], Graham W. Johnson, PhD[a,b,c], Dario J. Englot, MD, PhD[a,b,c,d,e,f],*

KEYWORDS

- Connectomics • Epilepsy surgery • SEEG • iEEG • fMRI • DTI • Connectivity

KEY POINTS

- Despite improvements in technology, many patients evaluated for epilepsy surgery are not deemed to be candidates, often due to an incomplete hypothesis.
- Connectomics can be implemented into epilepsy surgery evaluations.
- Connectomics may help expand surgical options for patients who were previously not candidates.
- Prospective evaluations of connectomics methods and partnerships between academia and industry are necessary to bring connectomics to the clinic.

INTRODUCTION

Epilepsy is a common neurologic disorder affecting approximately 1% of the global population.[1] Approximately 40% of patients do not respond to medical treatment alone. Patients with drug-resistant epilepsy can be treated surgically through resection, ablation, or neuromodulation and between 65% and 70% of patients can achieve seizure freedom.[2,3] Surgical treatment of epilepsy is predicated on the successful localization of the area thought to be generating seizures, the seizure onset zone (SOZ).[4,5] However, localization is a complex process that can differ across institutions and does not always result in a clear surgical plan.[6] In fact, nearly 50% of those evaluated for epilepsy surgery are not candidates for surgery and the principle reason is the lack of a

hypothesis for SOZ localization (**Fig. 1**).[7] Despite this difference, surgical cases have been stable. Therefore, it has been proposed that the complexity of epilepsy being evaluated for surgery has increased in recent years.[7]

Shifts in patient complexity have occurred before. From the early to late twentieth century, the surgical treatment of epilepsy vastly expanded because physicians were able to better localize the SOZ. Originally, epilepsy surgery was limited to only Jacksonian focal epilepsy syndromes. The clinical features combined with intraoperative stimulation to localize the "spasming center" were the only localizing methodologies available.[8–10] The addition of electroencephalography (EEG) along with more advanced intraoperative stimulation spurred the expansion of epilepsy surgery to temporal lobectomies.[11] Localization was improved

[a] Department of Biomedical Engineering, Vanderbilt University, PMB 351631, 2301 Vanderbilt Place, Nashville, TN 37235, USA; [b] Vanderbilt University Institute of Imaging Science (VUIIS), 1161 21st Avenue South, Medical Center North AA-1105, Nashville, TN 37232, USA; [c] Vanderbilt Institute for Surgery and Engineering (VISE), 1161 21st Avenue South, MCN S2323, Nashville, TN 37232, USA; [d] Department of Neurological Surgery, Vanderbilt University Medical Center, 1161 21st Avenue South, T4224 Medical Center North, Nashville, TN 37232, USA; [e] Department of Electrical and Computer Engineering, Vanderbilt University, PMB 351824, 2301 Vanderbilt Place, Nashville, TN 37235, USA; [f] Department of Radiological Sciences, Vanderbilt University Medical Center, 1161 21st Avenue South, Nashville, TN 37232, USA
* Corresponding author.
E-mail address: dario.englot@vumc.org

Neurosurg Clin N Am 35 (2024) 61–72
https://doi.org/10.1016/j.nec.2023.09.001
1042-3680/24/© 2023 Elsevier Inc. All rights reserved.

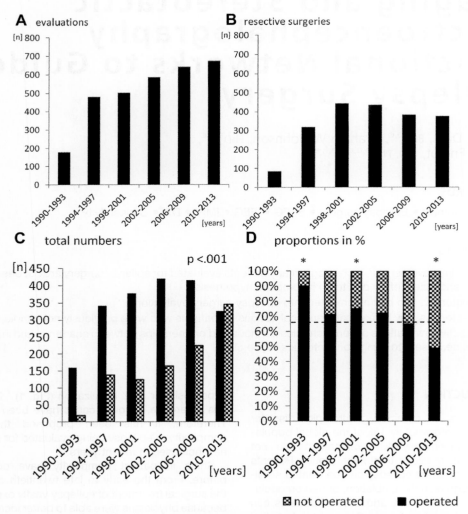

Fig. 1. Epilepsy surgery evaluations are increasing but resection trends are stable, and the most cited reason is the lack of a hypothesis. (*A*) Panel shows the number of presurgical evaluations across different timepoints. (*B*) Panel shows the number of resective surgeries during the same timepoints. (*C*) Panel shows the percentage of rejected cases by patient/parent or neurologist. (*D*) Panel shows the breakdown of reason for rejection, with the most common being risks and no hypothesis. *Significant deviation from estimated grand mean (*p* <0.05) using GLM. GLM, generalised linear model. (*Adapted from* Cloppenborg et al[7]; with permission.)

further by intracranial EEG (iEEG) and neuroimaging such as MRI.[12–14] Although challenging, the earlier paradigm shift led to one of the most effective operations in neurosurgery.[9,10] Just as historical approaches to epilepsy surgery shifted their paradigm from the "spasming center" to the SOZ, the modern epilepsy surgery paradigm has shifted from the SOZ to the seizure network.

The "network revolution" in epilepsy has shifted the paradigm of epilepsy surgery toward localization strategies that quantify the network and treatment plans that disrupt the network (**Fig. 2**A).[15–18] The seizure network can be disrupted by resection, ablation, neuromodulation, or a

combination of modalities (**Fig. 2**B–D). However, the network must first be discovered, quantified, and then treated. Representing the brain as a network relies on examining the connectivity, or relation of signals between areas of the brain. Structural connectivity (SC) represents white matter connections between regions. Functional connectivity (FC) represents neural communication between areas in the brain, with high FC representing a strong connection and low FC representing a weak connection. These measures are often derived from diffusion-weighted imaging (DWI), functional MRI (fMRI), and iEEG. Discovery of the seizure network may be completed

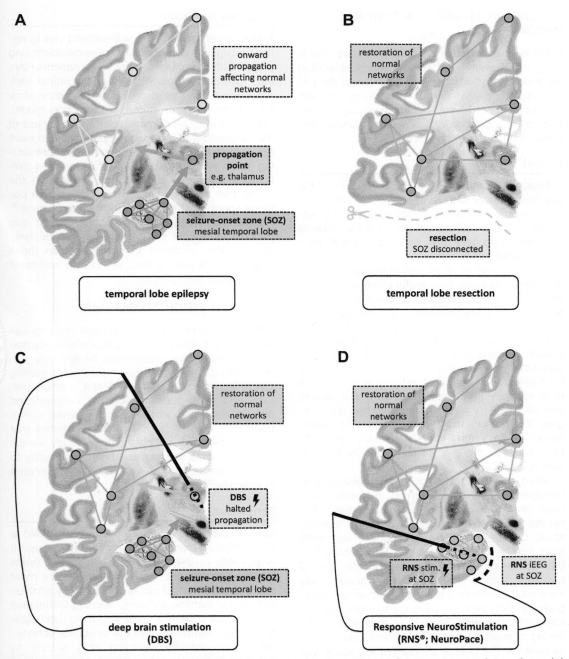

Fig. 2. Conceptual depiction of how various treatment modalities may disrupt the seizure network in epilepsy. (*A*) Panel depicts normal networks, propagation networks, and the seizure network. (*B*) Panel demonstrates how resection is thought to disrupt the seizure network. (*C*) Panel demonstrates how DBS is thought to disrupt the seizure network. (*D*) Panel demonstrates how RNS is through to disrupt the seizure network. RNS, responsive neurostimulation. (*Adapted from* Piper et al[15]; with permission.)

noninvasively through neuroimaging techniques such as DWI and fMRI. DWI and fMRI have shown promise in the lateralization of the epileptic network as well as the prediction of seizure freedom after surgery. Localization of the network can be completed with iEEG. The addition of connectivity-based studies may be a missing link in identifying and treating the seizure network in patients previously not considered epilepsy surgery candidates.

FUNCTIONAL MAGNETIC RESONANCE IMAGING

FMRI is a noninvasive imaging technique that is being increasingly used in the presurgical workup for epilepsy for lateralization and localization of language and memory.[19,20] However, network studies with fMRI may benefit epilepsy surgery through lateralization of the seizure network and prediction of seizure freedom.

Lateralization

Lateralization of the epileptic network is one of the key predictors of seizure freedom.[5,21,22] Although conventional methods can lateralize seizure networks in most patients, more complex patients are difficult to lateralize and may benefit from fMRI augmented lateralization.[23]

FC abnormalities in mesial temporal networks have been relatively successful in lateralizing epilepsy.[24] However, the exact connections vary between studies. Narasimhan and colleagues used FC between mesial temporal structures and the default mode network to lateralize patients with mesial temporal lobe epilepsy (mTLE).[25] Morgan and colleagues sought to improve lateralization by splitting their cohort of patients with temporal lobe epilepsy (TLE) into those who are seizure free after surgery versus not seizure free after surgery. The authors found that FC from the hippocampi to the ventral lateral nucleus of the right thalamus was the best differentiator for left TLE versus right TLE.[26]

Given these slight disparities in lateralization hypotheses, machine learning methods have been used to improve epilepsy lateralization but results have been mixed. A machine learning study by Gholipour and colleagues used fMRI data from a multicenter cohort to lateralize TLE but achieved an accuracy below that of FC methods alone.[27] Deep learning models may improve this accuracy but they must remain interpretable. Only recently have studies began using these methods with Luckett and colleagues publishing innovative work using a convolutional neural network.[28] A unique strength of this study was the interrogation of what anatomic areas the model used to classify left and right TLE, overcoming the "black box" nature of deep learning (**Fig. 3**). Similar to earlier FC studies, the authors found that resting state networks including the default mode network, medial temporal network, and dorsal attention network were all the strongest predictors of left versus right TLE (see **Fig. 3**). The overall accuracy was substantially greater than other methods but the generalizability is unknown.

Outcome Prediction

Prediction of patients who will respond well to epilepsy surgery may aid in surgical decision-making and provide insights into why some patients have less favorable outcomes. Although clinical variables have been used previously, FC may allow for a more accurate outcome prediction model. He and colleagues demonstrated that hubness of the thalamus was increased in patients who were not seizure free after surgery, perhaps representing more widespread epilepsy.[29] Guo and colleagues used dynamic FC and found that the states that seizure free and not seizure free patients spent most of their time in were different.[30] Additionally, Negishi and colleagues found that patients who were seizure free had connectivity abnormalities localized to one lobe than those who were not seizure free, which may represent a more localized epilepsy.[31]

DIFFUSION-WEIGHTED IMAGING

DWI is a method by which white matter tracts can be estimated. Tractography is typically performed in the preoperative assessment for epilepsy surgery and has historically been used for stratifying risk.[32] The risk of a visual field deficit, memory deficits, and naming deficits can all be predicted through localization of well-known white matter tracts.[33–37] Eartier study has demonstrated that SC is different in patients with epilepsy versus healthy controls and represents an opportunity to lateralize the seizure network and predict outcome in epilepsy.[38,39]

Lateralization

Lateralization of the seizure network with DWI is most helpful in ambiguous, nonlesional cases. It is possible to use common white matter tracts for this purpose but these approaches are most accurate with lesional cases of TLE.[40] The addition of machine learning and deep learning techniques on diffusion measures has improved lateralization.[41] The combination of the structural connectome and machine learning was shown to lateralize TLE accurately, agnostic to lesional and nonlesional cases.[42] Furthermore, the connections used by the network to lateralize were consistent with other studies of left versus right TLE, increasing interpretability of the network.

Outcome Prediction

It can be useful for surgical decision-making to know the chances of achieving seizure freedom after epilepsy surgery. Prediction of seizure freedom can aid in the decision process to proceed with

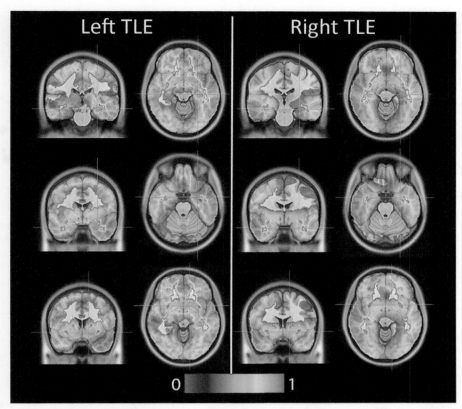

Fig. 3. Deep learning approaches to lateralize TLE can be used both as tools for epilepsy surgery and hypothesis generation. The displayed heatmap represents the spatial location of features used in a deep learning model. As can be seen, the right hemisphere is more important for classification of right TLE, and the left hemisphere is more important for classification of left TLE. (*From* Luckett et al[28]; with permission.)

epilepsy surgery, modify the surgical plan, or avoid surgery for those that are not candidates. Several scoring systems have been proposed based on clinical variables; however, a connectome-based approach may achieve more accurate outcome predictions.[43,44] SC has been particularly accurate in the prediction of seizure freedom after surgery. Increased ipsilateral SC abnormalities, especially those related to the ipsilateral mesial structures, are most often used.[45–47] One study examined seizure recurrence and found that more widespread SC abnormalities were associated with seizure recurrence (**Fig. 4**).[46] However, these studies were limited to anterior temporal lobectomies and to TLE.

Machine learning approaches have also been used for seizure outcome prediction.[48,49] However, it can be difficult to interpret what machine learning approaches use to stratify patients. One such example of this is a study by Johnson and colleagues where the authors reduced the features down to the connections that best stratified patients who were and were not seizure free.[49]

INTRACRANIAL ELECTROENCEPHALOGRAPHY
Neurostimulation

One of the first techniques for identifying the SOZ for resection in epilepsy was through intraoperative stimulation.[10] Stimulation has also been used for localization of eloquent cortex, both intraoperatively and preoperatively.[50,51] In the early twenty-first century, single pulse electrical stimulation (SPES) has been increasingly used after implantation of iEEG for the identification of epileptogenic tissue.[52] A prospective study by Valentin and colleagues demonstrated the effectiveness of SPES to identify epileptogenic tissue. They reported that when abnormal responses (delays and repetitive spiking) were present in the resected area, 96% of patients achieved an Engel I or II favorable seizure outcome.[53,54] The results of this study were promising for patients who had abnormal responses to SPES; however, nearly 40% of patients had no abnormal responses. Can we make use of this technique in more patients using a network-based approach?

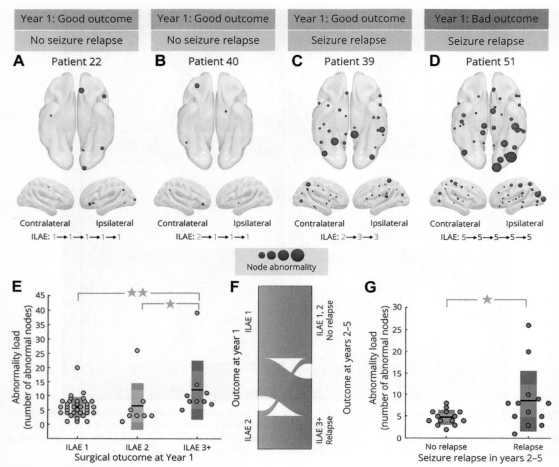

Fig. 4. More widespread structural abnormalities were present in patients with a poor outcome after epilepsy surgery. An example of these widespread abnormalities can be seen in panels (*C, D*). Examples of more localized abnormalities can be seen in panels (*A, B*). Four patients with their structural abnormalities are shown in panels (*A–D*). Panel (*E*) shows the structural abnormality for international league against epilepsy (ILAE) 1, 2, and 3+ patients. Significantly more abnormal nodes are present in ILAE 3+ vs ILAE 2 and ILAE 1 patients. Panel (*F*) shows the proportion ILAE 1 and ILAE 2 patients who relapsed (had seizure recurrence) at year 1. Panel (*G*) shows the abnormality load for patients who did and did not relapse in years 2-5. All patients included in panel G were ILAE 1 or 2. One star indicates *p* <0.05 and two stars indicate *p* <0.01. (*From* Sinha et al[46]; with permission.)

Network stimulation studies with SPES allow for directional information to be inferred, as a stimulus is delivered and responses are computed from all other contacts.[55,56] Two major thoughts have predominated in this field: (1) SOZs influence the entire network more so than other regions and (2) SOZs are more highly connected to itself.

The idea of SOZs influencing the network more so than other regions has been proposed and studied by several in the field, with SPES studies providing evidence.[57,58] Furthermore, these findings become even stronger when only contacts that were labeled as an SOZ and resected in patients with an Engel I outcome are analyzed.[59] In addition to influencing the network, SOZs have been shown to demonstrate increased within SOZ connections.[59,60] The finding of "hypercoupling" of SOZs may represent the seizure network and is most present in patients who were seizure free after surgery.[61]

Although the connectivity metrics used by earlier studies have performed relatively well, many were originally developed for use in iEEG grids. This allowed for the assumption of directionality of neurons. This can represent a limitation because more centers are using stereotactic EEG, which have varying directionality of pyramidal neurons. In order to overcome this limitation, one study used a deep learning model to analyze SPES responses, resulting in improvements in the accuracy of SOZ localization.[42]

Resting State Networks

Although ictal data acquired from iEEG are the gold standard for localization of the seizure network, interictal data have the potential to improve localization, especially in cases in which ictal localization fails. Interictal network approaches to iEEG have been used since the early 2000s. Initially, several studies reported that SOZs had increased connectivity to other SOZs.[62–67] With the addition of directional connectivity measures, Narasimhan and colleagues noted that SOZs had higher inward connectivity from all other regions in the brain in 2020.[68] This finding was also observed by Jiang and colleagues[69] More recent studies have noted that in addition to the increase in inward connectivity, there is a decreased outward connectivity from seizure networks, leading to the idea that seizure networks are suppressed at baseline.[70,71] One such study proposed the Interictal Suppression Hypothesis (ISH), which postulated that SOZs had higher inward connectivity and lower outward connectivity during the resting state, suggesting that SOZs are suppressed at rest to prevent seizures (**Fig. 5**).[71] Other group has described a similar "Sources and Sinks" phenomenon, suggesting that inward inhibition of the SOZ may aid presurgical localization.[70] Although these network-based approaches seem valuable, they have yet to be prospectively evaluated.

MULTIMODAL

The combination of SC and FC has been shown to improve the accuracy of outcome prediction.[71–73] One such approach is to combine SC and FC to develop a connectivity profile of seizure free patients. Such a fingerprint can then be compared with a patient's connectome to predict seizure freedom with an accuracy of 100% in one study (**Fig. 6**).[72,73]

Others have had success expanding the combination of SC and FC to combine iEEG and DWI. Due to the difference in sampling between iEEG and neuroimaging methods, this can be a technical challenge. To overcome this, Johnson and colleagues developed an algorithm for subsampling whole-brain tractography with iEEG near-field dynamic localization, thus allowing for the computation of SC in the same areas sampled by iEEG.[71] By combining the ISH findings of increased inward FC and decreased outward FC along with SC, the authors found that they were able to better differentiate SOZs, propogative zones (PZs) and non-involved zones (NIZs) (**Fig. 7**).

DISCUSSION

Despite an increase in surgical evaluations, there has not been an increase in surgical treatments.[7]

Interictal Suppression Hypothesis (ISH) in Focal Epilepsy

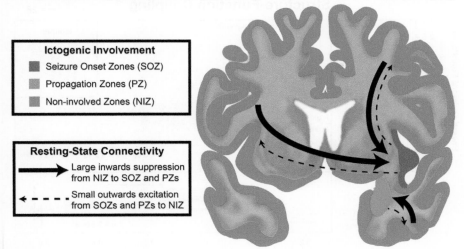

Fig. 5. The ISH is a novel conceptualization that may localize the seizure network. The ISH proposes that at baseline, the seizure network is suppressed by regions not involved in the seizure network. The noninvolved zones can be seen in blue, the propagation zones can be seen in orange, and the seizure onset zones can be seen in red. (*From* Johnson et al[71]; with permission.)

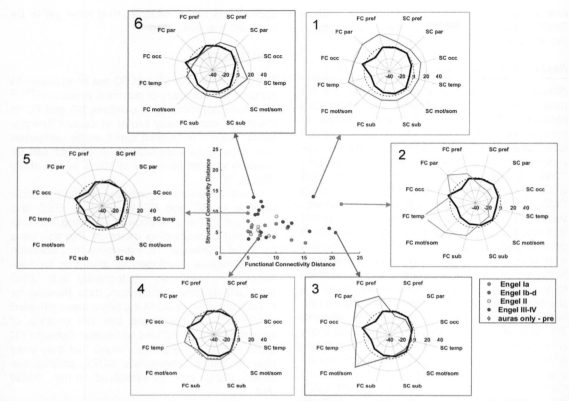

Fig. 6. SC and FC profiles can be used to accurately predict outcomes from epilepsy surgery. Both FC and SC were used to develop a "network fingerprint" of patients who were seizure free. Connectivity profiles of 6 example patients with their corresponding outcome data are depicted. dashed line, zero denoting age-matched control. FC, functional connectome distance; mot/som, motor and sensory/motor lobe; occ, occipital lobe; par, parietal lobe; pref, prefrontal lobe; SC, structural connectome distance; sub, subcortical structures (all ipsilateral to seizure focus); temp, temporal lobe. (*Adapted from* Morgan et al[73]; with permission.)

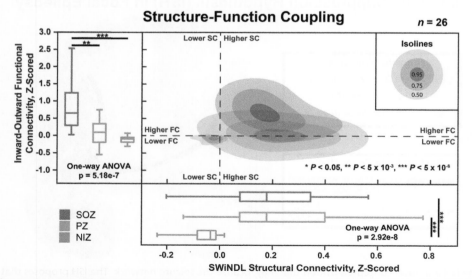

Fig. 7. The combination of the ISH FC and SC can more accurately differentiate the seizure network than functional or SC alone. SOZs are depicted in red, PZs are depicted in orange, and NIZs are depicted in blue. SC is on the x-axis and inward-outward connectivity is on the y-axis. (*Adapted from* Johnson et al[71]; with permission.)

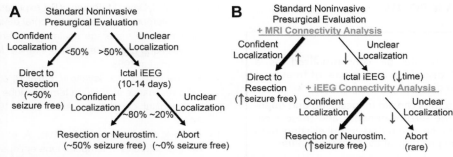

Fig. 8. How the addition of network studies could influence the presurgical evaluation for epilepsy surgery. The typical presurgical evaluation is depicted in panel (*A*). The proposed network augmented evaluation is depicted in panel (*B*). (*From* Johnson et al[76]; with permission.)

The reason most cited for patients not being surgical candidates is lack of a localization hypothesis. Why are we increasingly unable to understand the seizure network in patients when we have access to more technology than before?[4,6] Some suggest increasingly complex patients are being evaluated for epilepsy surgery.[7] Roadblocks such as these have been present in epilepsy surgery before and they were overcame with a paradigm shift, moving from "the spasming point" to the SOZ that if removed would result in seizure freedom. Now, the paradigm has shifted from a SOZ to a seizure network that can be treated with resection, ablation, neuromodulation, or a combination.[5,15,74–76]

There are limitations to network evaluations of epilepsy, and it is paramount to remember that network studies are a tool to augment clinical decision-making. DWI and fMRI network studies are useful for lateralization and outcome prediction but accurate localization of the seizure network with MRI connectivity alone has been more challenging. Network studies with iEEG have demonstrated promise in localizing and identifying the seizure network. However, a strong hypothesis must be developed due to the sparse sampling intrinsic to iEEG. A further limitation is the variability of processing methods between groups, creating challenges in generalizability. Thus, even with published methods and similar data acquisition between centers, connectomics can be difficult to implement. A further challenge is the paucity of prospective studies evaluating network measures for epilepsy surgery. However, the few studies published changed decision-making in 58% of cases and increased epilepsy surgery candidacy by 26%.[77]

Currently, the largest gap in epilepsy surgery is the lack of translation from the laboratory to the clinic. Despite the need for new ways to treat more complex epilepsy patients, the promising results from network studies, and several proposed implementation paths such as the one depicted in **Fig. 8**, few have used network approaches to augment presurgical evaluations.[76] Therefore, the next steps in this process require prospective evaluation of localization methodologies along with academic–commercial partnerships to bring the research from theoretic to practical. One could envision a network evaluation software package that is simple to use, repeatable, and clinically useful. Such an approach may allow for localization of a patient's seizure network and identification of key areas for multimodal treatment.

SUMMARY

The paradigm of epilepsy surgery has shifted to that of a network disorder.[15–18,74–76] This shift in the paradigm of epilepsy surgery may allow for the localization of seizure networks that were previously unable to be localized and the treatment of epilepsies, which were previously thought not to be surgical candidates. Connectivity can be evaluated with fMRI, DWI, and iEEG. FMRI and DWI connectivity studies have demonstrated the most success in lateralization of the seizure network and outcome prediction, whereas iEEG connectivity patterns have shown value in localizing the seizure network. Multimodal connectivity analyses, such as those combining SC and FC, have demonstrated the most success. However, translating connectomics from the laboratory to the clinic has been challenging. There is a need for improvement in localization and treatment of epilepsy. The field has taken a half measure in discussion and research of these methods but there is a need for action in the form of prospective evaluations of connectomics and partnerships between industry and academia to bring connectomics to all centers.

CLINICS CARE POINTS

- Epilepsy should be conceptualized as a network disorder with the goal of treatment being to disrupt the seizure network.
- Connectomics can aid in localizing and quantifying the seizure network and these measures can be computed using existing data from the presurgical evaluation pipeline.

DISCLOSURE

The authors declare no financial or commercial conflict of interest. This study was supported by the National Institutes of Health, United States (grant nos. T32GM007347, T32EB021937, F31NS120401, and R01NS112252).

REFERENCES

1. Beghi E. The epidemiology of epilepsy. Neuroepidemiology 2020;54(2):185–91.
2. Ryvlin P, Cross JH, Rheims S. Epilepsy surgery in children and adults. Lancet Neurol 2014/11/01/2014;13(11):1114–26.
3. Téllez-Zenteno JF, Dhar R, Wiebe S. Long-term seizure outcomes following epilepsy surgery: a systematic review and meta-analysis. Brain 2005;128(5):1188–98.
4. Baumgartner C, Koren JP, Britto-Arias M, et al. Presurgical epilepsy evaluation and epilepsy surgery. F1000Res 2019;8. https://doi.org/10.12688/f1000research.17714.1.
5. Vakharia VN, Duncan JS, Witt JA, et al. Getting the best outcomes from epilepsy surgery. Ann Neurol 2018;83(4):676–90.
6. Englot DJ. A modern epilepsy surgery treatment algorithm: incorporating traditional and emerging technologies. Epilepsy Behav 2018;80:68–74.
7. Cloppenborg T, May TW, Blümcke I, et al. Trends in epilepsy surgery: stable surgical numbers despite increasing presurgical volumes. J Neurol Neurosurg Psychiatry 2016;87(12):1322–9.
8. Krause F. Surgery of the brain and spinal cord: based on personal experiences. vol 2. Rebman; 1912.
9. Meador KJ, Loring DW, Flanigin HF. History of epilepsy surgery. J Epilepsy 1989;2(1):21–5.
10. Feindel W, Leblanc R, De Almeida AN. Epilepsy surgery: historical highlights 1909–2009. Epilepsia 2009;50(s3):131–51.
11. GIBBS FA, LENNOX WG, Gibbs EL. The electroencephalogram in diagnosis and in localization of epileptic seizures. Arch Neurol Psychiatr 1936;36(6):1225–35.
12. Talairach J, David M, Tournoux P. L'exploration chirurgicale stéréotaxique du lobe temporal dans l'épilepsie temporale: repérage anatomique stéréotaxique et technique chirurgicale. Paris, France: Masson & Cie, Editeurs; 1958.
13. Kuznieky R, de la Sayette V, Ethier R, et al. Magnetic resonance imaging in temporal lobe epilepsy: pathological correlations. Ann Neurol 1987;22(3):341–7.
14. Berkovic SF, Andermann F, Olivier A, et al. Hippocampal sclerosis in temporal lobe epilepsy demonstrated by magnetic resonance imaging. Ann Neurol 1991;29(2):175–82.
15. Piper RJ, Richardson RM, Worrell G, et al. Towards network-guided neuromodulation for epilepsy. Brain 2022;145(10):3347–62.
16. Sinha N, Johnson GW, Davis KA, et al. Integrating network neuroscience into epilepsy care: progress, barriers, and next steps. Epilepsy Curr 2022;22(5):272–8.
17. Scott RC, Menendez de la Prida L, Mahoney JM, et al. The many facets of epilepsy networks. Epilepsia 2018;59(8):1475–83.
18. Davis KA, Jirsa VK, Schevon CA. Wheels within wheels: theory and practice of epileptic networks. Epilepsy Curr 2021;21(4). https://doi.org/10.1177/15357597211015663. 15357597211015663.
19. Sidhu MK, Duncan JS, Sander JW. Neuroimaging in epilepsy. Curr Opin Neurol 2018;31(4):371–8.
20. Szaflarski JP, Gloss D, Binder JR, et al. Practice guideline summary: Use of fMRI in the presurgical evaluation of patients with epilepsy: report of the guideline development, dissemination, and implementation subcommittee of the american academy of neurology. Neurology 2017;88(4):395–402.
21. Téllez-Zenteno JF, Hernández Ronquillo L, Moien-Afshari F, et al. Surgical outcomes in lesional and non-lesional epilepsy: a systematic review and meta-analysis. Epilepsy Res. May 2010;89(2–3):310–8.
22. Krucoff MO, Chan AY, Harward SC, et al. Rates and predictors of success and failure in repeat epilepsy surgery: A meta-analysis and systematic review. Epilepsia 2017;58(12):2133–42.
23. Bien CG, Szinay M, Wagner J, et al. Characteristics and surgical outcomes of patients with refractory magnetic resonance imaging-negative epilepsies. Arch Neurol. Dec 2009;66(12):1491–9.
24. Bettus G, Bartolomei F, Confort-Gouny S, et al. Role of resting state functional connectivity MRI in presurgical investigation of mesial temporal lobe epilepsy. J Neurol Neurosurg Psychiatry 2010;81(10):1147–54.
25. Narasimhan S, González HFJ, Johnson GW, et al. Functional connectivity between mesial temporal and default mode structures may help lateralize surgical temporal lobe epilepsy. J Neurosurg 2022;137(6):1571–81.

26. Morgan VL, Sonmezturk HH, Gore JC, et al. Lateralization of temporal lobe epilepsy using resting functional magnetic resonance imaging connectivity of hippocampal networks. Epilepsia. Sep 2012;53(9):1628–35.

27. Gholipour T, You X, Stufflebeam SM, et al. Common functional connectivity alterations in focal epilepsies identified by machine learning. Epilepsia 2022;63(3):629–40.

28. Luckett PH, Maccotta L, Lee JJ, et al. Deep learning resting state functional magnetic resonance imaging lateralization of temporal lobe epilepsy. Epilepsia 2022;63(6):1542–52.

29. He X, Doucet GE, Pustina D, et al. Presurgical thalamic "hubness" predicts surgical outcome in temporal lobe epilepsy. Neurology 2017;88(24):2285–93.

30. Guo D, Feng L, Yang Z, et al. Altered temporal variations of functional connectivity associated with surgical outcomes in drug-resistant temporal lobe epilepsy. Front Neurosci 2022;16:840481.

31. Negishi M, Martuzzi R, Novotny EJ, et al. Functional MRI connectivity as a predictor of the surgical outcome of epilepsy. Epilepsia 2011;52(9):1733–40.

32. Duncan JS, Winston GP, Koepp MJ, et al. Brain imaging in the assessment for epilepsy surgery. Lancet Neurol 2016;15(4):420–33.

33. Piper RJ, Yoong MM, Kandasamy J, et al. Application of diffusion tensor imaging and tractography of the optic radiation in anterior temporal lobe resection for epilepsy: a systematic review. Clin Neurol Neurosurg 2014;124:59–65.

34. Yogarajah M, Focke NK, Bonelli S, et al. Defining Meyer's loop–temporal lobe resections, visual field deficits and diffusion tensor tractography. Brain 2009;132(6):1656–68.

35. Papagno C, Casarotti A, Comi A, et al. Long-term proper name anomia after removal of the uncinate fasciculus. Brain Struct Funct 2016;221(1):687–94.

36. McDonald CR, Leyden KM, Hagler DJ, et al. White matter microstructure complements morphometry for predicting verbal memory in epilepsy. Cortex 2014;58:139–50.

37. Middlebrooks EH, Yagmurlu K, Szaflarski JP, et al. A contemporary framework of language processing in the human brain in the context of preoperative and intraoperative language mapping. Neuroradiology 2017;59(1):69–87.

38. Bernhardt BC, Fadaie F, Liu M, et al. Temporal lobe epilepsy. Hippocampal pathology modulates connectome topology and controllability 2019;92(19):e2209–20.

39. Yu Y, Chu L, Liu C, et al. Alterations of white matter network in patients with left and right non-lesional temporal lobe epilepsy. Eur Radiol 2019;29(12):6750–61.

40. García-Pallero MA, Hodaie M, Zhong J, et al. Prediction of laterality in temporal lobe epilepsy using white matter diffusion metrics. World Neurosurg 2019;128:e700–8.

41. Gleichgerrcht E, Munsell BC, Alhusaini S, et al. Artificial intelligence for classification of temporal lobe epilepsy with ROI-level MRI data: a worldwide ENIGMA-Epilepsy study. Neuroimage Clin 2021;31:102765.

42. Johnson GW, Cai LY, Doss DJ, et al. Localizing seizure onset zones in surgical epilepsy with neurostimulation deep learning. J Neurosurg 2023;138(4):1002–7.

43. Jehi L, Yardi R, Chagin K, et al. Development and validation of nomograms to provide individualised predictions of seizure outcomes after epilepsy surgery: a retrospective analysis. Lancet Neurol. Mar 2015;14(3):283–90.

44. Dugan P, Carlson C, Jetté N, et al. Derivation and initial validation of a surgical grading scale for the preliminary evaluation of adult patients with drug-resistant focal epilepsy. Epilepsia 2017;58(5):792–800.

45. Bonilha L, Jensen JH, Baker N, et al. The brain connectome as a personalized biomarker of seizure outcomes after temporal lobectomy. Neurology 2015;84(18):1846–53.

46. Sinha N, Wang Y, Moreira da Silva N, et al. Structural brain network abnormalities and the probability of seizure recurrence after epilepsy surgery. Neurology 2021;96(5):e758–71.

47. Chen X, Wang Y, Kopetzky SJ, et al. Connectivity within regions characterizes epilepsy duration and treatment outcome. Hum Brain Mapp 2021;42(12):3777–91.

48. Gleichgerrcht E, Munsell B, Bhatia S, et al. Deep learning applied to whole-brain connectome to determine seizure control after epilepsy surgery. Epilepsia 2018;59(9):1643–54.

49. Johnson GW, Cai LY, Narasimhan S, et al. Temporal lobe epilepsy lateralisation and surgical outcome prediction using diffusion imaging. J Neurol Neurosurg Psychiatry 2022;93(6):599–608.

50. DuanYu N, GuoJun Z, Liang Q, et al. Surgery for perirolandic epilepsy: Epileptogenic cortex resection guided by chronic intracranial electroencephalography and electric cortical stimulation mapping. Clin Neurol Neurosurg 2010;112(2):110–7.

51. Alarcon G, Nawoor L, Valentin A. Electrical Cortical Stimulation: Mapping for Function and Seizures. Neurosurg Clin N Am 2020;31(3):435–48.

52. Trébuchon A, Chauvel P. Electrical Stimulation for Seizure Induction and Functional Mapping in Stereoelectroencephalography. J Clin Neurophysiol 2016;33(6):511–21.

53. Valentín A, Alarcón G, Honavar M, et al. Single pulse electrical stimulation for identification of structural abnormalities and prediction of seizure outcome after epilepsy surgery: a prospective study. Lancet Neurol 2005;4(11):718–26.

54. Engel J. Surgical treatment of the epilepsies. New York: Raven Press; 1987.

55. Matsumoto R, Kunieda T, Nair D. Single pulse electrical stimulation to probe functional and pathological connectivity in epilepsy. Seizure 2017;44:27–36.

56. Prime D, Rowlands D, O'Keefe S, et al. Considerations in performing and analyzing the responses of cortico-cortical evoked potentials in stereo-EEG. Epilepsia 2018;59(1):16–26.

57. Hays MA, Coogan C, Crone NE, et al. Graph theoretical analysis of evoked potentials shows network influence of epileptogenic mesial temporal region. Hum Brain Mapp 2021;42(13):4173–86.

58. Zhao C, Liang Y, Li C, et al. Localization of Epileptogenic Zone Based on Cortico-Cortical Evoked Potential (CCEP): A Feature Extraction and Graph Theory Approach. Front Neuroinform 2019;13:31.

59. van Blooijs D, Leijten FSS, van Rijen PC, et al. Evoked directional network characteristics of epileptogenic tissue derived from single pulse electrical stimulation. Hum Brain Mapp 2018;39(11):4611–22.

60. Boido D, Kapetis D, Gnatkovsky V, et al. Stimulus-evoked potentials contribute to map the epileptogenic zone during stereo-EEG presurgical monitoring. Hum Brain Mapp 2014;35(9):4267–81.

61. Guo Z-h, Zhao B-t, Toprani S, et al. Epileptogenic network of focal epilepsies mapped with cortico-cortical evoked potentials. Clin Neurophysiol 2020; 131(11):2657–66.

62. Mormann F, Lehnertz K, David P, et al. Mean phase coherence as a measure for phase synchronization and its application to the EEG of epilepsy patients. Phys Nonlinear Phenom 2000;144(3):358–69.

63. Bettus G, Ranjeva JP, Wendling F, et al. Interictal functional connectivity of human epileptic networks assessed by intracerebral EEG and BOLD signal fluctuations. PLoS One 2011;6(5):e20071.

64. Bartolomei F, Bettus G, Stam CJ, et al. Interictal network properties in mesial temporal lobe epilepsy: a graph theoretical study from intracerebral recordings. Clin Neurophysiol 2013;124(12):2345–53.

65. Lagarde S, Roehri N, Lambert I, et al. Interictal stereotactic-EEG functional connectivity in refractory focal epilepsies. Brain 2018;141(10):2966–80.

66. Paulo DL, Wills KE, Johnson GW, et al. SEEG Functional Connectivity Measures to Identify Epileptogenic Zones: Stability, Medication Influence, and Recording Condition. Neurology 2022;98(20):e2060–72.

67. Goodale SE, González HFJ, Johnson GW, et al. Resting-State SEEG May Help Localize Epileptogenic Brain Regions. Neurosurgery 2020;86(6): 792–801.

68. Narasimhan S, Kundassery KB, Gupta K, et al. Seizure-onset regions demonstrate high inward directed connectivity during resting-state: An SEEG study in focal epilepsy. Epilepsia 2020; 61(11):2534–44.

69. Jiang H, Kokkinos V, Ye S, et al. Interictal SEEG Resting-State Connectivity Localizes the Seizure Onset Zone and Predicts Seizure Outcome. Adv Sci (Weinh) 2022;9(18):e2200887.

70. Gunnarsdottir KM, Li A, Smith RJ, et al. Source-sink connectivity: a novel interictal EEG marker for seizure localization. Brain 2022;145(11):3901–15.

71. Johnson GW, Doss DJ, Morgan VL, et al. The Interictal Suppression Hypothesis in focal epilepsy: network-level supporting evidence. Brain 2023; awad016. https://doi.org/10.1093/brain/awad016.

72. Morgan VL, Englot DJ, Rogers BP, et al. Magnetic resonance imaging connectivity for the prediction of seizure outcome in temporal lobe epilepsy. Epilepsia 2017;58(7):1251–60.

73. Morgan VL, Sainburg LE, Johnson GW, et al. Presurgical temporal lobe epilepsy connectome fingerprint for seizure outcome prediction. Brain Commun 2022;4(3):fcac128.

74. Engel J Jr, Thompson PM, Stern JM, et al. Connectomics and epilepsy. Curr Opin Neurol 2013;26(2).

75. Zijlmans M, Zweiphenning W, van Klink N. Changing concepts in presurgical assessment for epilepsy surgery. Nat Rev Neurol 2019;15(10):594–606.

76. Johnson GW, Doss DJ, Englot DJ. Network dysfunction in pre and postsurgical epilepsy: connectomics as a tool and not a destination. Curr Opin Neurol 2022;35(2).

77. Boerwinkle VL, Mirea L, Gaillard WD, et al. Resting-state functional MRI connectivity impact on epilepsy surgery plan and surgical candidacy: prospective clinical work. J Neurosurg: Pediatrics PED 2020; 25(6):574–81.

Interpretation of the Intracranial Electroencephalogram of the Human Hippocampus

Vasileios Kokkinos, CNIM, NA-CLTM, PhD, PhD, PhD

KEYWORDS

• Epilepsy • Epilepsy surgery • Intracranial EEG • Hippocampus

KEY POINTS

- Understanding what constitutes an abnormal feature/pattern in the intracranial electroencephalogram (iEEG) is inherently linked to the understanding of its normal constituents.
- Stereo-electroencephalography (sEEG) contacts in hippocampal space are picking up the surrounding neuronal activity with finer spectral detail, due to the lack of major white matter filtering.
- sEEG contacts in the hippocampus record high-amplitude surrounding neuronal activity due to a combination of strong electric fields in the transverse and anterio-posterior directions.
- Intermittent delta activity in the hippocampal iEEG is a normal property and should not be interpreted as a marker of hippocampal epileptogenicity or other pathologic condition.
- Near-continuous delta, lack of higher frequencies in the background, reduced foreground spindles and barques, and interictal activity abundance, constitute hallmarks of abnormal hippocampal iEEG.

INTRODUCTION

Stereo-electroencephalography (sEEG) allowed epileptologists and neurophysiologists in the epilepsy field to record the intracranial electroencephalogram (iEEG) from regions of the human brain previously unreachable by subdural electrodes.[1] The most recent introduction of robotic technology in the operating room setting, along with the development of multimodal imaging platform for surgical planning, has further increased the accuracy of sEEG targeting.[2,3] Our experience from studying nonepileptic regions of the human brain has revealed that not all brain structures generate the same iEEG because their spectral constituents differ across regions and brain states.[4–6] Consequently, the interpretation of the iEEG signal derived by sEEG requires individualized approaches, depending on the anatomic structure being recorded.[7–9]

In this article, the main aspects for the interpretation of the hippocampal iEEG will be presented, namely normal background features and foreground elements, as well as characteristics of the abnormal background of the hippocampus because of established epileptogenicity. A special paragraph will be devoted to the notably increased amplitude of the hippocampal iEEG, which may render some foreground iEEG elements more aggressive than they actually are. The terms "sEEG" (implemented by depth electrodes) and "electrocotricography" ("ECoG"; implemented by subdural grid and strip electrodes) will be used

Comprehensive Epilepsy Center, Northwestern Memorial Hospital, 675 North Street Clair Street, Galter 7-109, Chicago, IL 60611, USA
E-mail address: vasileios.kokkinos@nm.org

Neurosurg Clin N Am 35 (2024) 73–82
https://doi.org/10.1016/j.nec.2023.08.004
1042-3680/24/© 2023 Elsevier Inc. All rights reserved.

hereby as subcategories of the broader term "iEEG" because they constitute distinct modalities of recording the intracranial electric fields of the brain.[10]

INTERPRETATION OF THE HIPPOCAMPAL INTRACRANIAL ELECTROENCEPHALOGRAM
Understanding the Intracranial Electroencephalogram Amplitude in the Hippocampus

In his classic '85 article, Pierre Gloor described the manner in which synchronized population pyramidal neuron-generated postsynaptic potentials give rise to electric fields of different orientations depending on their position across the gyral-sulcal continuum.[11] Modeling the neuronal sources that generate the ECoG signal, he described how the disk-shaped subdural electrode contacts placed on the cortical surface are primarily sensitive to electric fields of the gyral crown. This is due to the vertical orientation of the electric fields to the electrode contact surface. He also described that the subdural electrode disks are secondarily sensitive to electric fields generated in the sulcal walls and minimally sensitive to electric fields originating toward the bottom of the sulci. As such, the subdural ECoG signal is primarily representing activity of neocortical gyral surface, with mild representation of sulcal activity. Because the subdural iEEG approach has been the dominant in the twentieth century, the epilepsy surgery community is familiar with the above concept.[12] However, as sEEG has progressively spread worldwide only since the first 2 decades of the twenty-first century, it is imperative to understand the respective neuronal contributions to the iEEG signal in order to provide clinically meaningful interpretations.

The distinct geometry of sEEG electrodes and their contacts renders the acquired signal also distinct from the subdural electrode-derived ECoG signal in terms of neocortical representation. Understanding the geometry of iEEG recording by both subdural and sEEG electrodes is the first step in understanding the neuronal distribution represented by each recording modality. Because the subdural disk electrodes are primarily sensitive to vertical electric fields in a single-dimension fashion, the cylindrical shape of the sEEG electrode contacts render them sensitive to vertically oriented electric fields but in a 2-dimensional fashion (2D). In other words, although subdural contacts are optimally picking up the neuronal activity of the surface they are placed on, sEEG contacts are optimally sensitive to proximal electric fields generated at the same

horizontal plane all around each contact.[13] The volume of a subdural grid provides a multiplicity of 1-dimensional ECoG recording points, thereby generating a 2D overview of the brain's electrical activity. The multiple contacts of a single sEEG electrode provide a multiplicity of 2D recording planes, thereby allowing for a 3-dimensional (3D) overview of the electrical activity throughout the surrounding brain; a 3D representation enhanced by the presence of multiple sEEG electrodes.[14–18]

Because of the geometric differences, the iEEG signal recorded by a sEEG electrode going through a neocortical gyrus (**Fig. 1**A, B) represents a different portion of the gyral electric activity compared with the iEEG recorded by a subdural electrode on the same gyrus. A subdural electrode at the top of the gyrus is highly sensitive to synchronized neuronal activity representing cortical-subcortical interaction (mainly neocortical layers 5 and 6), which generate electric fields of vertical orientation with respect to the gyral surface.[11] However, the sEEG signal at the gyral crown is more sensitive to synchronized neuronal activity generated at the entry point plane that represents cortico-cortical interactions (primarily neocortical layers 2, 3, and 4) because they generate electric fields of vertical orientation to the cylindrical surface of the sEEG contacts[13] (see **Fig. 1**B). However, as the cortico-cortical interaction can create electric fields of opposite direction, the iEEG signal at the horizontal gyral plane is prone to cancellation among surrounding neuronal populations, thereby rendering the sEEG signal of lower amplitude than that of a subdural disk where most neuronal populations generating the ECoG signal have the same orientation. Further contribution to the sEEG signal comes from electric fields generated from the walls and the bottom of the surrounding sulci (see **Fig. 1**A). These electric fields can represent both cortico-subcortical and cortico-cortical interactions depending on the orientation of the wall and the bottom with respect to the sEEG electrode; the deepest their generator neuronal populations reside, the more unlikely they can be picked up by a surface subdural contact. However, the volume of white matter that often resides between the sEEG contacts and the neocortical generators is a confounding factor that affects the amplitude as well as the content of the recorded iEEG signal.[19] A sEEG electrode passing in parallel but distant to a sulcal wall will record an iEEG signal of lower amplitude and poorer in high-frequency content than one that passes close to the inner surface of the sulcus wall. For that reason, one of the main goals of sEEG implantation planning is to increase the number of contacts passing through or very close

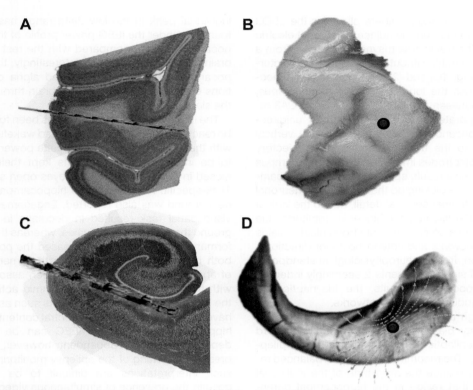

Fig. 1. Electric fields in neocortex and archicortex architectures. (*A*) An sEEG electrode passing through a hemispheric gyrus (coronal section) is recording moderate neocortical activity from the gyral crown entry point. The sEEG contacts are picking up vertically oriented electric fields from the proximal walls of the 2 adjacent sulci, although the signal is often high-passed filtered because of the white matter residing in between. The red isoelectric lines represent fields generated along the cron and the walls of a typical neocortical gyrus. (*B*) The main electric fields that constitute the sEEG signal at the entry point (lateral cortical view) are generated by cortico-cortical connections. However, although these electric fields are vertical to the cylindrical sEEG surface, they can be opposing in direction and partially cancel each other because of the multidirectional neocortical connections, thereby resulting in an overall moderate-amplitude neocortical sEEG signal. The green isoelectric lines represent fields generated across the neocortical surface because of cortico-cortical interactions. (*C*) An sEEG electrode passing through the hippocampal parenchyma (coronal section) is picking up more immediate neuronal activity due to its increased proximity to the trisynaptic circuit constituent regions (CA1–4 and dentate gyrus) and the reduced white matter (mossy fibers) volume around it. The red isoelectric lines represent fields generated along the transverse cross-section of the hippocampus. (*D*) In addition to the electric fields in the transverse axis, sEEG contacts implanted in the hippocampus also pick up high amplitude unidirectional electric fields forming across longitudinal networks of the CA1 and CA3 regions (lateral view of the hippocampal surface). The green isoelectric lines represent fields generated across the longitudinal axis of the hippocampus.

to gray matter structures on their way to their target. Overall, the combination of the above confounding factors, that is, the electric field cancellations at the gyral crown and the parenchymal white matter that surrounds the sEEG electrode, result in an iEEG signal of moderate although fair amplitude and often appearing as low-pass filtered.

It is clear that the geometric features of the brain parenchyma surrounding the sEEG electrodes play a significant role in the iEEG signal recorded, in terms of both quality and anatomic representation. It is thereby conceivable that the archicortical densely folded 3-layered environment of the

hippocampus will result in an iEEG signal of different qualitative and quantitative features compared with the 6-layered sparsely folded neocortical structures. Indeed, the iEEG from sEEG electrodes residing in hippocampal space presents with high amplitude and wide frequency range (toward both lower and higher frequencies), thereby overshadowing the rest of the nonhippocampal contacts of the implantation coverage when looking at the full reviewing montage. There are 2 reasons for the distinct hippocampal sEEG signal: (1) the dense folding of the hippocampal CA1-4 regions and the dentate around the hilus space and the mossy fibers allow for the sEEG contacts to pick-up the adjacent neuronal electric fields of the transverse trisynaptic circuit[20] from a closer proximity, without major white matter interference (**Fig. 1**C) and (2) the longitudinal connections across the long axis of the hippocampus, formed between neurons of the CA1 and CA3 regions separately,[21–25] generate strong unidirectional noncanceling electric fields of vertical direction to the traditional orthogonal trajectory of sEEG electrodes implanted in the hippocampus (**Fig. 1**D). As a result, sEEG contacts in hippocampal space are picking up the surrounding neuronal activity with finer spectral detail, due to the lack of white matter filtering, and higher in amplitude, due to receiving a combination of strong electric fields in the transverse and anterio-posterior directions. In addition, from a neurophysiological standpoint, the sEEG signal represents 2 seemingly independent hippocampal circuits, the trisynaptic and the longitudinal CA3/CA1 networks.

The high amplitude of the hippocampal sEEG signal may bias the iEEG interpretation toward interictal epileptic activity and archicortical epileptogenicity. The recommendation for a balanced review is to reduce the amplitude of the individual contacts that reside in the hippocampal parenchyma (because they are determined by the post-implantation CT fused with a preoperative MRI) so as their background iEEG level is comparable to that of the lateral temporal neocortical contacts of the same electrode (typically a 3 or 4 times reduction is sufficient). Moreover, note that before interpreting the hippocampal iEEG, the presence of the sEEG contacts in the hippocampal parenchyma has to be verified by an accurate 3D electrode reconstruction; a low amplitude iEEG, lacking the variety of high-frequency features, may suggest that the sEEG electrode intended to record from the hippocampus failed to reach its target.

The Normal Intracranial Electroencephalogram Background of the Hippocampus

There is only a handful of studies investigating the normal profile of the iEEG of the human hippocampus, despite the fact that sEEG has been used to target the mesio-temporal structures for more than 70 years. The consistent presence of beta oscillatory activity in the hippocampus has been confidently established,[26] as well as the occasional presence of gamma.[27] The presence of prominent, although irregular, delta and theta activities in the hippocampus has been reported by early iEEG recordings.[28] More recently, an individual peak in the low-delta range has been found to render the iEEG power profile of the hippocampus unique compared with the rest of the brain during wakefulness.[4,6] Interestingly, the hippocampus presents with reduced alpha oscillations compared with the rest of brain throughout the sleep–wake cycle.[6]

The iEEG of the hippocampus has been found to be reactive to simple tasks of relaxed wakefulness, with the background theta and delta power found to be increased when patients kept their eyes closed in comparison with the eyes open state.[29] Task-specific reactivity of the hippocampal iEEG background was also reported. Engagement in a visuospatial task resulted in decrease in background theta and delta activities, whereas the performance of a verbal task increased the power in both bands.[29,30] Tasks requiring the emergence of spatial navigation skills have been associated with the presence of ~3 Hz rhythmic activity in the human hippocampus.[31] Results such as these have demonstrated that the spectral content of the hippocampal background iEEG can be state-dependent and task-dependent; however, in the presurgical setting of the epilepsy monitoring unit such interpretations are difficult to be made, despite the presence of simultaneous video.

During sleep, the prominence of delta activity persists in the hippocampus throughout the non-rapid eye-movement (NREM) phase.[32] A detailed whole-brain study of iEEG spectral profiles across the sleep stages showed that the hippocampus presents with significant power peaks in the mid-delta range during NREM II and slow wave sleep (SWS).[5] The overall dominance and stability of hippocampal delta during NREM sleep is significant, considering that the iEEG in rest of the temporal lobe becomes progressively slower as the sleep deepens.[6] This phenomenon suggests that the level of sleep deepening has a higher limit in the archicortex than the surrounding neocortex. In other words, the hippocampus is maintaining a steady level of sleep, lighter than that of the neocortex during SWS. A similar counterintuitive phenomenon was observed during rapid eye-movement (REM) sleep, where the hippocampus also presents with increased delta power.[5,33,34] This finding was interpreted in the context of the hippocampus belonging to a group of brain regions (namely the primary visual, auditory, and motor regions) that do not share the cortical high-frequencies and mixed-frequencies iEEG profile brought on by the emergence of REM.[35] Another interesting observation is that theta activity during REM seems rather reduced compared with wakefulness—a feature not observed in the rest of the brain.[35] These findings reveal an iEEG sleep profile of the hippocampal archicortical formation that is distinct and independent from the concurrently manifested neocortical one. A typical sample of normal iEEG from a patient with a non-epileptogenic left hippocampus (**Fig. 2**) during NREM II is shown in **Fig. 3**.

It is also important to note that although focal delta activity has been typically associated with underlying focal brain lesions,[36,37] its presence in the hippocampal iEEG has been demonstrated to be a normal property and should not be interpreted as a marker of hippocampal epileptogenicity or other pathologic condition.

The Normal Intracranial Electroencephalogram Foreground Elements of the Hippocampus

The hippocampal spindles

The presence of spindles in the hippocampus has been reported since the first intracranial recordings in epilepsy patients.[28] Despite the fact that they were given their name due to their morphologic similarity with the sleep spindles recorded on scalp EEG—they are both waxing and waning sinusoidal oscillations—studies have shown that they occur independently.[38,39] In other words, there is no temporal correlation between the spindles generated in the archicortex of the hippocampus and the spindles appearing on scalp EEG during NREM sleep intervals; apparently, the latter are paced by thalamo-cortical interactions.[40] Therefore, it is recommended that we refer to the spindles of the hippocampal iEEG as "hippocampal spindles," so to avoid confusion with their scalp doppelgangers. Hippocampal spindles, being exclusively generated in hippocampal space, are spatially restricted in the brain compared with the scalp sleep spindles that seem more diffuse,[39]

and typically oscillate at 12 to 13 Hz.[5] The hippocampal spindles constitute a normal element of the hippocampal iEEG because they are met rather equally in epileptogenic and nonepileptogenic hippocampi, at percentages of ~90% and ~80%, respectively.[41] However, their frequency of occurrence in the iEEG background can be reduced inversely proportionally to the increase of interictal activity in epileptogenic hippocampi.[42] Hippocampal spindles are not specific to either the left or the right hippocampus, and they can manifest both independently and at times in synchrony between the 2 hippocampi.[41] An example of background iEEG with prominent hippocampal spindle activity is shown in **Fig. 4**.

The hippocampal barques

Hippocampal barques are the intracranial correlate of the well documented "14&6/sec positive spikes" normal variant that appears on scalp EEG.[43,44] They manifest as series of high-amplitude ~14 Hz spikes following a "'ramping-up/often ramping-down" profile that may be overlaid on lower amplitude ~6 Hz slow waves. Three barque subtypes have been identified: (1) The 14 Hz-only subtype that presents as a series of 14 Hz high-amplitude spikes; (2) The mixed 14 and 6 Hz subtype that presents as a series of 14 Hz high-amplitude spikes overlaid by 6 Hz slow waves or followed by 6 Hz spike-over-slow wave complexes; (3) The 6 Hz-only subtype that manifests as a series of 6 Hz high-amplitude spike-over-slow wave complexes (**Fig. 5**).[41,44] Although they manifest with negative polarity within the hippocampus parenchyma, they reverse their phase outside the hippocampal volume to positive, thereby generating the positive spikes profile of their scalp 14&6/sec manifestations.[45]

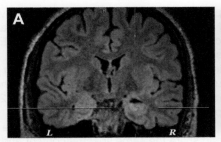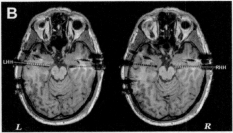

Fig. 2. A patient with temporal lobe epilepsy who underwent bilateral temporal sEEG to establish laterality of seizure origin. (*A*) Coronal FLAIR section showing hyperintensity in the right hippocampal region. (*B*) sEEG electrode reconstruction over a postoperative T1. The left (LHH) and right (RHH) sEEG electrodes implanted in an orthogonal fashion from the middle temporal gyrus targeting the respective hippocampi in the anterior/head region (LHH: left hippocampus head; RHH: right hippocampus head). This intracranial investigation confirmed the potential of the right hippocampus to generate the typical seizures of the patient, and showed no ictal involvement of the left hippocampus. The iEEG samples shown in the following **Figs. 3–6** are derived from this sEEG investigation.

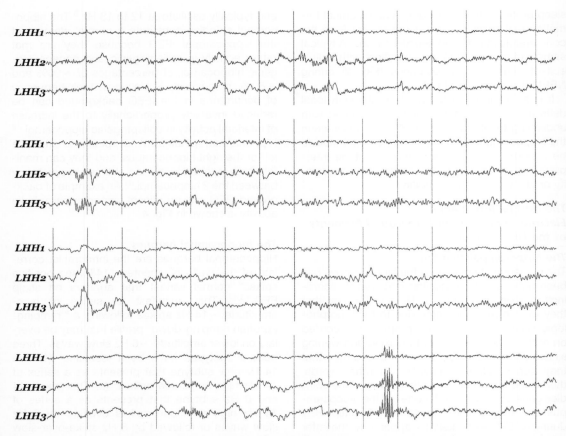

Fig. 3. Typical normal hippocampal iEEG sample from the nonepileptogenic anterior left hippocampus of our **Fig. 2** patient during NREM II stage of sleep (4 consecutive intervals of 15 s each, total 1 min). Contacts 1 to 3 were in the anterior hippocampus parenchyma. Note: (1) The intermittent and prominent background delta activity, manifesting with either moderate-amplitude prolonged delta wave sequences or high-amplitude brief delta waves. (2) The high frequencies, mostly in the beta range, constantly present in the hippocampal iEEG background, often overlaying intermittent delta waves. (3) The frequent occurrence of hippocampal spindles. (4) The occasional occurrence of hippocampal barques. Vertical lines represent 1-s intervals. The montage is referential to a midline scalp electrode.

Their high-amplitude spiky morphology has often been the reason that barques have been misinterpreted as paroxysmal (**Fig. 6**; barque activity in the nonepileptogenic left hippocampus can be interpreted as polyspike activity), and thereby as markers of hippocampal epileptogenicity, in the past.[46,47] However, the hippocampal barques, similar to hippocampal spindles, are normal variants of the hippocampal iEEG because they occur rather equally in epileptogenic and nonepileptogenic hippocampi, at percentages of ~20% and ~35%, respectively, with the higher incidence in the latter suggesting a tendency to increase their presence in the absence of epileptogenic substrates.[41] Barques manifest either exclusively or with higher amplitude in the posterior hippocampus.[45] Hippocampal barques occur

predominantly, although not exclusively, during NREM II and SWS stages of sleep, with rare to occasional occurrences in NREM I and REM sleep stages, as well as the wakefulness state. Interestingly, hippocampal barque density (count per minute) can be found increased during SWS compared with NREM II (Kokkinos et al., 2023, unpublished data).

As spindles and the 14 Hz-only barque subtype can share the same spectral content and assume similar morphologies, 3 criteria were developed to tell them apart: (1) Amplitude: Barques present on iEEG with moderate-amplitude to high-amplitude profiles while spindles present with low-amplitude to moderate-amplitude profiles; the amplitude criterion has only within-patient validity due to the high variability of hippocampal

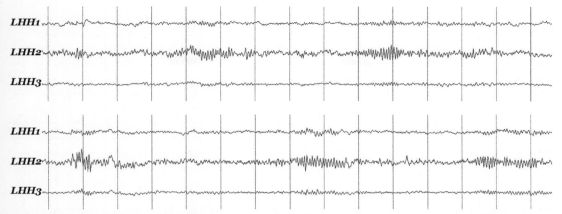

Fig. 4. Normal hippocampal iEEG sample of prominent spindle activity from the nonepileptogenic anterior left hippocampus of our **Fig. 2** patient during NREM II stage of sleep (2 consecutive intervals of 15 s each, total 30 s). Note that hippocampal spindles can be brief (<1 s) or prolonged (>1 s), often overlaid on slow delta/theta waves and occur every 4 to 6 s. Vertical lines and montage as in **Fig. 3**.

iEEG waveform amplitudes across subjects because of respective variability in sEEG contact locations and impedances. (2) Symmetry: Barques are highly asymmetric waveforms, with a high-amplitude negative phase and a moderate-amplitude to low-amplitude positive phase, whereas spindles are relatively symmetric as sinusoidal oscillations. (3) Paroxysmality: Barques manifest as spiky waveforms, whereas spindles are rather smooth/blunt sinusoids.

The Abnormal Background Intracranial Electroencephalogram of the Hippocampus

Understanding what constitutes an abnormal feature/pattern in the iEEG is inherently linked to the understanding of its normal constituents. Although there have been no focused studies investigating the abnormal features of the hippocampal background iEEG, some empirical observations are hereby outlined, based on our current knowledge of the hippocampus' normal background iEEG properties.

1. An iEEG background with abundant, near-continuous or continuous delta wave activity, that may or may not be rhythmic, is more likely to be abnormal. As described previously, delta activity is prominent in the hippocampus but is mostly intermittent, allowing for iEEG intervals of higher frequency profile (such as the interval with hippocampal spindle predominance of **Fig. 4**).

2. An iEEG background lacking high-frequency components, such as transient and/or irregular low-amplitude elements in the beta and low gamma range, and thereby presenting as a suppressed iEEG background, is more likely to be abnormal. The normal background, as one can tell from the samples of **Figs. 3** and **4**, is rich in low-amplitude mixed frequencies of variable duration and distribution.

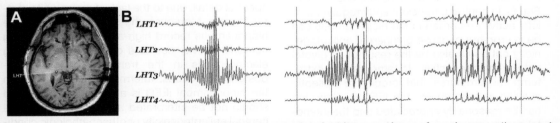

Fig. 5. Short samples of normal hippocampal iEEG demonstrating the 3 barque subtypes from the nonepileptogenic posterior left hippocampus of our patient in **Fig. 2**. (*A*). Barques are best recorded from the tail of the hippocampus (LHT: left hippocampus tail). (*B*) Left: The 14 Hz-only subtype that presents as a series of 14 Hz high-amplitude spikes; Middle: The mixed 14 and 6 Hz subtype that presents as a series of 14 Hz high-amplitude spikes overlaid by 6 Hz slow waves or followed by 6 Hz spike-over-slow wave complexes; Right: The 6 Hz only subtype that manifests as a series of 6 Hz high-amplitude spike-over-slow wave complexes. Vertical lines and montage as in **Fig. 3**.

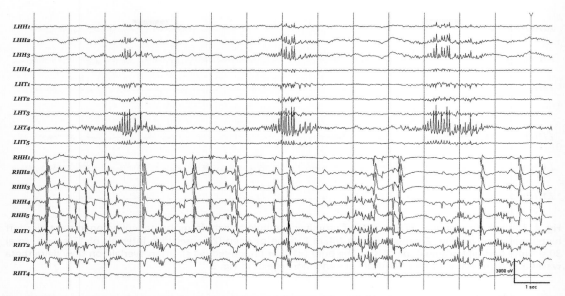

Fig. 6. Bilateral hippocampal iEEG from the patient of **Fig. 2**, with each hippocampus targeted in the anterior/head and the posterior/tail regions (LHH: left hippocampus head; LHT: left hippocampus tail; RHH: right hippocampus head; RHT: right hippocampus tail). The series of hippocampal barques, maximum in the left hippocampus tail (LHT1-5), can be easily misinterpreted as paroxysmal activity, namely polyspikes. The abundance of interictal spiking activity in the right anterior hippocampus (RHH1-5) is overwhelming the iEEG background and renders it hardly appreciable. The tail of the right hippocampus (RHH1-4) presents with mixed local barque/spindle activity and propagated interictal spikes from the ipsilateral anterior hippocampus. Note that the interictal activity of the sclerotic and epileptogenic right hippocampus does not infiltrate the iEEG of the nonepileptogenic left hippocampus.

3. An iEEG background lacking or presenting with notable reduction in distinctive foreground elements, such as hippocampal spindles and/or barques, is more likely to be abnormal. The occurrence of hippocampal spindles has been shown to be inversely affected by the volume of interictal activity during sleep,[42] and hippocampal barques appear less often in the epileptogenic hippocampal population.[41]

4. An iEEG background overwhelmed by interictal activity to the degree that the background itself is hardly discernible and appreciable, is most likely abnormal (see the right hippocampus of **Fig. 6**). In contrast, transient and irregular interictal activity recorded in the hippocampus can be interpreted because of inherent epileptogenicity but could also be the result of its pivotal networking connectivity to temporal and extratemporal structures that propagate epileptic activity; in both cases, the iEEG background can be reasonably appreciated and the interictal activity recorded does not constitute a definite marker of hippocampal epileptogenicity.

Note that 2 and 3 can be a result of the sEEG electrode missing the hippocampus and residing either in ventricular space or white matter space surrounding the hippocampus. It is imperative that electrode and contact locations are verified in the hippocampal parenchyma by accurate 3D electrode reconstruction for a confident and meaningful iEEG interpretation to be carried out.

SUMMARY

Understanding what constitutes an abnormal feature/pattern in the iEEG is inherently linked to the understanding of its normal constituents. The sEEG contacts in hippocampal space are picking up the surrounding neuronal activity with finer spectral detail, due to the lack of major white matter filtering. Moreover, the sEEG contacts in the hippocampus record high-amplitude surrounding neuronal activity due to a combination of strong electric fields in the transverse and anterioposterior directions. Intermittent delta activity in the hippocampal iEEG is a normal property and should not be interpreted as a marker of hippocampal epileptogenicity or other pathologic conditions. Hippocampal spindles and barques are normal constituents of the hippocampal iEEG foreground activity. However, a constellation of near-continuous delta, lack of higher frequencies in the background, reduced foreground spindles and barques, and interictal activity abundance, constitute hallmarks of an abnormal hippocampal iEEG.

DISCLOSURE

The author has no conflict of interest to disclose.

REFERENCES

1. Jobst BC, Bartolomei F, Diehl B, et al. Intracranial EEG in the 21st Century. Epilepsy Curr 2020;20(4): 180–8.
2. Bourdillon P, Châtillon CE, Moles A, et al. Effective accuracy of stereoelectroencephalography: robotic 3D versus Talairach orthogonal approaches. J Neurosurg 2018;1–9.
3. Bottan JS, Rubino PA, Lau JC, et al. Robot-Assisted Insular Depth Electrode Implantation Through Oblique Trajectories: 3-Dimensional Anatomical Nuances, Technique, Accuracy, and Safety. Oper Neurosurg (Hagerstown) 2019. https://doi.org/10.1093/ons/opz154. pii: opz154.
4. Frauscher B, von Ellenrieder N, Zelmann R, et al. Atlas of the normal intracranial electroencephalogram: neurophysiological awake activity in different cortical areas. Brain 2018;141(4):1130–44.
5. von Ellenrieder N, Gotman J, Zelmann R, et al. How the human brain sleeps: direct cortical recordings of normal brain activity. Ann Neurol 2020;87(2): 289–301.
6. Kalamangalam GP, Long S, Chelaru MI. A neurophysiological brain map: Spectral parameterization of the human intracranial electroencephalogram. Clin Neurophysiol 2020;131(3):665–75.
7. Bulacio JC, Chauvel P, McGonigal A. Stereoelectroencephalography: Interpretation. J Clin Neurophysiol 2016;33(6):503–10.
8. Bartolomei F, Nica A, Valenti-Hirsch MP, et al. Interpretation of SEEG recordings. Neurophysiol Clin 2018;48(1):53–7.
9. Kokkinos V. Interpretation of the Intracranial Stereoelectroencephalography Signal. Neurosurg Clin N Am 2020;31(3):421–33.
10. Mercier MR, Dubarry AS, Tadel F, et al. Advances in human intracranial electroencephalography research, guidelines and good practices. Neuroimage 2022;260:119438.
11. Gloor P. Neuronal generators and the problem of localization in electroencephalography: application of volume conductor theory to electroencephalography. J Clin Neurophysiol 1985;2:327–54.
12. Graf M, Niedermeyer E, Schiemann J, et al. Electrocorticography: information derived from intraoperative recordings during seizure surgery. Clin Electroencephalogr 1984;15:83–91.
13. Carvallo A, Modolo J, Benquet P, et al. Biophysical Modeling for Brain Tissue Conductivity Estimation Using SEEG Electrodes. IEEE Trans Biomed Eng 2019;66(6):1695–704.
14. Isnard J, Taussig D, Bartolomei F, et al. French guidelines on stereoelectroencephalography (SEEG). Neurophysiol Clin 2018;48(1):5–13.
15. Chassoux F, Navarro V, Catenoix H, et al. Planning and management of SEEG. Neurophysiol Clin 2018;48(1):25–37.
16. Talairach J, Bancaud J, Bonis A, et al. Functional stereotaxic exploration of epilepsy. Confin Neurol 1962;22:328–31.
17. Bancaud J, Angelergues R, Bernouilli C, et al. Functional stereotaxic exploration (SEEG) of epilepsy. Electroencephalogr Clin Neurophysiol 1970;28(1): 85–6.
18. Munari C, Bancaud J. The role of stereo-electroencephalography (SEEG) in the evaluation of partial epileptic patients. In: The epilepsies. London: Butterworths; 1987. p. 267–306.
19. Mercier MR, Bickel S, Megevand P, et al. Evaluation of cortical local field potential diffusion in stereotactic electro-encephalography recordings: A glimpse on white matter signal. Neuroimage 2017;147: 219–32.
20. Andersen P. The Hippocampus. Boston, MA: Springer US; 1975. p. 155–75.
21. Lorente de Nò R. Studies on the structure of the cerebral cortex II. Continuation of the study of the ammonic system. J Psychol Neurol 1934;46:113–7.
22. Miles R, Traub RD, Wong RK. Spread of synchronous firing in longitudinal slices from the CA3 region of the hippocampus. J Neurophysiol 1988;60(4): 1481–96.
23. Amaral DG, Witter MP. The three-dimensional organization of the hippocampal formation: a review of anatomical data. Neuroscience 1989;31(3): 571–91.
24. Li X-G, Somogyi P, Ylinen A, et al. The hippocampal CA3 network: an in vivo intracellular labeling study. J Comp Neurol 1994;339(2):181–208.
25. Amaral DG, Ishizuka N, Claiborne B. Neurons, numbers and the hippocampal network. Prog Brain Res 1990;83:1–11.
26. Hirai N, Uchida S, Maehara T, et al. Beta-1 (10–20 Hz) cortical oscillations observed in the human medial temporal lobe. Neuroreport 1999;10:3055–9.
27. Hirai N, Uchida S, Maehara T, et al. Enhanced gamma (30–150 Hz) frequency in the human medial temporal lobe. Neuroscience 1999;90:1149–55.
28. Brazier MA. Studies of the EEG activity of limbic structures in man. Electroencephalogr Clin Neurophysiol 1968;25:309–18.
29. Meador KJ, Thompson JL, Loring DW, et al. Behavioral state-specific changes in human hippocampal theta activity. Neurology 1991;41:869–72.

30. Huh K, Meador KJ, Lee GP, et al. Human hippocampal EEG: effects of behavioral activation. Neurology 1990;40:1177–81.

31. Watrous AJ, Lee DJ, Izadi A, et al. A comparative study of human and rat hippocampal low-frequency oscillations during spatial navigation. Hippocampus 2013;23(8):656–61.

32. Moroni F, Nobili L, De Carli F. Slow EEG rhythms and inter-hemispheric synchronization across sleep and wakefulness in the human hippocampus. Neuroimage 2012;60:497–504.

33. Bódizs R, Kántor S, Szabó G, et al. Rhythmic hippocampal slow oscillation characterizes REM sleep in humans. Hippocampus 2001;11:747–53.

34. Ferrara M, Moroni F, De Gennaro L, et al. Hippocampal sleep features: relations to human memory function. Front Neurol 2012;3:57.

35. Kalamangalam GP, Long S, Chelaru MI. Neurophysiological brain mapping of human sleep-wake states. Clin Neurophysiol 2021;132(7):1550–63.

36. Gloor P, Ball G, Schaul N. Brain lesions that produce delta waves in the EEG. Neurology 1977;27(4):326–33.

37. Huppertz HJ, Hof E, Klisch J, et al. Localization of interictal delta and epileptiform EEG activity associated with focal epileptogenic brain lesions. Neuroimage 2001;13(1):15–28.

38. Nakabayashi T, Uchida S, Maehara T, et al. Absence of sleep spindles in human medial and basal temporal lobes. Psychiatry Clin Neurosci 2001;55(1):57–65.

39. Frauscher B, von Ellenrieder N, Dubeau F, et al. Scalp spindles are associated with widespread intracranial activity with unexpectedly low synchrony. Neuroimage 2015;105:1–12.

40. Schreiner T, Kaufmann E, Noachtar S, et al. The human thalamus orchestrates neocortical oscillations during NREM sleep. Nat Commun 2022;13(1):5231.

41. Kokkinos V, Hussein H, Frauscher B, et al. Hippocampal spindles and barques are normal intracranial electroencephalographic entities. Clin Neurophysiol 2021;132(12):3002–9.

42. Frauscher B, Bernasconi N, Caldairou B, et al. Interictal hippocampal spiking influences the occurrence of hippocampal sleep spindles. Sleep 2015;38(12):1927–33.

43. Kokkinos V, Zaher N, Antony A, et al. The intracranial correlate of the 14&6/sec positive spikes normal scalp EEG variant. Clin Neurophysiol 2019;130(9):1570–80.

44. Kokkinos V, Richardson RM, Urban A. The Hippocampal Barque: An Epileptiform but Non-epileptic Hippocampal Entity. Front Hum Neurosci 2020;14:92.

45. Kokkinos V, Urban A, Frauscher B, et al. Barques are generated in posterior hippocampus and phase reverse over lateral posterior hippocampal surface. Clin Neurophysiol 2022;136:150–7.

46. Montplaisir J, Leduc L, Laverdiere M, et al. Sleep spindles in the human hippocampus: normal or epileptic activity. Sleep 1981;4:423–8.

47. Malow BA, Carney PR, Kushwaha R, et al. Hippocampal sleep spindles revisited: physiologic or epileptic activity. Clin Neurophysiol 1999;110(4):687–93.

Evolution of SEEG Strategy
Stanford Experience

Vivek P. Buch, MD[a],*, Josef Parvizi, MD, PhD[b]

KEYWORDS

- StereoEEG • SEEG • Stereotactic electroencephalography • Intracranial epilepsy monitoring
- Epilepsy networks

KEY POINTS

- Overall stereoelectroencephalography (SEEG) has a better risk profile and patient tolerability compared with subdural electrodes.
- Innovations in percutaneous and robotic platforms has greatly enhanced the efficiency, precision, and safety of SEEG placement.
- SEEG has enabled novel understanding of epilepsy as a three-dimensional network disease.
- Novel thalamic propagation mapping during SEEG developed by our group may provide unique insights into future personalized treatments for refractory epilepsy.

TECHNOLOGICAL AND METHODOLOGICAL CHANGES IN INVASIVE MONITORING

At its onset, stereoelectroencephalography (SEEG)-style depth electrode implantation began for the specific purpose of targeting the mesial temporal lobe in combination with subdural electrodes for concomitant broad frontoparietotemporal cortical coverage.[1] In these initial periods, only frame-based stereotactic platforms were available. Combining a surgical procedure using a frame for depth electrode implantation along with a craniotomy for subdural electrode coverage was logistically challenging. With the advent of neuronavigation, stereotactic techniques with a more favorable intraoperative workflow emerged.

These platforms, such as Medtronic Stealth Vertek device (Medtronic Inc, Minneapolis, MN) suffered from potentially lower accuracy compared with the frame.[2] However, the primary goal for intracranial monitoring at the time was gross regional anatomic localization. Therefore, stereotactic platforms with lower accuracy (approximately 2–4 mm), but with an easier intraoperative workflow when used in combination with open craniotomy, were preferred and considered acceptable.[3]

Over time, however, it became clear that the depth electrodes enabled interesting evaluation of not just regional but perhaps network-level involvement of seizure onset and propagation patterns. Therefore, as centers began experimenting with multidepth electrode SEEG, our understanding of epilepsy diagnosis and treatment evolved into much more of a network-centric as opposed to region-centric approach, which further reinforced the utility of SEEG.[4] Because the adoption increased, clear evidence mounted for an overall favorable morbidity profile of SEEG compared with craniotomy.[5]

Simultaneously, advancements in robotic implantation platforms such as ROSA (Zimmerbiomet, Warsaw, IN) enabled a final push toward creating highly precise and efficient operative workflows for SEEG.[6] Thus, as the desire to understand the three dimensionality of epileptic networks became more relevant, along with the technological advancements for safe, precise, and efficient intraoperative placement, the adoption of SEEG increased to the point of becoming the dominant approach in invasive monitoring.

Early adoption of robot-assisted SEEG at our institution started immediately after the US Food

a Stanford University, 453 Quarry Road Room 245C, Palo Alto, CA 94304, USA; b Stanford University, 213 Quarry Road MC 5957 Fl 2, Palo Alto, CA 94304, USA
* Corresponding author.
E-mail address: vpbuch@stanford.edu

Neurosurg Clin N Am 35 (2024) 83–85
https://doi.org/10.1016/j.nec.2023.08.003
1042-3680/24/© 2023 Elsevier Inc. All rights reserved.

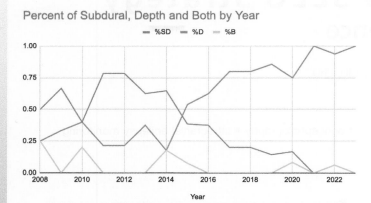

Percent of Subdural, Depth and Both by Year

— %SD   — %D   — %B

Fig. 1. Evolution of invasive epilepsy monitoring strategy over time at Stanford. SD, Subdural; D, Depth, B, Both.

and Drug Administration approval in 2015. Before this, only 30% to 50% of cases were either using SEEG style depths or combination subdural electrodes with depths. However, after we purchased our robotic platform, SEEG quickly became the dominant modality at our institution, approaching 90% to 100% of cases by 2021 (**Fig. 1**). Robot-assisted SEEG enabled a safe and precise method for us to understand the critical importance of nontemporal subcortical and deep mesial regions in limbic/temporal-lobe-mimic epilepsies. Regions such as insula, anterior cingulate gyrus, and posterior medial cortex (encompassing the retrosplenial, posterior cingulate, and precuneal subregions) were inadequately sampled with historical approaches. Epilepsies that may have been previously diagnosed as temporal lobe or frontal lobe seizures based on invasive subdural monitoring were perhaps actually originating from these subcortical or deep regions, leading to suboptimal therapeutic response to treatment such as temporal lobectomy.

Now, at our institution, the primary utility of subdural electrodes is for intraoperative mapping epileptic and/or functional activity around cortical or superficial lesions before resection. We have also used subdural grids for phase II monitoring in some of these cases where there was a desire for seizure or functional mapping before resection. However, even in these cases, we have still found that the most common seizure onset zone comes not from the superficial cortex but the fundus of sulci surrounding the lesion, and thus we always combine subdural grids with surrounding SEEG depths to map both the superficial cortical and deep sulcal regions around the region of interest. These types of insights have altered our therapeutic approach in many cases for SEEG-guided resection, ablation, or responsive neurostimulation (RNS).

EVOLUTION IN INVASIVE MONITORING STRATEGY

These advancements in phase II monitoring capabilities have enabled a significant amount of insight to be derived from deep regions of the brain. The shift from region-centric to network-centric evaluation has also led to a shift in therapeutic options such as thalamic deep brain stimulation (DBS)[7,8] and RNS.[9,10] However, despite the overall good efficacy of thalamic stimulation, there remains variability in these outcomes.

Because we know that the thalamus is a central node in seizure propagation pathways, and we know that modulation of certain thalamic nuclei can significantly improve seizure burden, we believed that further evaluation of multinuclear thalamic involvement during SEEG monitoring could result in significant new and beneficial insights. Therefore, we pioneered a safe approach to extend electrodes sampling desired cortical and subcortical targets into multiple sites in the thalamus spanning anterior, middle, and posterior nuclear groups.[11] Having access to data about the modes and extent of thalamic involvement during seizure propagation, at the individual patient level, could be used to improve SOZ localization or prognosticate the potential success of resective or ablative procedures. Further, as noted extant literature suggests that a significant proportion of epilepsy patients is not benefitted from anterior nucleus of thalamus (ANT) stimulation, and one reason for failure of neuromodulation in these patients may be due to impersonal thalamic targeting, that is, targeting a nucleus of the thalamus that is not the primary propagation node—as we have recently shown.[11] Therefore, multisite thalamic sampling could help determine optimal, personalized thalamic modulation target if a resectable or ablatable focus is not identified during the phase II.

Despite its extremely informative potential, a detailed discussion of risks is required before undertaking SEEG. The primary risk is hemorrhage, with approximately 0.5% to 1.5% per lead rate across both implantation and explantation.[12] These are almost always asymptomatic and self-resolve. Careful planning of avascular trajectories helps mitigate risk of bleeding although it does not prevent it. Further, use of best-practice stereotactic technique, with fine back-and-forth movements, frequent pauses, and slow/deliberate motion when passing instrumentation intracranially, is critical to ensuring safety. In addition, because each lead has an independent risk of hemorrhage, it is also critical to have a strong hypothesis-driven plan. Surgically, we advocate for trying to combine superficial and deep targets into the same electrode when possible. This includes using a fewer number of diagonal trajectories instead of multiple direct perpendicular approaches, as well as maximizing desired coverage with combination of vertical and horizontal trajectories when helpful for such regions as insula, cingulate, and orbitofrontal gyri.

SUMMARY

Thus, overall, SEEG has favorable risk profile, patient tolerability, and superior investigative capability of individualized three-dimensional seizure onset activity over subdural electrodes. Further, our recent surgical approach to safely enable multinuclear thalamic propagation mapping can only be performed with SEEG. For these reasons, SEEG has become the gold standard of phase II monitoring at our institution, and we believe the ability to develop precision network-centric approaches to therapy will be critical to enhance our ability to care for medically refractory, and importantly, even complex multifocal, generalized, or surgically refractory epilepsy patients.

DISCLOSURE

The authors have nothing to disclose.

REFERENCES

1. Crandall PH, Walter RD, Rand RW. Clinical applications of studies on stereotactically implanted electrodes in temporal-lobe epilepsy. J Neurosurg 1963;20:827–40.

2. Rodionov R, O'Keeffe A, Nowell M, et al. Increasing the accuracy of 3D EEG implantations. J Neurosurg 2019;133:35–42.

3. Narváez-Martínez Y, García S, Roldán P, et al. [Stereoelectroencephalography by using O-Arm® and Vertek® passive articulated arm: Technical note and experience of an epilepsy referral centre]. Neurocirugia (Astur) 2016;27:277–84.

4. Kramer MA, Cash SS. Epilepsy as a disorder of cortical network organization. Neuroscientist 2012; 18:360–72.

5. Tandon N, Tong BA, Friedman ER, et al. Analysis of Morbidity and Outcomes Associated With Use of Subdural Grids vs Stereoelectroencephalography in Patients With Intractable Epilepsy. JAMA Neurol 2019;76:672–81.

6. González-Martínez J, Bulacio J, Thompson S, et al. Technique, Results, and Complications Related to Robot-Assisted Stereoelectroencephalography. Neurosurgery 2016;78:169–79.

7. Fisher R, Salanova V, Witt T, et al. Electrical stimulation of the anterior nucleus of thalamus for treatment of refractory epilepsy. Epilepsia 2010;51:899–908.

8. Dalic LJ, Warren AEL, Bulluss KJ, et al. DBS of Thalamic Centromedian Nucleus for Lennox-Gastaut Syndrome (ESTEL Trial). Ann Neurol 2022; 91:253–67.

9. Nair DR, Laxer KD, Weber PB, et al. Nine-year prospective efficacy and safety of brain-responsive neurostimulation for focal epilepsy. Neurology 2020;95:E1244–56.

10. Razavi B, Rao VR, Lin C, et al. Real-world experience with direct brain-responsive neurostimulation for focal onset seizures. Epilepsia 2020;61:1749–57.

11. TQ W, et al. Multisite thalamic recordings to characterize seizure propagation in the human brain. Brain 2023;139:16–7.

12. Triano MJ, Schupper AJ, Ghatan S, et al. Hemorrhage Rates After Implantation and Explantation of Stereotactic Electroencephalography: Reevaluating Patients' Risk. World Neurosurg 2021;151:e100–8.

Evolution of Stereo-Electroencephalography at Massachusetts General Hospital

Pranav Nanda, MD, MPhil[a,b,]*, R. Mark Richardson, MD, PhD[a,b]

KEYWORDS

- Epilepsy surgery • Seizure networks • Stereo-electroencephalography • Local field potentials
- Epilepsy

KEY POINTS

- Stereo-electroencephalography (sEEG) is an effective means to parse patients' seizure networks.
- Thalamic sEEG informs treatment strategies in select cases.
- A hypothesis-driven approach is critical in planning sEEG implantations.

INTRODUCTION AND HISTORY

An estimated 70 million people are affected by epilepsy worldwide,[1] and of these patients, more than 30% are thought to have intractable and drug-resistant disease according to the criteria of the International League Against Epilepsy.[2,3] Patients with refractory epilepsy endure significant levels of morbidity and mortality, and their recurrent seizures bear a high burden on patients, their families, and their health care systems.[4–7] Given that data demonstrate the limited benefit of adding additional adjunctive antiepileptic drugs to patients' medication regimens,[8,9] epilepsy surgery is central to the management of these patients, and it provides them with a possible therapeutic avenue toward relieving the steep toll that drug-resistant epilepsy takes on quality of life.

However, the efficacy of epilepsy surgery is contingent upon understanding the nature and pattern of a patient's specific form of epilepsy, both to determine if they are a candidate for surgery and to select and tailor the most appropriate and targeted intervention.[10] A variety of noninvasive techniques—including MRI, PET, scalp electroencephalography (EEG), ictal single-photon emission computed tomography, functional MRI, magnetoelectroencephalography, neuropsychological batteries, and careful review of patient seizure semiology—are regular components of presurgical evaluation, and they may provide sufficient information to confidently ascertain surgical candidacy and guide surgical treatment.[11] However, in other cases where noninvasive modalities are inconclusive or discordant, invasive monitoring may be necessary to more conclusively and precisely define a patient's epilepsy in order to determine the next steps.[11,12]

Long-term monitoring using intracranial EEG for the guidance of epilepsy surgery was first performed using epidural electrodes in 1939 at the Montreal Neurologic Institute as a product of the collaboration between Penfield and Jasper.[13,14] In the late 1940s, Hayne and Meyers used stereotactically implanted depth electrodes for epilepsy, targeting the thalamus to describe the relationship between cortical and subcortical seizure activity, although their methodology lacked sufficient patient-specific accuracy for broader uptake and application.[15,16] As Talairach revolutionized the

a Department of Neurosurgery, Massachusetts General Hospital, Boston, MA 02114, USA; b Department of Neurosurgery, Harvard Medical School, Boston, MA 02115, USA
* Corresponding author.
E-mail address: pnanda@mgh.harvard.edu

Neurosurg Clin N Am 35 (2024) 87–94
https://doi.org/10.1016/j.nec.2023.09.007
1042-3680/24/© 2023 Elsevier Inc. All rights reserved.

techniques of stereotaxy at St Anne Hospital in Paris in the 1950s, Bancaud and he pioneered the use of stereotactic implantations of depth electrodes to precisely map out the spatiotemporal characteristics of patients' seizures, a process formalized in 1962 as stereo-EEG (sEEG).[17,18] Although subdural grid and strip electrodes were developed in the same time frame, they became increasingly popular only in the 1980s, in part because of their ability to cover large swaths of cortex with high local resolution and in part because of lower technical requirements, expertise, and cost than sEEG.[14] Other simplified approaches were also developed, including foramen ovale electrodes, which were developed by Wieser and Yaşargil and implemented as a method to confirm and lateralize mesial temporal lobe epilepsy.[14,19] Although sEEG remained the preferred method of invasive monitoring for epilepsy surgery evaluation in France, Canada, and Italy, grid and strip electrode implantations predominated investigations in the United States until the 2000s, possibly both due to incomplete penetrance of sEEG literature in the American epilepsy community and due to burdensome technical requirements for sEEG.[20] However, with the advent of frameless and robotic methods which expedite safe implantation[21] and with increased international discourse around sEEG,[22] its use has risen dramatically in the United States as well.[14,20,23]

IMPLICATIONS OF A SEIZURE NETWORK APPROACH

At Massachusetts General Hospital (MGH), invasive monitoring has involved recording intracranial EEG using all of these various modalities, occasionally in combination. The strategies for intracranial EEG implantations at MGH have evolved in parallel to the evolution of the surgical epilepsy field's approach to seizures as network phenomena.

Increasingly, epilepsy is understood as a network disorder in which the normal connectivity of the brain is altered and specific aberrant networks undergird the onset and propagation of seizures.[24–27] Spencer described epilepsy in 2002 as a disorder of specific sets of large-scale cortical and subcortical neuronal networks, identifying 3 such networks using clinical observation, intracranial EEG, PET, anatomy, and treatment response.[24] Subsequent research analyzing structural imaging, functional imaging, and electrophysiologic studies has similarly supported the epilepsy network framework, with various studies demonstrating abnormalities in structural and connectivity measures distant to the presumed epileptogenic zone.[28–36] Treatment response to traditional resective procedures has also been observed to vary depending on distributed graph theoretic metrics,[37–40] indicating the clinical relevance of epilepsy's network characteristics. Furthermore, new and effective neuromodulatory procedures such as thalamic deep brain stimulation (DBS) and responsive neurostimulation (RNS) rely on the network properties of epilepsy in order to have benefit.

This perspective on epilepsy as a network disorder informs surgical evaluation because it expands the purview of epilepsy surgery beyond seizure focus resection, and it reframes epilepsy surgery as, at its core, disrupting pathologic seizure networks by the most effective and safest means available.[41] While removing epileptogenic zones remains a major component of this concept, the door is also open to other modes of network modulation. For instance, the power of this reframing of epilepsy surgery has been amplified by the introduction of new technologies—including laser interstitial thermal therapy (LITT), RNS, and DBS—which provide effective tools for seizure network disruption that can be used independently or in conjunction.[25] As a consequence, adopting a seizure network approach shifts the goal of surgical epilepsy evaluation away from hunting for a seizure onset zone to defining the spatiotemporal characteristics of a patient's seizure network in order to identify critical nodes amenable to treatment.

IMPLEMENTING THE SEIZURE NETWORK APPROACH AT MASSACHUSETTS GENERAL HOSPITAL

In the practice of invasive monitoring for surgical epilepsy evaluation at MGH, there was an inflection point at the start of 2020, as the strategy toward intracranial EEG implantations shifted from an emphasis on singularly finding epileptogenic zones for the purpose of resection to an increasingly hypothesis-driven epileptic network approach.[42] Of note, this inflection point occurred when novel neuromodulatory techniques were becoming available for epilepsy, as DBS of the anterior nucleus of the thalamus was approved by the Food and Drug Administration in 2018[43] and the first successful reports of RNS of the centromedian nucleus began emerging in 2020.[44–46] Review of all 159 invasive monitoring cases at MGH from April 2016 through June 2023 reveals how this paradigm shift toward seizure networks concretely took form. This evolution is clarified by comparing cases in the focus era (66 cases) and network era (93 cases) occurring before and after January 2020, respectively.

Of the 66 cases performed in the focus era, 27 involved sEEG depth electrodes (41%), 25 foramen ovale electrodes (38%), 9 grid and strip electrodes (14%), and 5 combination implantations (8%). Conversely, of the 93 cases performed in the subsequent network era, 89 involved sEEG depth electrodes (96%), 2 foramen ovale electrodes (2%), 1 grid and strip electrodes, and 1 combined implantation (1%), representing a dramatic and significant increase in the proportion of invasive investigations using sEEG (**Fig. 1**A–B). This change in practice reflects the way in which sEEG implantations facilitate network investigation. Because sEEG enables the acquisition of electrophysiological activity from disparate parts of the brain, including deep cortical and subcortical structures, and because it produces data with high temporal resolution, it is optimized for revealing the complex spatiotemporal dynamics of seizures.[47] In comparison specifically to grid and strip electrodes, sEEG investigations offer increased spatial flexibility—in terms of both depth and diversity of electrodes—and they offer a favorable safety profile.[48,49]

Of note, while sEEG bears advantages of versatility, it inherently comes with the limitation of sparse spatial coverage. Although implantation is relatively safe, the additive risk of implanting additional electrodes is nontrivial, with some studies estimating intracerebral hemorrhage rate as approximately 1.5% per electrode,[50] and so it is critical to be thoughtful about restricting the number of electrodes to those which are needed (typically limited to a maximum of 18 per implantation at MGH), necessitating a hypothesis-driven approach. As invasive monitoring strategies have more explicitly involved primary and alternative hypotheses in the network era at MGH, the number of implanted electrodes and contacts have significantly decreased (**Fig. 2**A–D). The mean number of electrodes and the mean number of contacts in the focus era were 14.3 and 195.3, respectively

(standard deviations 3.0 and 43.7), and in the network era, they were 13.1 and 159.9 (standard deviations 3.5 and 45.3). The length of implantations has also significantly decreased from a mean of 13.2 days in the focus era (standard deviation 5.7) to a mean of 9.7 days in the network era (4.2 standard deviation) (**Fig. 3**A–B). Direct testing of hypotheses may have contributed to this decrease in length of implantation, which may also be related to the introduction of a bedside lead removal system, in place of waiting for the availability of operating room and anesthesia resources for lead removal. The emphasis on hypothesis testing also led to an increase in asymmetric implantations (see **Fig. 3**C–D). In the focus era, there were 17 symmetric implantations with equal number of leads in each hemisphere (53%), 11 partially asymmetric implantations (34%), and 4 unilateral implantations (13%). Conversely, in the network era, there were 24 symmetric implantations (27%), 29 partially asymmetric implantations (32%), and 37 unilateral implantations (41%).

During the network era, the average age of patients undergoing sEEG at MGH has significantly decreased. The mean age at sEEG during the focus era was 35.4 years (standard deviation 12.9 years) while the mean age at sEEG during the network era has been 29.2 years (standard deviation 15.0 years) (**Fig. 4**A–B). Whereas 1 pediatric patient (age<18 years) underwent sEEG in the focus era, sEEG has been performed on 22 pediatric patients in the network era (youngest: 3.4 years). The increase in pediatric sEEG implantations may be partially attributable to an increasing comfort with implanting young patients both locally and globally.[51,52] It is also likely related to the inclusion of certain pediatric patients, such as patients with multifocal periventricular nodular heterotopia and complex porencephalic cysts, as targeted surgical candidates within the seizure network paradigm.

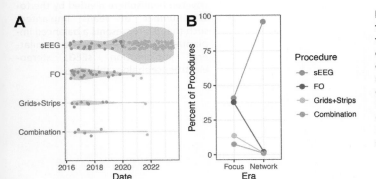

Fig. 1. Intracranial investigations over time at Massachusetts General Hospital. (*A*) Each point represents an intracranial investigation for presurgical epilepsy workup (focus era—red; network era—blue), and the shaded region represents a violin plot. (*B*) Percent of intracranial investigations comprised by the indicated procedure. FO, foramen ovale electrodes; sEEG, stereo-electroencephalography.

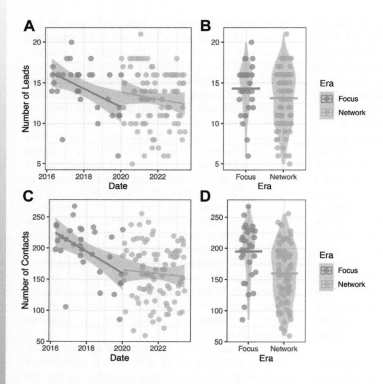

Fig. 2. Number of leads and contacts per investigation. (*A,C*) Each point represents an sEEG implantation, lines are linear trend lines within era, and the shaded region is 95% confidence interval. (*B,D*) Each point represents an sEEG implantation, the shaded region represents a violin plot, and the line represents the mean within era. sEEG, stereo-electroencephalography.

The network era at MGH has been characterized by an increasing number of thalamic implantations, with 30 implantations including leads targeting the thalamus (33%) (see **Fig. 4**C–D). As has been previously described, the presence of early thalamic involvement in a patient's ictal propagation pattern informs surgical decision-making at MGH in a pre-defined set of patients, particularly in assessing the value of RNS or DBS systems targeting specific thalamic nuclei.[25] Moreover, the risk of thalamic

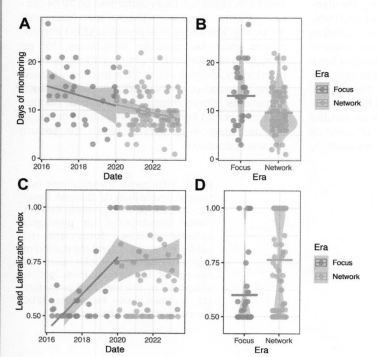

Fig. 3. Length and symmetry of implantation. (*A,C*) Each point represents an sEEG implantation, lines are linear trend lines within era, and the shaded region is 95% confidence interval. (*B,D*) Each point represents an sEEG implantation, the shaded region represents a violin plot, and the line represents the mean within era. The lead lateralization index for an implantation refers to the number of implanted leads on the more densely covered hemisphere divided by the total number of leads implanted, such that 0.5 represents a balanced implantation and 1.0 represents a unilateral implantation. sEEG, stereo-electroencephalography.

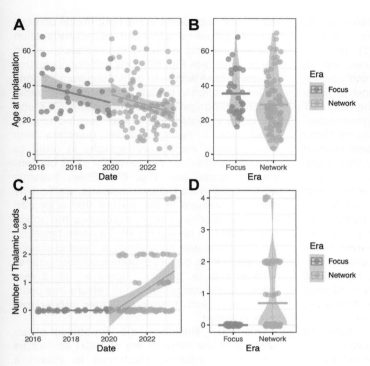

Fig. 4. Age at implantation and thalamic implantations. (*A,C*) Each point represents an sEEG implantation, lines are linear trend lines within era, and the shaded region is 95% confidence interval. (*B,D*) Each point represents an sEEG implantation, the shaded region represents a violin plot, and the line represents the mean within era. sEEG, stereo-electroencephalography.

depth electrodes is similar to the risk incurred for a cortical sEEG electrode, and this risk is minimized by targeting the thalamus by extending an electrode that was intended to be implanted regardless, as has been previously described.[25,53] In select situations, implantations at MGH include multiple thalamic nuclei which are hypothesized to be involved in the seizure network and which could be targeted for neuromodulation.

The profile of treatments offered after sEEG has changed during the network era. Most notably, significantly fewer are not offered any surgical option after sEEG, as 7 patients were not offered surgical intervention in the focus era (22%), whereas 3 were not offered surgical intervention in the network era (3%) (**Fig. 5**A–B). Because the goal

of epilepsy surgery under the seizure network approach is disruption of a patient's seizure network rather than specifically excising the seizure onset zone, patients have more options for treatment, especially with the development of new neuromodulatory technologies. Indeed, while the proportion of patients not offered treatment declined in the network era, an increasing number of patients were offered RNS, combined RNS/resection, or ablation by LITT.

ILLUSTRATIVE CASE

In 2020, a 9-year-old boy presented for surgical epilepsy evaluation, having had refractory seizures since 19 months of age. He had 3 primary

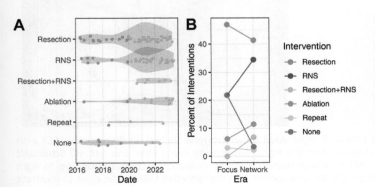

Fig. 5. Surgical interventions offered after sEEG. (*A*) Each point represents a surgical intervention offered after sEEG (focus era—red; network era—blue), and the shaded region represents a violin plot. (*B*) Percent of offered interventions comprised by the indicated procedure. RNS, responsive neurostimulation; sEEG, stereo-electroencephalography.

types of seizures: (1) a left gaze preference with left hand and arm clonic activity frequently progressing to status epilepticus, (2) frequent staring episodes lasting 1 to 2 minutes, and (3) unresponsiveness with tachycardia and desaturation. MRI was notable for extensive right-sided polymicrogyria (**Fig. 6**A) whereas PET demonstrated extensive regions of hypermetabolism and hypometabolism, worse on the right than the left (see **Fig. 6**B). Video EEG demonstrated abundant high-amplitude right frontotemporal epileptiform discharges, generalized periodic discharges maximal at the vertex, 2 electroclinical seizures with generalized EEG onset but left focal motor semiology, and an episode of tachycardia and desaturation with left frontal lateralized periodic discharges late in the event. Given these data, it was hypothesized that the patient's epilepsy may have been related to the right-sided polymicrogyria or it might represent a bilateral process possibly with thalamic involvement. As such, he underwent sEEG implantation.

The patient's sEEG implantation included 12 right-sided electrodes and 4 left-sided electrodes, with electrodes targeting the centromedian nucleus of the thalamus bilaterally (see **Fig. 6**C). After 6 days, sufficient information was collected to make a surgical recommendation, and so the depth electrodes were explanted. Particularly, 3 electroclinical seizures were associated with onset in the right frontal operculum with diffuse temporal and insular propagation and with thalamic involvement a few seconds into the seizures (see **Fig. 6**D). One additional electroclinical seizure was seen originating from a poorly defined location in the left hemisphere with rapid thalamic propagation. After discussion in a multidisciplinary conference, it was decided to proceed with a right opercular resection with intraoperative electrocorticography in order to attempt to alleviate the patient's most burdensome seizures (see **Fig. 6**E). Given thalamic involvement in the patient's seizures, particularly early involvement in the seizure that appeared left-sided in origin, the group retained the option of implanting a bithalamic RNS system targeting the centromedian nucleus as a second-staged procedure if the patient experienced poor postresective seizure control. However, at 2-year follow-up, the patient remained seizure-free postoperatively, and therefore further procedures were obviated.

This case illustrates the hypothesis-driven strategy of the network era at MGH as well as the use of thalamic electrodes to inform a measured and flexible approach to neuromodulatory options. Moreover, it demonstrates that disrupting targeted nodes in a patient's broader delineated seizure network can yield an excellent clinical outcome.

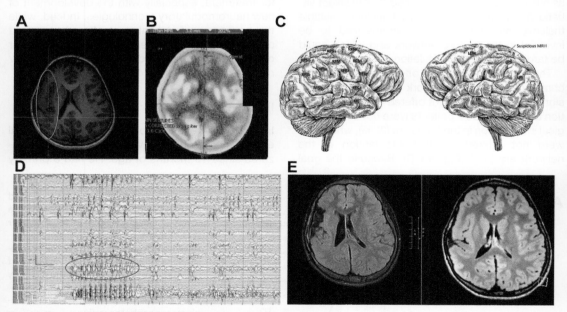

Fig. 6. Illustrative case. (*A*) Preoperative MRI with right-sided polymicrogyria circled. (*B*) Preoperative PET with diffuse hypermetabolism and hypometabolism, with the right abnormality worse than the left. (*C*) Schematic of sEEG implantation plan. (*D*) Sample sEEG data with seizure onset in circled contacts corresponding to right frontal operculum. (*E*) Postoperative MRI on the left and comparison preoperative MRI on the right to illustrate the extent of resection. sEEG, stereo-electroencephalography.

CLINICS CARE POINTS

- sEEG implantations can be designed to test hypotheses about patient's seizure networks that guide surgical decision making.
- Thalamic sEEG recordings can be used to inform neuromodulatory strategies for epilepsy management.
- The application of a seizure network paradigm expands the set of epilepsy patients who are candidates for surgical work-up and intervention.

SUMMARY

The MGH surgical epilepsy group's shift toward a seizure network paradigm has necessitated an evolution in the approach to invasive monitoring for presurgical workup. Implantations have been increasingly hypothesis driven, they are more dominated by sEEG depth electrodes, they serve a broader and younger population, and they more frequently target thalamic nuclei. In these ways, sEEG implantations are optimized for the delineation of patients' seizure networks and the critical nodes to be targeted in treatment.

DISCLOSURE

None of the authors have any conflicts of interest to disclose.

REFERENCES

1. Thijs RD, Surges R, O'Brien TJ, et al. Epilepsy in adults. Lancet 2019;393(10172):689–701.
2. Kalilani L, Sun X, Pelgrims B, et al. The epidemiology of drug-resistant epilepsy: A systematic review and meta-analysis. Epilepsia 2018;59(12):2179–93.
3. Sultana B, Panzini MA, Veilleux Carpentier A, et al. Incidence and Prevalence of Drug-Resistant Epilepsy. Neurology 2021;96(17):805–17.
4. Strzelczyk A, Griebel C, Lux W, et al. The Burden of Severely Drug-Refractory Epilepsy: A Comparative Longitudinal Evaluation of Mortality, Morbidity, Resource Use, and Cost Using German Health Insurance Data. Front Neurol 2017;8. https://doi.org/10.3389/fneur.2017.00712.
5. Thomas SV, Sarma PS, Alexander M, et al. Economic Burden of Epilepsy in India. Epilepsia 2001;42(8):1052–60.
6. Hong Z, Qu B, Wu XT, et al. Economic burden of epilepsy in a developing country: A retrospective cost analysis in China. Epilepsia 2009;50(10):2192–8.
7. Willems LM, Richter S, Watermann N, et al. Trends in resource utilization and prescription of anticonvulsants for patients with active epilepsy in Germany from 2003 to 2013 — A ten-year overview. Epilepsy Behav 2018; 83:28–35.
8. Luciano AL, Shorvon SD. Results of treatment changes in patients with apparently drug-resistant chronic epilepsy. Ann Neurol 2007;62(4):375–81.
9. Callaghan BC, Anand K, Hesdorffer D, et al. Likelihood of seizure remission in an adult population with refractory epilepsy. Ann Neurol 2007;62(4):382–9.
10. Ryvlin P, Cross JH, Rheims S. Epilepsy surgery in children and adults. Lancet Neurol 2014;13(11):1114–26.
11. Zumsteg D, Wieser HG. Presurgical Evaluation: Current Role of Invasive EEG. Epilepsia 2000;41(s3):S55–60.
12. Noachtar S, Borggraefe I. Epilepsy surgery: A critical review. Epilepsy Behav 2009;15(1):66–72.
13. Almeida AN, Martinez V, Feindel W. The First Case of Invasive EEG Monitoring for the Surgical Treatment of Epilepsy: Historical Significance and Context. Epilepsia 2005;46(7):1082–5.
14. Reif PS, Strzelczyk A, Rosenow F. The history of invasive EEG evaluation in epilepsy patients. Seizure 2016;41:191–5.
15. Hayne R, Meyers R, Knott JR. Characteristics of electrical activity of human corpus striatum and neighboring structures. J Neurophysiol 1949;12(3):185–96.
16. Hayne R, Meyers R. An Improved Model of a Human Stereotaxic Instrument. J Neurosurg 1950;7(5):463–6.
17. Bancaud J. Contribution of functional exploration by stereotaxic ways to the surgery of epilepsy; 8 case reports. Neurochirurgie 1959;5(1):55–112.
18. Talairach J, Bancaud J, Bonis A, et al. Functional Stereotaxic Exploration of Epilepsy. Stereotact Funct Neurosurg 1962;22(3–5):328–31.
19. Wieser HG, Elger CE, Stodieck SRG. The 'foramen ovale electrode': a new recording method for the preoperative evaluation of patients suffering from mesio-basal temporal lobe epilepsy. Electroencephalogr Clin Neurophysiol 1985;61(4):314–22.
20. Chabardes S, Abel TJ, Cardinale F, et al. Commentary: Understanding Stereoelectroencephalography: What's Next? Neurosurgery 2018;82(1):E15–6.
21. Serletis D, Bulacio J, Bingaman W, et al. The stereotactic approach for mapping epileptic networks: a prospective study of 200 patients. J Neurosurg 2014;121(5):1239–46.
22. Chassoux F. Stereoelectroencephalography in focal cortical dysplasia: A 3D approach to delineating the dysplastic cortex. Brain 2000;123(8):1733–51.
23. Gonzalez-Martinez J, Mullin J, Vadera S, et al. Stereotactic placement of depth electrodes in medically intractable epilepsy. J Neurosurg 2014;120(3):639–44.
24. Spencer SS. Neural Networks in Human Epilepsy: Evidence of and Implications for Treatment. Epilepsia 2002;43(3):219–27.
25. Richardson RM. Closed-Loop Brain Stimulation and Paradigm Shifts in Epilepsy Surgery. Neurol Clin 2022;40(2):355–73.

26. Schaper FLWVJ, Nordberg J, Cohen AL, et al. Mapping Lesion-Related Epilepsy to a Human Brain Network. JAMA Neurol 2023;80(9):891.

27. Kramer MA, Cash SS. Epilepsy as a Disorder of Cortical Network Organization. Neuroscientist 2012;18(4).

28. Laufs H. Functional imaging of seizures and epilepsy. Curr Opin Neurol 2012;25(2):194–200.

29. Centeno M, Carmichael DW. Network Connectivity in Epilepsy: Resting State fMRI and EEGâ€"fMRI Contributions. Front Neurol 2014;5. https://doi.org/10.3389/fneur.2014.00093.

30. Bernhardt BC, Hong S, Bernasconi A, et al. Imaging structural and functional brain networks in temporal lobe epilepsy. Front Hum Neurosci 2013;7. https://doi.org/10.3389/fnhum.2013.00624.

31. Richardson MP. Large scale brain models of epilepsy: dynamics meets connectomics. J Neurol Neurosurg Psychiatry 2012;83(12):1238–48.

32. van Diessen E, Diederen SJH, Braun KPJ, et al. Functional and structural brain networks in epilepsy: What have we learned? Epilepsia 2013;54(11):1855–65.

33. Englot DJ, Konrad PE, Morgan VL. Regional and global connectivity disturbances in focal epilepsy, related neurocognitive sequelae, and potential mechanistic underpinnings. Epilepsia 2016;57(10):1546–57.

34. Hatton SN, Huynh KH, Bonilha L, et al. White matter abnormalities across different epilepsy syndromes in adults: an ENIGMA-Epilepsy study. Brain 2020;143(8):2454–73.

35. Weiss SA, Pastore T, Orosz I, et al. Graph theoretical measures of fast ripples support the epileptic network hypothesis. Brain Commun 2022;4(3). https://doi.org/10.1093/braincomms/fcac101.

36. Larivière S, Bernasconi A, Bernasconi N, et al. Connectome biomarkers of drug-resistant epilepsy. Epilepsia 2021;62(1):6–24.

37. He X, Doucet GE, Pustina D, et al. Presurgical thalamic "hubness" predicts surgical outcome in temporal lobe epilepsy. Neurology 2017;88(24):2285–93.

38. Gleichgerrcht E, Munsell B, Bhatia S, et al. Deep learning applied to whole-brain connectome to determine seizure control after epilepsy surgery. Epilepsia 2018;59(9):1643–54.

39. Gleichgerrcht E, Keller SS, Drane DL, et al. Temporal Lobe Epilepsy Surgical Outcomes Can Be Inferred Based on Structural Connectome Hubs: A Machine Learning Study. Ann Neurol 2020;88(5):970–83.

40. Weiss SA, Fried I, Wu C, et al. Graph theoretical measures of fast ripple networks improve the accuracy of post-operative seizure outcome prediction. Sci Rep 2023;13(1):367.

41. Piper RJ, Richardson RM, Worrell G, et al. Towards network-guided neuromodulation for epilepsy. Brain 2022;145(10):3347–62.

42. Richardson RM. Decision making in epilepsy surgery. Neurosurg Clin N Am 2020 Jul;31(3):471–9.

43. Sitnikov AR, Grigoryan YA, Mishnyakova LP. Bilateral stereotactic lesions and chronic stimulation of the anterior thalamic nuclei for treatment of pharmacoresistant epilepsy. Surg Neurol Int 2018;9:137.

44. Kokkinos V, Urban A, Sisterson ND, et al. Responsive neurostimulation of the thalamus improves seizure control in idiopathic generalized epilepsy: a case report. Neurosurgery 2020;87(5):E578–83.

45. Welch WP, Hect JL, Abel TJ. Case report: responsive neurostimulation of the centromedian thalamic nucleus for the detection and treatment of seizures in pediatric primary generalized epilepsy. Front Neurol 2021;12. https://doi.org/10.3389/fneur.2021.656585.

46. Sisterson ND, Kokkinos V, Urban A, et al. Responsive neurostimulation of the thalamus improves seizure control in idiopathic generalised epilepsy: initial case series. J Neurol Neurosurg Psychiatry 2022;93(5):491–8.

47. McGonigal A, Bartolomei F, Regis J, et al. Stereoelectroencephalography in presurgical assessment of MRI-negative epilepsy. Brain 2007;130(12):3169–83.

48. Tandon N, Tong BA, Friedman ER, et al. Analysis of Morbidity and Outcomes Associated With Use of Subdural Grids vs Stereoelectroencephalography in Patients With Intractable Epilepsy. JAMA Neurol 2019;76(6):672.

49. Gonzalez-Martinez J, Bulacio J, Alexopoulos A, et al. Stereoelectroencephalography in the "difficult to localize" refractory focal epilepsy: Early experience from a North American epilepsy center. Epilepsia 2013;54(2):323–30.

50. McGovern RA, Ruggieri P, Bulacio J, et al. Risk analysis of hemorrhage in stereo-electroencephalography procedures. Epilepsia 2019;60(3):571–80.

51. Kennedy BC, Katz J, Lepard J, et al. Variation in pediatric stereoelectroencephalography practice among pediatric neurosurgeons in the United States: survey results. J Neurosurg Pediatr 2021;1–9. https://doi.org/10.3171/2021.1.PEDS20799.

52. Sacino MF, Huang SS, Schreiber J, et al. Is the use of Stereotactic Electroencephalography Safe and Effective in Children? A Meta-Analysis of the use of Stereotactic Electroencephalography in Comparison to Subdural Grids for Invasive Epilepsy Monitoring in Pediatric Subjects. Neurosurgery 2019;84(6):1190–200. https://doi.org/10.1093/neuros/nyy466.

53. Pizarro D, Ilyas A, Chaitanya G, et al. Spectral organization of focal seizures within the thalamotemporal network. Ann Clin Transl Neurol 2019;6(9):1836–48.

The Value of Stereo-electroencephalography in Temporal Lobe Epilepsy
Huashan Experience

Shize Jiang, MD[a,1], Yanming Zhu, MD[b,c,1], Jie Hu, MD, PhD[a,*]

KEYWORDS

- Temporal lobe epilepsy • Stereo-electroencephalography • MRI negative epilepsy
- Pseudo temporal lobe epilepsy • Temporal plus epilepsy

KEY POINTS

- Temporal lobe epilepsy (TLE) is one of the most common drug-refractory epilepsies; its treatment and diagnosis still need significant improvement due to the complex nature of its network.
- The authors' experience in treating TLE cases with stereo-electroencephalography (SEEG) evaluation during the past 10 years is summarized here.
- The authors demonstrate the value of SEEG in different types of TLE and discuss how SEEG may lead to improved treatment outcomes in TLE.

INTRODUCTION

Temporal lobe epilepsy (TLE) is the most common type of drug-refractory epilepsy and accounts for the majority of drug-resistant epilepsy in adults.[1,2] Surgical resection of the epileptogenic zone can effectively control epileptic seizures, with an effective rate of more than 70%.[3] However, whether the epileptogenic zone can be accurately located has become the key to the efficacy of surgical treatment for epilepsy.

In the 1950s, cortical electroencephalography (EEG) was the most accurate method for finding epileptogenic areas.[4] The predecessors of the Montreal School of Epilepsy, Penfield and Jasper, located epileptogenic foci based on interictal spikes and intraoperative cortical electrical stimulation techniques. Based on this, the standard anterior temporal lobe resection procedure was gradually established.[5]

The European school's concept of an epileptogenic focus was initially derived from the work of Talairach and Bancaud in the 1960s.[6] They attached great importance to the electrical-clinical information during a seizure, rather than interictal spikes. Careful attention was made to the analysis of seizure semiology, which could clarify the propagation of epileptiform discharges in the brain based on the evolution of clinical seizures. Based on this, Talairach and Bancaud created the stereo-electroencephalography (SEEG) methodology to study the anatomic structure of epileptogenic zones with individual cases. They defined the epileptogenic zone as "the site of the beginning of the epileptic seizures and their primary organization."[7] Therefore, the definition of the epileptogenic focus by the European school is an electro-clinical definition of the ictal period, which not only emphasizes the precise anatomic location of the initiation of the ictal discharge and the early spread of the ictal discharge but also highlights the electro-clinical relationship of the ictal discharge. With the development of contemporary SEEG and the maturity of technology,

[a] Department of Neurosurgery, Huashan Hospital, Fudan University, Shanghai, China; [b] Program in Speech and Hearing Bioscience and Technology, Harvard Medical School, Boston, MA, USA; [c] Department of Neurosurgery, Massachusetts General Hospital, 55 Fruit Street, Boston, MA 02114, USA
[1] Dr. Shize Jiang & Dr. Yanming Zhu have contributed equally to this work.
* Corresponding author.
E-mail address: hujietongli@sina.com

Neurosurg Clin N Am 35 (2024) 95–104
https://doi.org/10.1016/j.nec.2023.09.008
1042-3680/24/© 2023 Elsevier Inc. All rights reserved.

SEEG has more advantages than cortical EEG in locating temporal lobe epileptogenic areas.

SEEG technology was introduced into China by Professor Sinclair Liu and his colleagues in the 2010s. We, the Department of Neurosurgery of Huashan Hospital, started to conduct SEEG recordings in 2014. Our electrode implantation technology was initially the same as conventional deep brain stimulation (DBS) technology, using a Leksell stereotactic head frame. Electrodes were implanted with local anesthesia. However, this strategy faced certain limitations. For instance, the frame might block some electrode trajectories, which resulted in certain difficulties in formulating electrode implantation plans. In addition, with a stereotactic head frame, the coordinates need to be frequently changed when implanting different electrodes, resulting in increased workload and operative time.

As a result, we subsequently transitioned to using surgical robots (ROSA or SINO). The surgery was still performed under local anesthesia and fixed with a 3-pin head frame. However, we found that since the patient was awake during the operation, minor body movement could occur during the drilling procedure. As a result, implantation accuracy would decrease, and the target implantation error could reach 2 to 3 mm.

Currently, we use robot-assisted electrode implantation under general anesthesia. In comparison, the patient's comfort during general anesthesia has been improved, and the time efficiency of robot-assisted general anesthesia surgery has dramatically improved. The average time of each operation is about 1 to 2 hours. The implantation accuracy has also greatly improved compared with before, and the complication rate is reduced. We finally established our SEEG implantation protocol in our center, and the number of cases has increased steadily yearly.

So far, we have completed more than 200 SEEG cases, including about one-third of cases of TLE. Taking this opportunity, we will share our application in different types of TLE. The value summary is compiled into a document, hoping to provide a reference for others.

STEREO-ELECTROENCEPHALOGRAPHY IN UNILATERAL TEMPORAL LOBE EPILEPSY

For epilepsies caused by apparent temporal lobe lesions, including hippocampal sclerosis, tumors, vascular lesions, and so forth, if the anatomic electro-clinical symptoms are consistent, there is no difficulty in diagnosis, and we usually do not consider SEEG evaluation. However, in some exceptional cases, we may consider SEEG evaluation. For example, if the lesions are located in the dominant hemisphere close to the hippocampal formation, we may need SEEG to evaluate whether the hippocampal formation needs resection (**Fig. 1**A–F). Since the epileptogenic zone is not the same as the epileptogenic lesion, in many cases, the epileptogenic zone may exist close to or far away from the lesion. Therefore, when the lesion is close to an eloquent area, choosing the best surgical method can be challenging when decision-making is purely based on noninvasive information. Instead of lobectomy, in-depth evaluation should be carried out to clarify the location of the epileptogenic focus and balance the relationship between functional protection and epileptogenic focus resection to achieve the best outcome. In this case, we performed SEEG evaluation. We found that the seizure onset zone was restricted around the lesion and that the hippocampus was not initially involved. We performed resection surgery for this patient; he has been seizure-free for 3 years.

There are some other circumstances that may warrant SEEG investigation, such as dual pathology or multiple lesions. When the patient has an extratemporal lobe lesion but presents with TLE, we think it is reasonable to conduct SEEG evaluations (**Fig. 2**A) since the lesion may be misleading. As a result, we need to analyze the electro-clinical information to make further decisions carefully. We conducted SEEG recording (see **Fig. 2**B) for this patient and found seizures that were initiated from the mesial structures. We performed selective amygdalohippocampectomy (see **Fig. 2**C), and the patient has been seizure-free for 5 years.

STEREO-ELECTROENCEPHALOGRAPHY IN MRI-NEGATIVE TEMPORAL LOBE EPILEPSY

MRI-negative TLE is the most challenging type of TLE. MRI images play a decisive role in diagnosing temporal lobe pathology.[8,9] Accurately locating the epileptogenic focus of MRI-negative epilepsy is a considerable challenge. Because the brain is a complex network structure,[9–11] and there is significant heterogeneity between individuals, other causes will also produce different discharge characteristics. Therefore, lesions in the exact location may appear as distinct symptoms in different individuals. Symptoms pose a considerable challenge to the location of epileptogenic lesions. For such cases, it is often necessary to record multiple structures simultaneously, especially deep structures such as the hippocampus, amygdala, entorhinal cortex, and so forth. Subdural electrodes often cannot meet the requirements, and SEEG is the best choice for such cases.

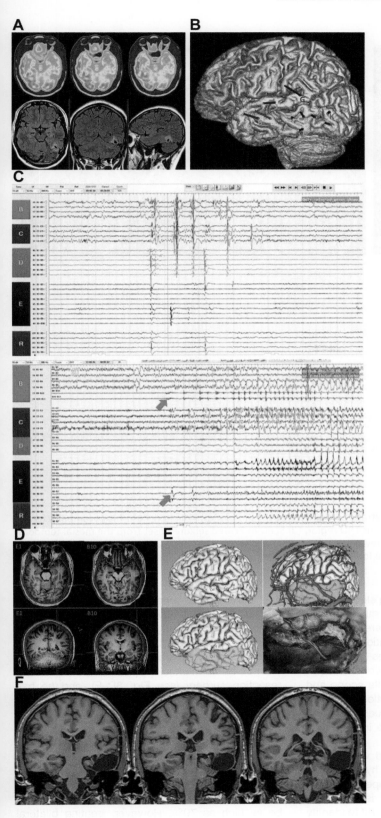

Fig. 1. SEEG exploration in TLE with lesion located adjacent to the hippocampus (*A*) MRI indicated the lesion located in the fusiform gyrus, and the PET scan indicated hypometabolism of the lesion and hippocampus (*B*) SEEG proposal indicating the location of the electrodes (*C*) Interictal SEEG indicated spikes in the hippocampus and the lesion. Ictal SEEG indicated initiated from the neocortex (*D*) The location of the electrodes corresponds to seizure onset (*E*) Surgical plan and intraoperative images (*F*) Postoperative MRI, which reveals the resection of the lesion and the preservation of the hippocampus. SEEG, stereoelectroencephalography; TLE, temporal lobe epilepsy.

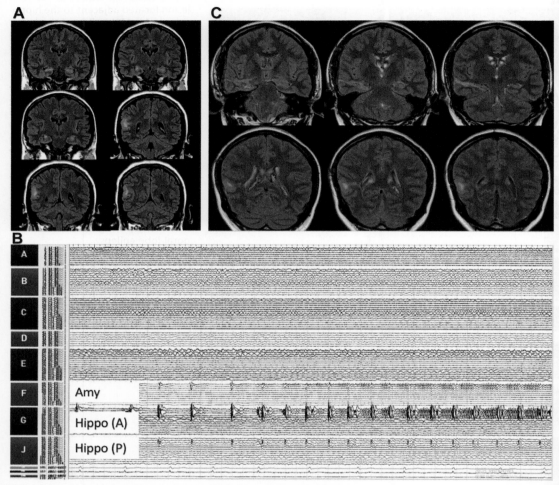

Fig. 2. SEEG exploration in TLE with extratemporal lesion (*A*) MRI images indicated right hippocampal sclerosis together with a lesion located in the right TPO region (*B*) SEEG indicated seizure onset from the mesial temporal region (*C*) Postoperative MRI, which reveals the resection of the hippocampus and amygdala. SEEG, stereo-electroencephalography; TLE, temporal lobe epilepsy; TPO, temporo-parieto-occipital junction.

At the same time, when designing electrode implantation plans, we need to keep in mind that TLE is a network disease and requires careful analysis of anatomic electro-clinical information to establish substantial clinical hypotheses and avoid "fishing expeditions".[11–13] We must consider evaluating the epileptogenic zone and its scope and clarify its relationship with the functional zone to guarantee the formulation of subsequent resection plans when designing the electrode implantation plan.

For example, a patient presented with normal MRI (**Fig. 3**A) but was found to have hypometabolism in the posterior part of the left superior temporal gyrus (see **Fig. 3**B), which is close to Wernicke's area. As a result, we needed to identify the boundary between the suspected epileptic foci

and the functional area. We conducted SEEG for this patient, mainly covering the left temporal and surrounding insular regions (see **Fig. 3**C). SEEG confirmed that the superior temporal gyrus contained the epileptic foci, and electrical stimulation did not cause Wernicke aphasia. We performed resection surgery (see **Fig. 3**D–E), and he has been seizure-free for 2 years.

STEREO-ELECTROENCEPHALOGRAPHY IN BILATERAL TEMPORAL LOBE EPILEPSY

The medical community has widely recognized the effectiveness of surgical treatment of unilateral TLE, and the seizure-free rate after surgery can be as high as 70%. However, treating bilateral TLE (BTLE) is still a thorny problem and an

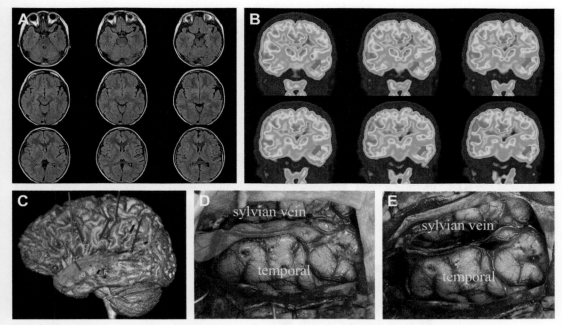

Fig. 3. SEEG exploration in MRI negative TLE (*A*) MRI images indicated no obvious lesion (*B*) PET scan shows hypometabolism in the left superior temporal gyrus (*C*) SEEG proposal indicating the location of the electrodes (*D*) Intraoperative images showing the epileptic foci identified with SEEG (*green*) (*E*) Intraoperative images after the resection of the epileptic foci. SEEG, stereo-electroencephalography; TLE, temporal lobe epilepsy.

essential reason for the failure of temporal lobe surgery.[14] Due to the low postoperative remission rate and the high proportion of severe impairment of memory function, the choice and method of surgical treatment of BTLE are still controversial in the surgical field.

In early studies, BTLE was judged only based on whether there were asynchronous bitemporal abnormal discharges in the interictal period of the scalp EEG.[15–17] Later, it was mainly based on the origin of seizures seen on EEG. BTLE was generally considered unsuitable for surgery, and most patients were not treated with surgical methods.[18,19] With the rapid development of neurosurgery technology and the deepening of understanding of TLE, we have gradually discovered bilateral independent discharges in the scalp EEG, clinical seizures with bilateral independent or simultaneous onset, bitemporal imaging changes, and other preoperative evaluation results.

Although BTLE is a commonly recognized phenomenon, there are no clear definitions or anatomic electro-clinical characteristics.[20] With an in-depth study of the anatomic electro-clinical relationships of BTLE, BTLE can be divided into 2 categories. The first category is bitemporal seizures of unknown side, which refers to the findings from video EEG (VEEG). In the VEEG or SEEG recording, at least 1 seizure involves both temporal lobes simultaneously or successively, and the

side of the seizure onset cannot be determined based on the clinical manifestations at the onset and during the seizure. The second category is seizures with bitemporal independent origins. As for the proportion of unilateral seizures in BTLE that must meet the criteria before surgery can be performed, each medical center's standards differ. Some studies have pointed out that unilateral ATL surgery can be achieved only when the ictal hemilateral ratio is at least 80%; some scholars have also suggested that the hemilateral ratio of bitemporal independent discharges during interictal periods must be greater than 90% in order for surgery to achieve satisfactory postoperative results.[21–23]

In our center, we believe SEEG examination is necessary for patients with suspected bilateral TLE after noninvasive evaluation. By performing SEEG, we seek to clarify the following questions. First, whether the patient has bilateral TLE; second, whether there is a clear dominant side of onset for the bilateral TLE. Among the cases we have treated, we have found that for patients with a history of encephalitis and presented with bilateral temporal lobe epilepsies, SEEG revealed that the probability of bilateral independent discharges is high. Resection surgery is often challenging to perform. Therefore, we recommend responsive neurostimulation or DBS so the patient can have a good prognosis. For those patients

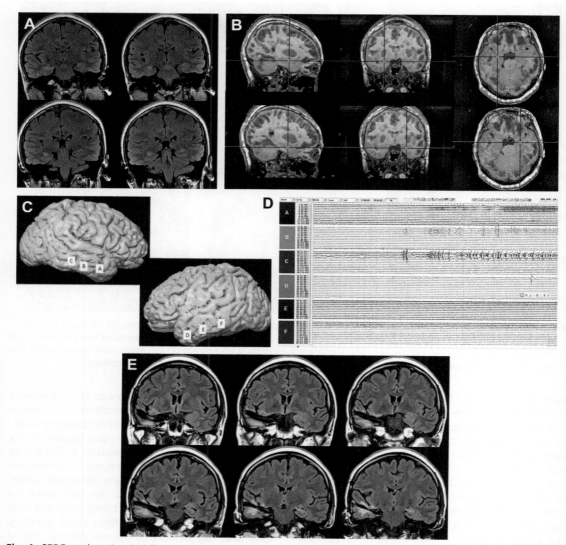

Fig. 4. SEEG exploration in bilateral TLE (*A*) MRI images indicated bilateral hippocampus atrophy together with hyper signal intensity (*B*) PET scan indicated hypometabolism of bilateral temporal regions (*C*) SEEG proposal exploring the bilateral temporal region (*D*) SEEG indicated seizure initiated from the right mesial temporal region (*E*) Postoperative MRI images indicated the resection of the right mesial temporal structures. SEEG, stereo-electroencephalography; TLE, temporal lobe epilepsy.

without a history of encephalitis, the probability of bilateral independent discharge is low if he/she only presented with bilateral hippocampal hyperintensity or atrophy (**Fig. 4**A–E). For such cases, we can use SEEG to evaluate the epileptogenic focus and ultimately assess whether there is an opportunity for resection.

STEREO-ELECTROENCEPHALOGRAPHY IN TEMPORAL PLUS EPILEPSY

Temporal plus epilepsy (TPE) is focal epilepsy in which the primary epileptogenic area extends

beyond the temporal lobe.[24] It involves the neighboring regions such as the insula, the suprasylvian opercular cortex, the orbitofrontal cortex, and the temporo-parieto-occipital junction. TPE is a type of multi-lobe epilepsy in the epilepsy network. The proposal for the additional syndrome of TPE is based on the failure of a typical temporal lobe resection in leading to seizure freedom.[25,26] As a result, SEEG could further verify this concept. While it has been characterized as being different from traditional TLE, TPE still has many unknowns in terms of its functional anatomy and electrophysiology. In particular, the clinical symptomatology of seizures in TPE may overlap with characteristics of known regions, making its definition more complex.

Ryvlin and Kahane pointed out that TLE plus syndrome is a particular type of multi-lobar epilepsy.[27] Its electro-clinical symptoms mainly reflect TLE. The MRI may have no apparent changes or may only present hippocampal sclerosis. Barba and colleagues further divided TPE into 3 subtypes: the temporo-frontal group, the temporo-sylvian group, and the temporo-parieto-occipital junction group.[28] However, it should be noted that electro-clinical symptomatology's localization significance is unclear, and the specificity is poor. In addition, the electro-clinical symptomatology locates the area where symptomatology occurs, not the epileptogenic zone, and the symptomatogenic zone does not always overlap with the epileptogenic zone. In addition, if the epileptogenic focus starts from the asymptomatic area, clinical symptoms will only occur after the abnormal discharge spreads to the symptomatogenic zone, which will also cause deviations in the localization of electro-clinical symptoms.

STEREO-ELECTROENCEPHALOGRAPHY IN PSEUDO TEMPORAL LOBE EPILEPSY

Pseudo temporal lobe epilepsy (PTLE) is another confusing type of epilepsy. Schneider first proposed the concept of PTLE in 1965.[29] The EEG during the seizure is often located in the temporal area, and the clinical seizure symptoms are also similar to temporal lobe seizures, especially medial temporal lobe seizures. Still, the epileptogenic area is outside the temporal lobe.[30] PTLE is challenging to diagnose. It is not easy to detect by scalp EEG. However, SEEG can detect the location of the epilepsy source area.[31,32] PTLE is almost always refractory to antiepileptic drugs, and temporal lobe resection alone is often ineffective.[32] Therefore, patients can often obtain effective results by resection of the epilepsy source area and symptom onset area.

It is essential to carefully identify the epileptogenic and symptomatogenic zones in diagnosing PTLE.[32] The epileptogenic zone is the area that produces epileptiform discharges. The seizure disappears after this area is removed, while the symptomatogenic site is the brain area activated by epileptiform discharges and results in symptoms.[33] Clinically, the symptomatogenic zone can be determined by the clinical characteristics and electroencephalogram pattern during the seizure. These 2 areas are not necessarily in the same brain area, especially when the epilepsy

source area is far from the functional cortex. The brain has many "silent areas" where epilepsy occurs, which spread to other brain areas to produce symptoms. As shown in **Fig. 5**A–E, the patient presented with typical TLE but had a small lesion in the right parietal-occipital region. Luckily, the patient complained of an occult visual aura before the seizure onset, which drew our attention. We conducted SEEG for this patient and found that the lesion located in the parietal-occipital region was the fundamental epileptic foci. This phenomenon is critical when performing resection treatment. It is challenging to diagnose PTLE without an abnormal MRI. At this time, the symptoms and EEG patterns during the seizure should be carefully analyzed. Those with MRI abnormalities outside the temporal lobe should also trigger a careful examination of the relationship between electro-clinical and MRI abnormalities. Intracranial electrodes, especially SEEG, play a decisive role in determining the epileptogenic zone in PTLE. The potential epileptogenic and symptomatogenic zones and essential nodes in the abnormal network should be considered when designing the surgical proposal.

DISCUSSION

SEEG technology is a lesion localization technology that has been increasingly used in refractory epilepsy recently. With an in-depth understanding of TLE and the development of SEEG recording, we have a deeper understanding of the epileptogenic network of TLE. Generally speaking, we now have fewer and fewer opportunities to use SEEG to evaluate focal TLE with anatomic electro-clinical anastomosis. However, for MRI-negative epilepsy and pseudo temporal lobe epilepsy, we are more inclined to use SEEG to describe its causes. In these cases, we find it important to characterize the epileptic network, explore the location of epileptogenic lesions, and ultimately assist in formulating surgical plans.

SEEG has some advantages over subdural EEG, especially for lesions in deeper structures or at sulcus depths. The spikes generated by structures such as the bottom of a sulcus or temporal pole adjacent to the hippocampus may spread easily to the hippocampus, and these may be challenging to record with strip electrodes, which can easily lead to the conclusion that the hippocampus is the origin. SEEG could record the electrophysiologic characteristics of those deep-seated regions of the brain in one time and one space, making the algorithm's derivation, evolution, and evolution process more 3-dimensional and

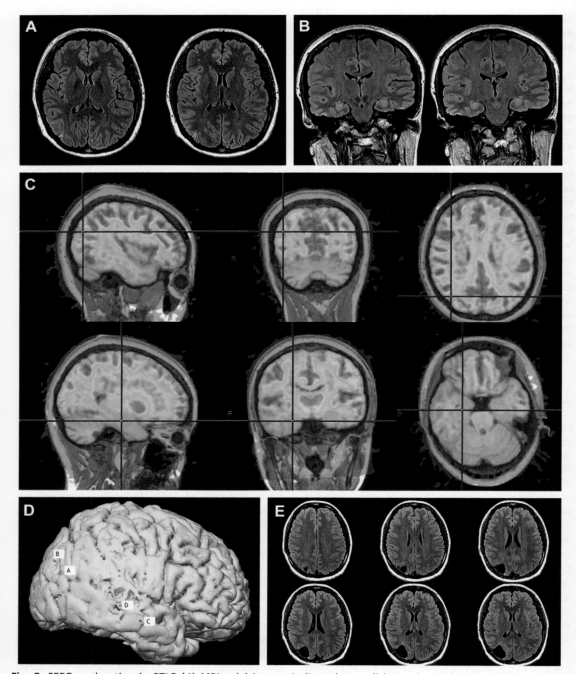

Fig. 5. SEEG exploration in PTLE (*A*) MRI axial images indicated a small lesion located in the right occipital-parietal region (*B*) MRI coronal images indicated slightly hyper signal intensity in the right hippocampus (*C*) PET scan indicated hypometabolism in the right occipital-parietal region and right temporal region (*D*) SEEG proposal exploring the right occipital-parietal region and right temporal region (*E*) Postoperative MRI images indicated the resection of the right occipital-parietal region. PTLE, pseudo temporal lobe epilepsy; SEEG, stereo-electroencephalography.

precise. Therefore, SEEG has been more widely promoted.

However, there are some limitations of SEEG technology. Most recorded EEG seizures of cortical origin spread radially, and SEEG may come with a limited number of electrodes in the cortical surface, primarily when insufficient electrode coverage exists. The information obtained during mapping may need to be more extensive when evaluating critical functional areas. In addition, head frame fixation is unsuitable for patients with large-area skull defects or relatively fragile skull development; for younger children, computed tomography scans should be performed to determine the thickness of the skull before surgery. Currently, SEEG electrodes are expensive in China, and some patients need help to afford surgery due to economic reasons.

In summary, SEEG has many advantages in locating the origin, conduction, and diffusion range of the epileptogenic zone in TLE and guiding the surgical plan. In addition, for epileptogenic foci recorded by SEEG that have deep origins, which are difficult to reach by surgery, or have essential functional areas, SEEG opens up the possibility of further treatment with thermal coagulation before electrode removal in order to reduce the surgical risk in these particular areas. Nevertheless, further clinical research will be needed to explore the utility of these applications.

CLINICS CARE POINTS

- Detailed preoperative evaluation is the guarantee for ensuring the efficacy of epilepsy surgery.
- When inconsistent anatomical-electro-clinical information appears in the non-invasive evaluation procedure, we may need SEEG assessment to assist in accurately locating the epileptogenic focus and clarifying the scope of the epileptogenic focus.
- For lesions very close to the functional area, SEEG will also provide critical information in helping us to make the surgical decision.

FUNDING INFORMATION

Science and Technology Commission of Shanghai Municipality (21Y21900600).

CONFLICTS OF INTEREST

All authors declare that we have no personal or institutional financial interest in drugs, materials, or devices described in their submissions.

REFERENCES

1. Thijs RD, Surges R, O'Brien TJ, et al. Epilepsy in adults. Lancet (London, England) 2019; 393(10172):689–701.

2. Sànchez J, Centanaro M, Solís J, et al. Factors predicting the outcome following medical treatment of mesial temporal epilepsy with hippocampal sclerosis. Seizure 2014;23(6):448–53.

3. West S, Nolan SJ, Newton R. Surgery for epilepsy: a systematic review of current evidence. Epileptic Disord 2016;18(2):113–21.

4. Feindel W. Development of surgical therapy of epilepsy at the Montreal Neurological Institute. The Canadian journal of neurological sciences Le journal canadien des sciences neurologiques 1991;18(4 Suppl):549–53.

5. Feindel W, Leblanc R, De Almeida AN. Epilepsy Surgery: Historical Highlights 1909–2009. Epilepsia 2009;50(s3):131–51.

6. Schijns OE, Hoogland G, Kubben PL, et al. The start and development of epilepsy surgery in Europe: a historical review. Neurosurg Rev 2015;38(3):447–61.

7. Kahane P, Landré E, Minotti L, et al. The Bancaud and Talairach view on the epileptogenic zone: a working hypothesis. Epileptic Disord : international epilepsy journal with videotape 2006;8(Suppl 2): S16–26.

8. Muhlhofer W, Tan YL, Mueller SG, et al. MRI-negative temporal lobe epilepsy-What do we know? Epilepsia 2017;58(5):727–42.

9. Vaughan DN, Rayner G, Tailby C, et al. MRI-negative temporal lobe epilepsy: A network disorder of neocortical connectivity. Neurology 2016;87(18):1934–42.

10. Bartolomei F, Cosandier-Rimele D, McGonigal A, et al. From mesial temporal lobe to temporoperisylvian seizures: a quantified study of temporal lobe seizure networks. Epilepsia 2010;51(10):2147–58.

11. Bartolomei F, Bettus G, Stam CJ, et al. Interictal network properties in mesial temporal lobe epilepsy: a graph theoretical study from intracerebral recordings. Clin Neurophysiol 2013;124(12):2345–53.

12. Van Gompel JJ, Noe K, Zimmerman RS. Intracranial EEG Monitoring. Epilepsy 2021;381–99.

13. Khoo HM, Hall JA, Dubeau F, et al. Technical Aspects of SEEG and Its Interpretation in the Delineation of the Epileptogenic Zone. Neurol Med -Chir 2020;60(12):565–80.

14. Joo EY, Lee EK, Tae WS, et al. Unitemporal vs Bitemporal Hypometabolism in Mesial Temporal Lobe Epilepsy. Arch Neurol 2004;61(7):1074–8.

15. Steinhoff BJ, So NK, Lim S, et al. Ictal scalp EEG in temporal lobe epilepsy with unitemporal versus bitemporal interictal epileptiform discharges. Neurology 1995;45(5):889–96.

16. Ergene E, Shih JJ, Blum DE, et al. Frequency of bitemporal independent interictal epileptiform discharges in temporal lobe epilepsy. Epilepsia 2000;41(2):213–8.

17. Asadi-Pooya AA, Farazdaghi M, Shahpari M. Clinical significance of bilateral epileptiform discharges in temporal lobe epilepsy. Acta Neurol Scand 2021; 143(6):608–13.

18. Chiang S, Fan JM, Rao VR. Bilateral temporal lobe epilepsy: How many seizures are required in chronic ambulatory electrocorticography to estimate the laterality ratio? Epilepsia 2022;63(1):199–208.

19. Dührsen L, Sauvigny T, Ricklefs FL, et al. Decision-making in temporal lobe epilepsy surgery based on invasive stereo-electroencephalography (sEEG). Neurosurg Rev 2020;43(5):1403–8.

20. Didato G, Chiesa V, Villani F, et al. Bitemporal epilepsy: A specific anatomo-electro-clinical phenotype in the temporal lobe epilepsy spectrum. Seizure 2015;31:112–9.

21. Aghakhani Y, Liu X, Jette N, et al. Epilepsy surgery in patients with bilateral temporal lobe seizures: A systematic review. Epilepsia 2014;55(12):1892–901.

22. Holmes MD, Miles AN, Dodrill CB, et al. Identifying potential surgical candidates in patients with evidence of bitemporal epilepsy. Epilepsia 2003; 44(8):1075–9.

23. Hirsch LJ, Spencer SS, Spencer DD, et al. Temporal lobectomy in patients with bitemporal epilepsy defined by depth electroencephalography. Ann Neurol 1991;30(3):347–56.

24. Kahane P, Barba C, Rheims S, et al. The concept of temporal 'plus' epilepsy. Rev Neurol (Paris) 2015; 171(3):267–72.

25. Barba C, Rheims S, Minotti L, et al. Surgical outcome of temporal plus epilepsy is improved by multilobar resection. Epilepsia 2022;63(4):769–76.

26. Barba C, Rheims S, Minotti L, et al. Temporal plus epilepsy is a major determinant of temporal lobe surgery failures. Brain 2015;139(2):444–51.

27. Ryvlin P, Kahane P. The hidden causes of surgery-resistant temporal lobe epilepsy: extratemporal or temporal plus? Curr Opin Neurol 2005;18(2):125–7.

28. Barba C, Barbati G, Minotti L, et al. Ictal clinical and scalp-EEG findings differentiating temporal lobe epilepsies from temporal 'plus' epilepsies. Brain 2007; 130(Pt 7):1957–67.

29. Schneider RC, Crosby EC, Farhat SM. Extratemporal lesions triggering the temporal-obe syndrome. J Neurosurg 1965;22:246–63.

30. Elwan SA, So NK, Enatsu R, et al. Pseudotemporal ictal patterns compared with mesial and neocortical temporal ictal patterns. J Clin Neurophysiol 2013; 30(3):238–46.

31. Aghakhani Y, Rosati A, Dubeau F, et al. Patients with temporoparietal ictal symptoms and inferomesial EEG do not benefit from anterior temporal resection. Epilepsia 2004;45(3):230–6.

32. Fish DR, Gloor P, Quesney FL, et al. Clinical responses to electrical brain stimulation of the temporal and frontal lobes in patients with epilepsy. Pathophysiological implications. Brain 1993;116(Pt 2):397–414.

33. Rosenow F, Lüders H. Presurgical evaluation of epilepsy. Brain 2001;124(9):1683–700.

Acute Effect of Vagus Nerve Stimulation in Patients with Drug-Resistant Epilepsy

A Preliminary Exploration via Stereoelectroencephalogram

Xiaoya Qin, PhD[a,b,1,2], Yuan Yuan, PhD[a,b,1,2], Huiling Yu, MD[b,2], Yi Yao, M.Med[c,d],*, Luming Li, PhD[b,e],*

KEYWORDS

• Vagus nerve stimulation • Acute stimulation • Weighted phase lag index • Desynchronization
• Stereoelectroencephalogram

KEY POINTS

- This study provided a valid and feasible experimental paradigm for characterizing the acute effect of vagus nerve stimulation (VNS).
- The ability of VNS to induce extensive desynchronization in different areas (especially epileptogenic regions) is important to its antiepileptic effect.
- The synchronization changes caused by VNS mainly occurred in the high-frequency bands such as low gamma and high gamma, which provided theoretic support for the search of potential biomarkers for patient screening.

INTRODUCTION

Vagus nerve stimulation (VNS) is an alternative surgical treatment approved by the Food and Drug Administration for patients with drug-resistant epilepsy (DRE). This method has been used in over 125,000 cases (including 35,000 children) worldwide until 2021.[1] The efficacy of VNS varies individually: 45% to 65% of the patients had a greater than 50% reduction in seizure frequency, and only 5% to 9% of patients achieved seizure freedom.[2-4]

The anti-seizure mechanism of VNS remains unclear, which poses a significant challenge in clinical use of VNS therapy. Three different temporal patterns have been considered in the antiepileptic

Funding: This article was supported by The National Key Research and Development Program of China (2021YFC2401205) and Shenzhen International Cooperation Research Project (GJHZ20180930110402104).

[a] Precision Medicine & Healthcare Research Center, Tsinghua-Berkeley Shenzhen Institute, Tsinghua University, Shenzhen, China; [b] National Engineering Research Center of Neuromodulation, School of Aerospace Engineering, Tsinghua University, Beijing, China; [c] Department of Functional Neurosurgery, Xiamen Humanity Hospital Affiliated to Fujian Medical University, Fujian, China; [d] Surgery Division, Epilepsy Center, Shenzhen Children's Hospital, Shenzhen, Guangdong, China; [e] IDG/McGovern Institute for Brain Research at Tsinghua University, Beijing, China

[1] These authors contributed equally to the manuscript: X. Qin and Y. Yuan were co-first authors of the study.
[2] Present address: Room 805, 8th Floor, Building C2, Zhiyuan, Nanshan District, Shenzhen, China 518071.
* Corresponding authors. N-204, Mengminwei Science and Technology Building, Tsinghua University, Beijing, P. R. China 100084.
E-mail addresses: tygnsjwk@163.com (Y.Y.); lilm@mail.tsinghua.edu.cn (L.L.)

effect of VNS[5–11]: (i) acute arrest effect, namely, the ongoing seizure can be directly prevented by VNS; (ii) acute preventive effect, wherein the seizure threshold is increased or the effect of seizure inducers is weakened with stimulation; and (iii) chronic progressive preventive effect, whereby the seizures frequency can be significantly reduced by chronic VNS. Among them, the acute preventive effect may be reflected by synchronously monitoring the impact of acute stimulation on brain activity. The efficacy of VNS is directly related to the response generated to the brain, and this response is highly likely to be reflected through electroencephalogram (EEG) changes caused by acute stimulation. In recent years, there has been an increasing interest in understanding the role of VNS in treating epilepsy through EEG characteristics.[12]

Some studies have found that acute VNS can significantly reduce whole-brain synchronization on scalp EEG in responders but not in nonresponders.[13,14] However, it is unclear whether the anti-seizure effect of VNS requires desynchronization of large-scale brain networks or simply the desynchronization of epileptogenic networks. Electrical signals from the epileptogenic areas, which can better reflect the effect of VNS against epilepsy, should be obtained to investigate the anti-seizure effect of VNS.

Recently, stereoelectroencephalography (SEEG) has been increasingly used to study the mechanism of VNS.[15–18] In clinical practice, SEEG allows monitoring of the actual origin and evolution of seizures by placing depth electrodes directly in intracranial regions.[19,20] Compared with scalp EEG, the SEEG electrode is implanted deep into the cerebral cortex and subcortical structures to directly acquire signals from the epileptogenic zone, providing a more comprehensive understanding of the effects of VNS on the brain.

In this study, 12 VNS device–implanted patients who underwent SEEG recordings were investigated. An acute VNS experiment was performed during SEEG monitoring to explore the regulation mechanism of VNS on epileptic network synchronization.

METHODS
Participants Recruitment

Twelve participants were recruited from Xiamen Humanity Hospital, Fujian Medical University and Shenzhen Children's Hospital between March 2020 and October 2022. Demographic characteristics are shown in **Table 1**.

The VNS was turned off at least 14 days before SEEG electrodes were implanted due to the poor efficacy of VNS or imaging examination. The VNS device was turned on if there was no complication such as intracranial edema and hemorrhage in the second or third days after implantation. Before the experiment, lead impedance was checked and functional integrity of system was validated. To accurately differentiate the "ON" and "OFF" stimulation periods, 2 additional electrodes were placed on the neck close to the scar and the thorax to capture the stimulation artifact from the VNS device.

This study was approved by the ethical committee of Xiamen Humanity Hospital, Fujian Medical University (code: AF-SOP-029–01.0) and the ethical committee of Shenzhen Children's Hospital (code: 202009302). A written informed consent was provided by all participants or their guardians.

Stereoelectroencephalography Data Acquisition and Grouping of Stereoelectroencephalography Channels

The Neuvo 64 to 512 Channel Long term EEG monitoring system (Compumedics Limited, Victoria, Australia) was used to collect SEEG data at a sampling rate of 2 kHz during stimulation with the optimal amplitude reported by the participants' guardians. For the participants whose optimal parameters were uncertain, the last amplitudes of VNS setting used before this study were taken into consideration as the optimal parameters. The other stimulation parameters were as follows: duty cycle, 23%; pulse width, 500 μs; and frequency, 30 Hz.

To prevent the cumulative effect of VNS, only the first 5 stimulations were selected and each had its own baseline (**Fig. 1**A). A period of equivalent duration to the subsequent ON period was selected as baseline to minimize the deviation caused by the spontaneous fluctuation of brain activity.

Bipolar montage was used to limit volume conduction effects and bias caused by common references.[21] Only contacts within the gray matter were selected. If more than 2 channels located in the same area, comparison was made and only the channel with the highest amplitude and least artifacts were selected. Then, the selected channels were grouped. According to epileptogenicity index (EI) proposed by Bartolomei and colleagues[22] and the prognosis of thermocoagulation or surgical resection, brain regions corresponding to selected channels of each participant were divided into 3 regions: epileptogenic zone (EZ), propagation zone (PZ), and noninvolved zone (NIZ). EI calculation was processed with AnyWave[23] (software available at http://meg.univ-amu.fr/wiki/AnyWave).

Table 1
Clinical characteristics of the participants

No./ Gender	Age at VNS Implantation/ Age at Enrollment	Etiology	MRI	Seizure Type	Seizure Onset	VNS Outcome	Treatment After SEEG Assessment (Engel Classification)
1/M	8/9.3	Missense mutation of DEPDC5 gene; Lennox-Gastaut syndrome	MRI negative	Tonic, spasm, myoclonic	Left hemisphere	Seizure frequency was reduced by about 50%, and status epilepticus happened more frequently when his VNS device was turned off.	Left hemisphere subtotal (IIIa)
2/M	5.6/6.8	MCD	Left temporo-parieto-occipital focal cortical dysplasia	Spasm, tonic, complex partial	Left temporo-parieto-occipita lobe	Seizure frequency was reduced by <25%; walking and language were slightly better than before.	Left temporo-parieto-occipital disconnection (Ia)
3/M	4/1.5	Infantile spasm; dysplasia of the left frontal and insular cortex	Left hemispheric volume reduction. Loss of gray white matter differentiation in left frontal lobe	Tonic, spasm, partial	Left hemisphere	Frequency of subtle seizure decreased by <25%; the duration of GTCS was shortened from 10 min–3 min.	Left frontal lobe disconnection (IVa)

(continued on next page)

Table 1
(continued)

No./ Gender	Age at VNS Implantation/ Age at Enrollment	Etiology	MRI	Seizure Type	Seizure Onset	VNS Outcome	Treatment After SEEG Assessment (Engel Classification)
4/M	3.8/8.2	Sequelae of encephalitis	Bilateral brain atrophy	Myoclonic, clonic, partial	Multiple lesions in both hemispheres, especially on the left.	The seizure frequency decreased by 90% at the sixth month of VNS therapy, but his seizure frequency began to increase gradually from the ninth month, and the current seizure frequency was about 30% lower than before VNS therapy.	RFTC in both hemispheres (Ia)
5/M	3.7/6.5	COL4A1 gene mutation; MCD	Abnormal shape of left frontal lobe and right parietal lobe, polycerebellar gyrus deformity with cerebral fissure deformity	Partial, spasm	Multiple lesions in both hemispheres.	No improvement in seizure frequency; slight improvement in cognition; being able to swallow solids.	RFTC in the left frontal lobe lesion and resection of the lesion in right parietal lobe (Ia)
6/M	4.2/5.3	Viral encephalitis	MRI negative	Tonic, complex partial	Bilateral fronto-temporo-insular lobe	No improvement in seizure frequency; the consciousness was recovered faster after GTCS than that before VNS, and the mouth twitching disappeared.	Left frontal lobe disconnection and left temporal lobectomy; RFTC in right frontal lobe, insular lobe, and temporal lobe (IIb)
7/M	8.3/10.7	Hypoglycemic encephalopathy; ulegyria in bilateral	Encephalopathy; ulegyria in bilateral	Partial	Multiple lesions in both hemispheres.	No improvement in seizure frequency.	RFTC in multiple lesions in both hemispheres (IIa)

8/M	1.5/2.3	Sequelae of acute necrotizing encephalopathy	Bilateral brain atrophy and bilateral hemispheric multifocal brain scar	Tonic-clonic, myoclonic	Multiple lesions in both hemispheres.	No improvement in seizure frequency	RFTC in multiple lesions in both hemispheres (IIIa)
9/M	1.6/2.9	TSC2 gene mutation; tuberous sclerosis complex	Many nodules of different sizes can be seen in both hemispheres.	Partial	Left frontal, parietal lobe, and right parietal lobe	No improvement in seizure frequency.	RFTC in left frontal, parietal lobe, and right parietal lobe (IIc)
10/M	4.5/5.8	FCD	Negative	Tonic, spam, partial	Medial side of left frontal lobe and paracentral lobule	More seizures in sleep; unable to walk with stimulation	RFTC in left frontal lobe and paracentral lobule (Ic)
11/F	0.5/4.1	MCD	Left hemisphere cortical dysplasia, right frontal polymicrogyria	Spasm, complex partial	Right frontal lobe	Frequency of spasm and subtle seizure both increased	RFTC in right frontal lobe (Ia)
12/M	3.3/5.7	Herpes simplex encephalitis	Bilateral insular, operculum, and mesial temporal lobe brain scar	Spasm, tonic, atypical absences, complex partial	Bilateral insular, operculum, and mesial temporal lobe	Frequency of spasm increased	Bilateral insular-operculum, and RFTC in mesial temporal lobe (IIb)

Abbreviations: F, female; FCD, focal cortical dysplasia; GTCS, generalized tonic-clonic seizures; M, male; MCD, malformations of cortical development; RFTC, radiofrequency thermocoagulation; SEEG, stereoelectroencephalography; VNS, vagus nerve stimulation.

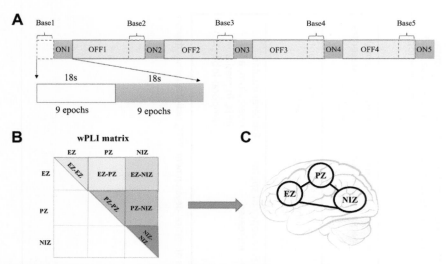

Fig. 1. (*A*) Timeline of the 5 acute stimulations. (*B*) The weighted phase lag index (wPLI) matrix. (*C*) The synchronization between and within epileptogenic zone (EZ), propagation zone (PZ), and noninvolved zone (NIZ) during the ON period and base period.

Synchronization Computation

All signals were segmented into 2-second epochs and band-pass filtered into 6 commonly used frequency bands: theta (3–7 Hz), alpha (7–13 Hz), beta 1 (14–20 Hz), beta 2 (21–30 Hz), low gamma (31–49 Hz), and high gamma (51–80 Hz). Synchronization of each band was assessed separately.

The weighted phase lag index (wPLI), proposed by Vinck and colleagues,[24] was used as an indicator of synchronization. The specific formula was as follows:

$$wPLI = \frac{|E\{\Im\{X\}sgn(\Im\{X\})\}|}{E\{|\Im\{X\}|\}}$$

where X was the cross spectrum of 2 time series, E was a function used to calculate the mean value, *sgn* was a function that extracts the sign of a real number, and $\Im\{X\}$ is the imaginary component of the cross spectrum.

The authors investigated all pairwise combinations of channels and built wPLI matrices accordingly (**Fig. 1**B). The mean wPLI values of all epochs for ON and base periods were assessed. Differences in synchronization matrices between ON and base periods were analyzed. The synchronization between and within the EZ, PZ, and NIZ during ON and base periods are given in **Fig. 1**C.

Segmentation, filtering, calculation of wPLI values, and statistical analysis were performed with custom scripts in MATLAB (MATrix LABoratory, MathWorks, Natick, Mass.).

Statistical Analysis

The wPLI values of each group during ON and base periods were tested for normality using Shapiro-Wilk test. If the normality test was passed, the wPLIs between ON period (including 5 wPLI: $wPLI_{ON1}$, $wPLI_{ON2}$, $wPLI_{ON3}$, $wPLI_{ON4}$, and $wPLI_{ON5}$) and base period (including 5 wPLI: $wPLI_{Base1}$, $wPLI_{Base2}$, $wPLI_{Base3}$, $wPLI_{Base4}$, and $wPLI_{Base5}$) were compared using paired t-test, otherwise, the Wilcoxon matched-pairs signed-rank test was employed.

At the group level, Kruskal-Wallis test was used and post hoc tests were performed using Dunn's multiple comparisons test in GraphPad Prism 9.5. A P-value less than 0.05 was considered to indicate a significant statistical difference.

RESULTS

Participants were ranked according to their clinical efficacy of VNS reported by their guardians from 1 to 12 in this study. The VNS efficacy of participant 1 was the best among all participants, whose seizure frequency was reduced by about 50% with VNS therapy, and status epilepticus happened more frequently when his VNS device was turned off. The seizure frequency of participants 2 and 3 decreased slightly with VNS therapy, both by less than 25%. The seizure frequency of the participant 4 decreased by 90% at the sixth month of VNS therapy, but his seizure frequency began to increase gradually from the ninth month. There was no improvement in seizure frequency of participants 5, 6, 7, 8, and 9 with VNS therapy. Participants 10, 11, and 12 were worse responders, whose seizure frequency increased when VNS devices were turned on.

Individual Changes in Synchronization Between and Within the Epileptogenic Zone, Propagation Zone, and Noninvolved Zone

Changes in synchronization within and between the EZ, PZ, and NIZ in all patients were investigated. As shown in **Fig. 2**, the authors found the following: (i) acute stimulation caused a significant decrease of wPLI values in participants 1, 2, 3, 4, and 5. However, the range of decrease differed among them. Significant decrease of wPLI values was seen in all regions in participant 1 when acute stimulation was applied. Meanwhile, it was only seen in 1 or 2 networks at beta 2 or gamma band in the other 3 participants; (ii) only participants 1, 2, 5, and 11 presented with significant changes of wPLI values in the EZ region during acute stimulation. The wPLI values of participants 1 and 2 decreased significantly at low-gamma band, and the wPLI values of participant 5 decreased significantly at high-gamma band. While the wPLI values of participant 11 increased significantly at low-gamma band; (iii) significant increase of wPLI values mainly were seen at the low-gamma and high-gamma bands of participants 11 and 12. The wPLI value within EZ at low-gamma band of participant 11 increased significantly, and the wPLI values within NIZ at low-gamma and high-gamma band of participant 12 increased significantly; and (iv) the proportion of networks with decreased wPLI value (including those with no statistical significance) in 36 networks (6 frequency bands $\times$ 6 networks) from participant 1 to participant 12 were 100%, 89%, 64%, 83%, 53%, 53%, 39%, 53%, 58%, 58%, 42%, and 17%, respectively.

The authors further explored the changes in the wPLI value of each channel at the low-gamma and high-gamma band during ON and base periods. **Figs. 3** and **4** show the average wPLI value of each channel during ON and base period at the low-gamma and high-gamma bands. The wPLI values of most channels were lower during ON period than base period in participant 1. The wPLI values of several channels increased in the participants with worse response to VNS, particularly in participant 12.

Group-level Changes in Synchronization Between and Within the Epileptogenic Zone, Propagation Zone, and Noninvolved Zone

Moreover, the authors compared the acute effect of VNS at the group level. All participants were divided into 3 groups based on their response to VNS: mild responder (MR, participant 1–participant 4) group, nonresponder (NR, participant 5–participant 9) group, and worse responder (WR, participant 10–participant 12) group. As shown in **Fig. 5**, there was a trend of increased $wPLI_{ON}$/$wPLI_{Base}$ ratios in the whole-brain network, EZ, EZ-PZ, and EZ-NIZ networks as the response changed from mild to worse. Although significant differences were found among the MR, NR, and WR groups, post hoc tests only revealed statistical differences between the MR and WR groups.

DISCUSSION

In this study, the authors explored the acute effects of VNS on the brain network synchronization of participants with different VNS efficacies and found that the complex antiepileptic effect of VNS was related to the desynchronization of the epileptogenic network as well as the desynchronization between the epileptogenic areas and other brain regions. In addition, the synchronization changes caused by acute VNS mainly occurred at high-frequency bands such as low-gamma (31–49 Hz) and high-gamma (51–80 Hz) bands, which may provide theoretic support for the search of potential biomarkers of VNS response.

Complex Desynchronization Mechanism of Vagus Nerve Stimulation

Taking advantage of the ability of SEEG to acquire signals from epileptogenic foci, the acute effect of VNS on the synchronization of the epileptogenic network and its propagation network were studied for the first time. Our results suggest that the ability of VNS to induce extensive desynchronization in the brain (especially epileptogenic regions) is essential to its antiepileptic efficacy. The epileptogenic network plays a pivotal role in the initiation and propagation of seizures. Modulating the synchronization of this network represents a promising approach to raise the seizure threshold, leading to a potential reduction in seizure frequency. The most widespread desynchronization caused by acute stimulation was observed in participant 1, who achieved the best response to VNS therapy among all participants. As the efficacy of VNS diminished in participants, its influence on the synchronization became less prominent. In some participants, VNS failed to elicit changes in the synchronization of networks. It is possible that the range of acute effects induced by VNS is related to whether the vagal ascending network still has extensive projections and the level of functional integrity of the vagal ascending network, such as the integrity of neurotransmitter systems correlated with VNS

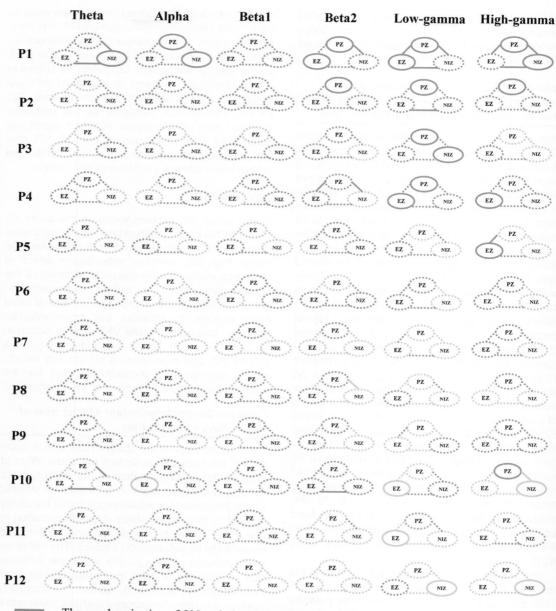

Theta | Alpha | Beta1 | Beta2 | Low-gamma | High-gamma

Fig. 2. Changes in synchronization within and between the epileptogenic zone (EZ), propagation zone (PZ), and noninvolved zone (NIZ) in all patients. The solid and dotted lines represent significant and nonsignificant differences, respectively.

The synchronization of ON period was significantly smaller than Base period (p<0.05)

The synchronization of ON period was smaller than Base period with no significant difference

The synchronization of ON period was significantly greater than Base period (p<0.05)

The synchronization of ON period was greater than Base period with no significant difference

mechanism,[25,26] or the abnormality of white matter bundles.

In addition to the extent of desynchronization of networks, specific frequency bands of brain activity affected by VNS was investigated in our study. Previous studies found that long-term VNS significantly modulated the synchronization of scalp EEG in the theta[27,28] and gamma (20–50 Hz)

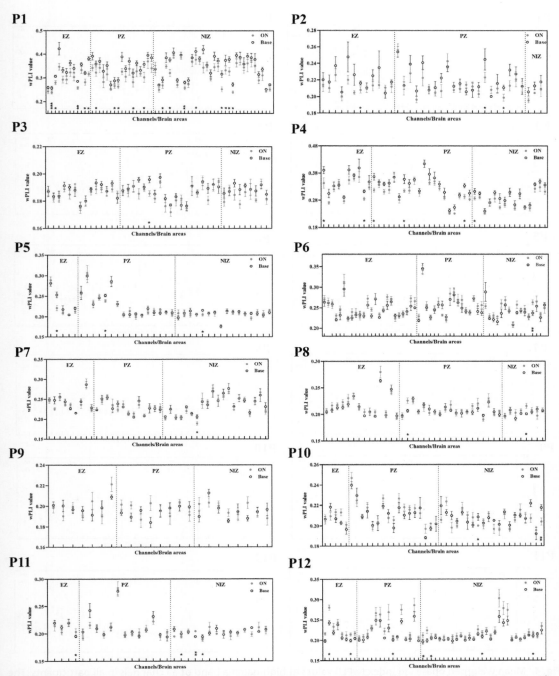

Fig. 3. Mean weighted phase lag index (wPLI) values at low-gamma band of all channels in all participants. The blue color represents the base period, and the red color indicates the ON period. *P<.05, **P<.01, ***P<.001.

bands.[28] For acute stimulation, Bodin and colleagues found that VNS could significantly decrease the synchronization of the broad band (1–48 Hz) and the delta band.[14] Sangare and colleagues revealed that short-term VNS significantly reduced the synchronization of the delta, theta,

and beta bands of VNS responders.[13] There was no consensus on the specific frequency band affected by VNS. Due to the low signal-to-noise ratio[29] and various kinds of artifacts contained in scalp EEG[30,31] most studies focused on analyzing lower frequency bands. There was only 1 study

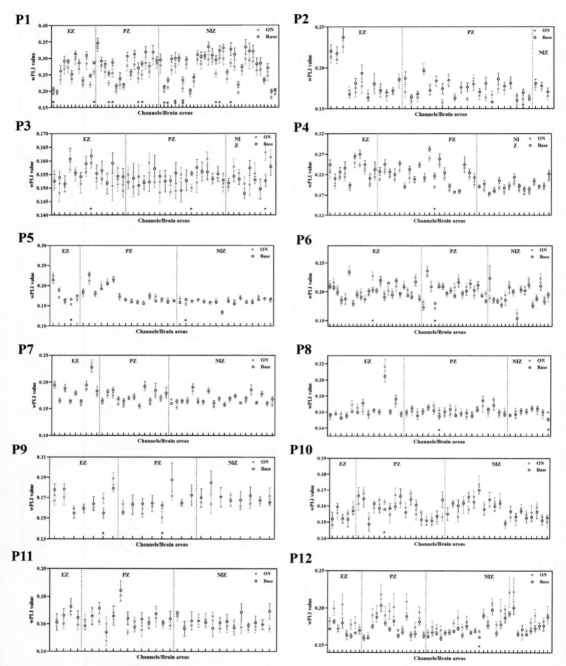

Fig. 4. Mean weighted phase lag index (wPLI) values at high-gamma band of all channels in all participants. The blue color represents the base period, and the red color indicates the ON period. *P<.05, **P<.01.

that included the analysis of the low-gamma band. In addition, whether signals in the high-frequency band (>30 Hz) can be obtained via scalp EEG remains controversial.[32] In our study, synchronization affected by acute stimulation was mainly at low and high gamma bands. This result provided evidence that VNS could induce synchronization changes at

gamma bands. The occurrence of gamma oscillation in the cerebral cortical network is attributed to the interaction between neurons and pyramidal cells in inhibitory γ-aminobutyric acid (GABA) energy efficiency and the abnormality of gamma oscillations has been reported in different neurologic diseases, such as epilepsy, autism, and

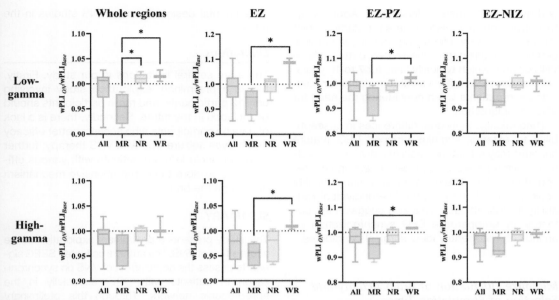

Fig. 5. Group-level comparisons of the acute effects of vagus nerve stimulation (VNS) in the low-gamma and high-gamma frequency bands. The asterisks (*) denote the results of pairwise comparisons in the post hoc test, indicating $P<.05$.

depression.[33,34] Previous studies have found that VNS can increase the $GABA_A$ receptor density (GRD), and the efficacy of VNS is significantly correlated with the normalization of GRD.[31]

The EEG desynchronization has been proposed as a possible mechanism underlying the antiepileptic effects of VNS in previous studies.[16,35–41] Through SEEG, our study also suggests that VNS likely exerts its anti-seizure effect through a widespread desynchronization effect, including epileptogenic networks, particularly at gamma band. Consequently, the reduction of cortical signal synchronization may prevent seizures and mitigate the spread of seizures within the brain. The specific brain structures affected by VNS should be explored through SEEG recordings in the future, such as the amygdala, hippocampus, and other nuclei in the limbic system, which will help to understand the anti-seizure mechanism of VNS more comprehensively.

Potential Biomarker of Vagus Nerve Stimulation Response

Presently, the clinical efficacy of VNS is primarily evaluated through self-reporting of changes in seizure frequency by patients or their guardians, which has inherent limitations in terms of subjectivity. Therefore, it is imperative to identify objective and measurable biomarkers that can reflect seizure severity, in order to facilitate the evaluation

of the effectiveness of VNS and other therapeutic interventions.

EEG changes have been observed to show parallelism or precedence with clinical outcomes, rendering them valuable as potential indicators of treatment response. Previous studies have shown that phase-based synchronization indicators are highly sensitive to the acute effect of VNS[13–15,27,42] and found significant VNS-induced changes of synchronization in VNS responders but not in nonresponders[13,14,27,42]. Invasive EEG studies showed that VNS induced acute effects in VNS nonresponders, including increasing h^2-based synchronization,[16] decreasing hemisphere synchronization in the alpha band during wakefulness and sleep,[15] and decreasing theta band synchronization during sleep.[15] However, these studies did not link these changes to VNS efficacy. According to our results, the acute effect of VNS varied greatly among individuals. In the authors' opinion, even after long-term therapy, VNS still has an acute effect on the brain activity of patients, but the degree and extent vary in individual cases with efficacy of VNS. This suggests the potential of synchronization as a biomarker for VNS response.

Investigating the effects of VNS on brain activity and exploring the relationship between VNS efficacy and electrophysiological characteristics can help to identify objective electrophysiological indicators for assessing the efficacy of VNS therapy and guiding parameter adjustments. Additionally, this approach may also serve as a starting point for preoperatively identifying the ideal surgical candidate. Considering the limited battery life of VNS device, which typically lasts for 7 to 10 years, such studies can offer valuable insights for clinicians and patients when considering the need for VNS reimplantation.

Theoretically, individual differences in susceptibility to external stimulus–induced EEG feature changes may reflect the basis of individual VNS efficacy differences between responders and nonresponders. The difference in this susceptibility could potentially underlie the inter-individual variability in VNS efficacy. This also suggests the potential for preoperative EEG synchronization as an indicator to identify ideal surgical candidates.

Minimize Fluctuation of Brain Activity and Selection of Stimulation Times

The effect of VNS is considered to be the result of both acute and long-term effects, but so far there is no fixed pattern for exploring the acute effects of VNS in both animal and human studies.

During SEEG analysis, the authors found that the impact of fluctuations of spontaneous brain activity cannot be ignored. To minimize this impact, the authors did not select SEEG data before the experiment as baseline, but specified the corresponding baseline period for each ON period.

In addition, it may take several VNS stimulations before the brain produces measurable electrophysiological responses, and the effects of VNS may gradually accumulate with ongoing stimulation. As VNS therapy progresses, the acute responses may become less noticeable or even disappear due to the emergence of a cumulative effect of VNS. The authors found that the most prominent acute responses were observed when VNS was administered 5 to 8 times. Therefore, the authors utilized data obtained from 5 stimulations for analyses. It is plausible that acute changes may not been detected in any of the patients if data of 20 stimulations were used. As for whether this optimal stimulation number of detecting acute effect is contingent on factors such as the neurophysiological profile of the patients, evaluation metrics, and stimulation parameters employed, it is worth further and comprehensive exploration. This underscores the imperative of determining the appropriate number of stimulations in relevant future studies.

Rational experimental design and data analysis methods are essential to explore the acute effects of VNS. Our study provides some reference for the experimental design of acute VNS studies in the future.

Limitations

There are several limitations in our study. Firstly, this is a preliminary exploration study involving only 12 participants, and more participants should be included in the future. Secondly, there is a lack of data on participants who achieve better efficacy or are even seizure-free with VNS therapy; further study will include more patients with various efficacies to explore the comprehensive mechanism of VNS on the brain.

SUMMARY

This study presents a preliminary exploration of the acute effect of VNS. The authors collected SEEG signals to assess the acute effect of VNS on synchronization in patients with DRE, especially in the epileptogenic network. Through this preliminary exploratory study, the authors found that the better the efficacy of VNS, the wider the spread of desynchronization assessed by wPLI at high-frequency bands caused by VNS. Future studies should focus on the association between the change in synchronization and the efficacy of VNS, exploring the possibility of synchronization as a biomarker for patient screening and parameter programming.

STATEMENT

The data that support the findings of this study, the specific *P* values, and more detailed methodologies (including the methods of selecting and grouping the channels, minimizing the fluctuation of brain activity, and selecting the stimulation times) are available from the corresponding author upon reasonable request.

CLINICAL CARE POINTS

- Individualized Parameter Programming: Tailoring VNS parameters based on the observed acute effects could enhance treatment efficacy.

- Clinicians should consider the correlation between desynchronization extent and VNS efficacy when programming parameters.

- Patient Screening Biomarkers: Clinicians should explore incorporating these biomarkers (synchronization changes, particularly in high-frequency bands) into the screening process for optimized patient selection.

ACKNOWLEDGMENTS

The authors would like to thank the entire team of researchers for their rigorous attitudes, professional skills, enthusiasm for the patients, and great efforts, including the nurses and staffs at Xiamen Humanity Hospital and Shenzhen Children's Hospital.

DISCLOSURE

The authors have nothing to disclose.

REFERENCES

1. LivaNova USA I. An Introduction to VNS Therapy® (English). 2021. Available at: https://www.livanova.com/epilepsy-vnstherapy/getmedia/36fdd6ad-1792-4139-9a81-d723b43fdc69/anz-vns-pt-intro-brochure.pdf.
2. Toffa DH, Touma L, El MT, et al. Learnings from 30 years of reported efficacy and safety of vagus nerve stimulation (VNS) for epilepsy treatment: A critical review. Seizure 2020;83:104–23.
3. Haneef Zulfi and Skrehot Henry C. Neurostimulation in generalized epilepsy: A systematic review and meta-analysis, Epilepsia, 64;(4):811-20.
4. Morris GL, Gloss D, Buchhalter J, et al. Evidence-based guideline update: vagus nerve stimulation for the treatment of epilepsy: report of the Guideline Development Subcommittee of the, American Academy of Neurology. Neurology 2013;81(16):1453–9.
5. Ben-Menachem E. Vagus-nerve stimulation for the treatment of epilepsy. Lancet Neurol 2002;1(8):477–82.
6. Elliott RE, Morsi A, Kalhorn SP, et al. Vagus nerve stimulation in 436 consecutive patients with treatment-resistant epilepsy: long-term outcomes and predictors of response. Epilepsy Behav 2011;20(1):57–63.
7. Henry TR. Therapeutic mechanisms of vagus nerve stimulation. Neurology 2002;59(6 Suppl 4):S3–14.
8. Raedt R, Clinckers R, Mollet L, et al. Increased hippocampal noradrenaline is a biomarker for efficacy of vagus nerve stimulation in a limbic seizure model. J Neurochem 2011;117(3):461–9.
9. De Herdt V, De Waele J, Raedt R, et al. Modulation of seizure threshold by vagus nerve stimulation in an animal model for motor seizures. Acta Neurol Scand 2010;121(4):271–6.
10. Henry TR, Votaw JR, Pennell PB, et al. Acute blood flow changes and efficacy of vagus nerve stimulation in partial epilepsy. Neurology 1999;52(6):1166–73.
11. Naritoku DK, Morales A, Pencek TL, et al. Chronic vagus nerve stimulation increases the latency of the thalamocortical somatosensory evoked potential. Pacing Clin Electrophysiol 1992;15(10 Pt 2):1572–8.
12. Workewych AM, Arski ON, Mithani K, et al. Biomarkers of seizure response to vagus nerve stimulation: A scoping review. Epilepsia 2020;61(10):2069–85.
13. Sangare A, Marchi A, Pruvost-Robieux E, et al. The effectiveness of vagus nerve stimulation in drug-resistant epilepsy correlates with vagus nerve stimulation-induced electroencephalography desynchronization. Brain Connect 2020;10(10):566–77.
14. Bodin C, Aubert S, Daquin G, et al. Responders to vagus nerve stimulation (VNS) in refractory epilepsy have reduced interictal cortical synchronicity on scalp EEG. Epilepsy Res 2015;113:98–103.
15. Ilyas A, Toth E, Pizarro D, et al. Modulation of neural oscillations by vagus nerve stimulation in posttraumatic multifocal epilepsy: case report. J Neurosurg 2018;1–7.
16. Bartolomei F, Bonini F, Vidal E, et al. How does vagal nerve stimulation (VNS) change EEG brain functional connectivity? Epilepsy Res 2016;126:141–6.
17. Schuerman WL, Nourski KV, Rhone AE, et al. Human intracranial recordings reveal distinct cortical activity patterns during invasive and non-invasive vagus nerve stimulation. Sci Rep 2021;11(1):22780.
18. Yokoyama R, Akiyama Y, Enatsu R, et al. The Immediate Effects of Vagus Nerve Stimulation in Intractable Epilepsy: An Intra-operative Electrocorticographic Analysis. Neurol Med -Chir 2020;60(5):244–51.
19. Chassoux F, Navarro V, Catenoix H, et al. Planning and management of SEEG. Neurophysiol Clin 2018;48(1):25–37.
20. Talairach J, Bancaud J, Szikla G, et al. [New approach to the neurosurgery of epilepsy. Stereotaxic methodology and therapeutic results. 1. Introduction and history]. Neurochirurgie 1974;20(Suppl 1):1–240.
21. Lagarde S, Roehri N, Lambert I, et al. Interictal stereotactic-EEG functional connectivity in refractory focal epilepsies. Brain 2018;141(10):2966–80.
22. Bartolomei F, Chauvel P, Wendling F. Epileptogenicity of brain structures in human temporal lobe epilepsy: a quantified study from intracerebral EEG. Brain 2008;131(Pt 7):1818–30.
23. Colombet B, Woodman M, Badier JM, et al. AnyWave: a cross-platform and modular software for visualizing and processing electrophysiological signals. J Neurosci Methods 2015;242:118–26.
24. Vinck M, Oostenveld R, van Wingerden M, et al. An improved index of phase-synchronization for electrophysiological data in the presence of volume-conduction, noise and sample-size bias. Neuroimage 2011;55(4):1548–65.
25. Aston-Jones G, Cohen JD. An integrative theory of locus coeruleus-norepinephrine function: adaptive gain and optimal performance. Annu Rev Neurosci 2005;28:403–50.

26. Fornai F, Ruffoli R, Giorgi FS, et al. The role of locus coeruleus in the antiepileptic activity induced by vagus nerve stimulation. Eur J Neurosci 2011;33(12):2169–78.

27. Fraschini M, Demuru M, Puligheddu M, et al. The reorganization of functional brain networks in pharmaco-resistant epileptic patients who respond to VNS. Neurosci Lett 2014;580:153–7.

28. Marrosu F, Santoni F, Puligheddu M, et al. Increase in 20-50 Hz (gamma frequencies) power spectrum and synchronization after chronic vagal nerve stimulation. Clin Neurophysiol 2005;116(9):2026–36.

29. Haufe S, DeGuzman P, Henin S, et al. Elucidating relations between fMRI, ECoG, and EEG through a common natural stimulus. Neuroimage 2018;179:79–91.

30. Islam MK, Rastegarnia A, Yang Z. Methods for artifact detection and removal from scalp EEG: A review. Neurophysiol Clin 2016;46(4–5):287–305.

31. Marrosu F, Serra A, Maleci A, et al. Correlation between GABA(A) receptor density and vagus nerve stimulation in individuals with drug-resistant partial epilepsy. Epilepsy Res 2003;55(1–2):59–70.

32. Michel CM, Murray MM. Discussing gamma. Brain Topogr 2009;22(1):1–2.

33. Struber D, Herrmann CS. Modulation of gamma oscillations as a possible therapeutic tool for neuropsychiatric diseases: A review and perspective. Int J Psychophysiol 2020;152:15–25.

34. Kayarian FB, Jannati A, Rotenberg A, et al. Targeting Gamma-Related Pathophysiology in Autism Spectrum Disorder Using Transcranial Electrical Stimulation: Opportunities and Challenges. Autism Res 2020;13(7):1051–71.

35. Chase MH, Sterman MB, Clemente CD. Cortical and subcortical patterns of response to afferent vagal stimulation. Exp Neurol 1966;16(1):36–49.

36. Chase MH, Nakamura Y, Clemente CD, et al. Afferent vagal stimulation: neurographic correlates of induced EEG synchronization and desynchronization. Brain Res 1967;5(2):236–49.

37. Carron R, Roncon P, Lagarde S, et al. Latest views on the mechanisms of action of surgically implanted cervical vagal nerve stimulation in epilepsy. Neuromodulation 2022;26(3):498–506.

38. Vespa S, Heyse J, Stumpp L, et al. Vagus nerve stimulation elicits sleep EEG desynchronization and network changes in responder patients in epilepsy. Neurotherapeutics 2021;18(4):2623–38.

39. Collins L, Boddington L, Steffan PJ, et al. Vagus nerve stimulation induces widespread cortical and behavioral activation. Curr Biol 2021;31(10):2088–98.e3.

40. Hachem LD, Wong SM, Ibrahim GM. The vagus afferent network: emerging role in translational connectomics. Neurosurg Focus 2018;45(3):E2.

41. Jaseja H. EEG-desynchronization as the major mechanism of anti-epileptic action of vagal nerve stimulation in patients with intractable seizures: clinical neurophysiological evidence. Med Hypotheses 2010;74(5):855–6.

42. Fraschini M, Puligheddu M, Demuru M, et al. VNS induced desynchronization in gamma bands correlates with positive clinical outcome in temporal lobe pharmacoresistant epilepsy. Neurosci Lett 2013;536:14–8.

Section III: Cutting Edge Technologies

Sensing-Enabled Deep Brain Stimulation in Epilepsy

Jimmy C. Yang, MD[a,b,*], Andrew I. Yang, MD[b], Robert E. Gross, MD, PhD[b,c]

KEYWORDS

• Neuromodulation • Deep brain stimulation • Epilepsy

KEY POINTS

- A new generation of deep brain stimulation devices allows for monitoring of local field potentials around the deep brain stimulator lead implant site.
- While data on local field potentials at deep brain stimulation sites have been adopted in a clinical capacity in movement disorders, its application in epilepsy is not yet well-defined.
- Specific biomarkers at deep brain stimulation sites will need to be identified in order to allow tracking of clinical response in patients with epilepsy.

INTRODUCTION

For patients with drug-resistant epilepsy who are not ideal candidates for resective or ablative procedures, neuromodulation has emerged as an important treatment option. The Stimulation of the Anterior Nucleus of the Thalamus in Epilepsy (SANTE) trial, published in 2010, demonstrated the efficacy of deep brain stimulation (DBS) of the anterior nucleus of the thalamus (ANT) in reducing seizure frequency.[1] Ultimately, in 2018, the United States Food and Drug Administration approved ANT DBS for the treatment of drug-resistant focal- onset epilepsy.

In both clinical trials and real-world reports, ANT DBS has proven to be effective a reducing seizure frequency as well as reducing rates of sudden unexpected death in epilepsy.[1–5] The SANTE randomized controlled trial demonstrated that after a randomized 3-month period of either stimulation on or off, subjects with stimulation on had a median 40.4% decrease in seizure frequency as compared to the control group that had a median 14.5% decrease in seizure frequency.[1] Long-term follow-up of subjects in the trial has revealed that at 7 years, participants had a median 75% seizure frequency reduction.[6] In addition, 9% of the subjects at the year 7 timepoint or at discontinuation were seizure free for greater than 6 months.[6] These findings have been similarly reflected in real-world studies.

However, while widespread adoption of ANT DBS for epilepsy has led to benefits for patients, clinicians have faced limitations with implementation of the technology. As patient reports of seizure frequency can be unreliable, clinicians have sought to better understand whether specific objective biomarkers can be used to track seizure activity. In addition, these biomarkers may also provide answers to another area of investigation, as to whether brain networks exhibit changes in response to stimulation. Recent clinical introduction of a device that can monitor local field potentials (LFPs) at the DBS electrode site may be able to provide clarity in these areas, though use of this

a Department of Neurological Surgery, The Ohio State University College of Medicine, Columbus, OH, USA;
b Department of Neurosurgery, Emory University, 1365 Clifton Road NE, Suite B6200, Atlanta, GA 30322, USA; c Department of Neurology, Emory University School of Medicine, 1365 Clifton Road NE, Suite B6200, Atlanta, GA 30322
* Corresponding author. Department of Neurological Surgery, The Ohio State University Wexner Medical Center, Center for Neuromodulation, 480 Medical Center Drive, Columbus, OH 43210.
E-mail address: Jimmy.Yang@osumc.edu

technology has largely been exploratory and anecdotal thus far.

ANTERIOR NUCLEUS OF THE THALAMUS INVOLVEMENT IN EPILEPSY NETWORKS

Characterization of epilepsy as a network disorder has led to hypothesis that the mechanism of action of ANT DBS lies in its ability to change pathologic connectivity, rather than interfering at seizure foci themselves. The ANT is believed to be connected to multiple areas of cortex via limbic circuits, primarily with its location within the circuit of Papez. While many of its connections are reciprocal, it receives cortical inputs from the retrosplenial cortex, the mammillary bodies via the mammillothalamic tracts, and the subiculum via the fornix, and its outputs reach the anterior cingulate, medial prefrontal lobe and subiculum.[7–9]

While the mechanisms of ANT DBS remain unknown, DBS can lead to both activation and inhibition of neural networks, depending on distance from the electrode and the underlying substrate, and DBS is thought to function by overriding neural circuitry or pathologic signaling.[9] Initial models have implicated the thalamus as either being directly recruited by cortical circuits, initiating seizure activity through excitatory thalamocortical networks, and/or propagating seizure activity to additional cortical regions through thalamocortical projections.[10,11]

Efforts to understand the neurophysiological role of the ANT in epilepsy have more recently used stereoelectroencephalography (SEEG) to sample the ANT to understand its connectivity with seizure onset zones. Supporting the hypothesis of the ANT's links to seizure onset zones in the hippocampus, a study by Yu and colleagues demonstrated that both hippocampal–thalamic and reciprocal thalamic–hippocampal evoked potentials can be seen.[12] Recent studies using SEEG approaches have also demonstrated that seizure activity can be detected at the ANT.[13–15]

ANT seizure activity may have unique properties based on its connectivity with seizure onset zones. One study that sampled the ANT in both temporal and extratemporal epilepsies demonstrated that in 83.3% of the 19 patients, the ANT was characterized as being involved in the seizure network.[13] This study also revealed different onset patterns at the ANT, in which the ANT could either be involved immediately at seizure onset or in a delayed fashion; interestingly, there was no clear difference between onset patterns of temporal versus extratemporal seizure onset zones.[13] In addition, different seizure types may have unique spectral features as they engage the ANT.[14]

Several studies have suggested that ANT stimulation can result in desynchronization of the epilepsy network. Initial studies investigating ANT involvement in seizure activity used surface *electroencephalography* (EEG) and suggested that ANT stimulation could induce changes in cortical networks.[16,17] In a SEEG-based study that sampled the ANT and the hippocampus, Yu and colleagues demonstrated that high-frequency stimulation of the ANT can result in desynchronization of the epileptic network.[12]

Based on these studies, seizure activity may be measured at the ANT, which would likely be reflected in changes in the power spectra, and network-based changes from ANT stimulation may potentially be detected. As a result, a DBS system that can record LFP ("sensing") may be of clinical utility.

DEEP BRAIN STIMULATION SENSING TECHNOLOGY IN EPILEPSY

The initial developement of DBS devices that could record LFPs from DBS electrode sites were investigational and used in research settings.[18,19] In the context of epilepsy, Gregg and colleagues used the investigational Medtronic Activa RC + S system and implanted DBS leads into the bilateral ANT and hippocampi in 4 subjects with temporal lobe epilepsy.[20] By analyzing interictal and ictal recordings from the ANT and examining different frequency bands, an optimal LFP-based seizure detector was determined to have a 7 Hz center frequency, 5 Hz bandwidth, and 10 second epoch duration.[20] However, the study was not designed to determine whether changes in LFP correlated with stimulation or clinical changes in seizure frequency, as the analyzed data were obtained during a baseline stimulation-off period.

The Medtronic Percept system was commercially introduced in 2020, making use of features previously restricted to investigational devices.[21] The device can monitor LFP signals across pairs of 2 contacts.[5] This bipolar referencing allows for sensing during stimulation, but only in cases of monopolar stimulation. The device has specific features that allow for live streaming of LFP activity.[22] While the device is able to store up to 60 days of data, these data are limited to average power of a pre-set 5 Hz frequency band over 10 min time windows.[22] Using these features, the Percept system may be able to detect changes in power spectra that correlate with seizure activity.[23] One report of responsive neurostimulation with leads implanted in the ANT demonstrated that seizure activity can be identified in the thalamus using an implanted device, which also supports the concept that LFP changes may be tracked chronically.[24]

Few studies have investigated the potential clinical relevance of the Percept system in epilepsy. An initial study that examined data from 1 epilepsy patient with the Percept system was able to perform broadband LFP recording during different types of seizures, which revealed unique signatures at specific frequencies.[25] In addition, when these frequencies were tracked over time, LFP power appeared to decrease when there was concomitant clinical improvement in seizure frequency.[25] However, while prior studies using the investigational system suggested 10 second epoch lengths as the optimal settings for detection, this is not feasible on the current generation of Percept systems.[5,20] In another report of 1 patient, LFP data from the Percept system were used to find unique signatures of the ANT in order to assist with electrode contact localization, which may inform the choice of the active (stimulating) contact during DBS programming.[26]

INSTITUTIONAL EXPERIENCE WITH DEEP BRAIN STIMULATION SENSING IN EPILEPSY

The authors' experience with sensing technology in epilepsy patients has been variable. Prior to programming, imaging is used to identify the contact closest to the junction of the ANT and the mammillothalamic tract for stimulation. The sensing contacts are the 2 surrounding this stimulating contact. Sensing is only possible with monopolar stimulation, and it is generally turned on at the time of implantation, prior to initiation of stimulation, at which time the frequency band selected for monitoring is the default 8 to 12 Hz band based on prior data from Medtronic.[27] During subsequent follow-up visits, interictal recordings can be streamed in clinic to identify patient-specific frequency bands that emerge as peaks in the power spectra displayed on the clinician tablet. Patients are also encouraged to use the device to mark seizure events, which trigger the device to compute and save power spectra from a 30 second segment of LFP data. Narrowband power that is continuously tracked by the device is also transferred to clinician tablets for review during follow-up visits.

The authors have observed varying success in identifying associations between changes in Percept tracked narrowband power at the default frequency band and clinical outcomes. In some patients, clinical benefit and narrowband device–averaged power appear to correlate (Fig. 1A), with a decrease in power being observed when clinical seizure frequency decreases. However, this has not been a consistent finding, as some patients who experience reductions in clinical seizure frequency have not had noteworthy trends in narrowband power (Fig. 1B).

In fact, there are multiple limitations associated with tracking narrowband power. First, the monitoring frequency band is initially arbitrarily selected, which may not be suitable in a heterogeneous

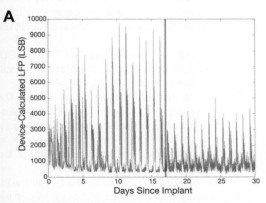

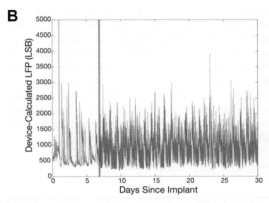

Fig. 1. Examples of Percept-calculated narrowband power. Sensing was turned on at the time of implantation, and red line indicated the timepoint at which stimulation was turned on. (A) Frequency band being monitored had a center frequency of 9.77 Hz. Stimulation was initiated at 1 mA amplitude, 90 μs pulse width, 145 Hz frequency, with cycled stimulation (1 minute on, 5 minutes off). After stimulation was turned on, the patient reported a 70% reduction in seizure frequency over baseline. Device-averaged narrowband power displayed a visible decrease in power of the tracked frequency band. (B) Frequency band being monitored had a center frequency of 8.79 Hz. Stimulation was initiated at 0.5 mA amplitude, 90 μs pulse width, 145 Hz frequency, with cycled stimulation (1 minute on, 5 minutes off). After stimulation was turned on, the patient reported a 50% reduction in seizure frequency over baseline. However, in this case, no visible change was seen in the power of the tracked frequency band. LFP, local field potential; LSB, least significant bit.[27,29,30]

disease process such as epilepsy. The optimal frequency band may in fact vary within the same patient (eg, across seizure types) and across patients (eg, depending on epilepsy type or coincident pathology). Second, the parameters that are used for chronically monitoring LFP signals (eg, temporal window of averaging, bandwidth) cannot be independently adjusted or configured. Third, identification of patient-specific frequency bands by simple visual inspection of power spectra, without statistical analysis, as displayed on the clinician tablet may be misleading. Fourth, current strategies for mitigating artifacts (eg, stimulation, patient motion, cardiac) remain limited.

Finally, seizures are characterized by complex changes across multiple frequency bands through their time course,[28] and tracking oscillatory power in a singular narrowband may not be a reliable and generalizable indicator of seizure activity. Non-oscillatory components of thalamic LFP activity, such as the 1/f slope of the power spectra, are alternative features that are being explored at authors' institution (Yang A, et al; under review). Although aperiodic LFP features such as the 1/f slope cannot be continuously tracked by the current Percept device, narrowband activity in the lower frequencies, which can be tracked by the device, may represent covarying metrics.

SUMMARY

Ultimately, ongoing questions remain regarding whether it will be possible to create a closed-loop DBS system that is able to not only monitor epileptiform activity at DBS sites and but also implement changes in therapy. While the Percept system allows interpretation of recorded narrowband power, it does not alter therapy based on these data and relies on clinician interpretation. As a result, the system is not truly closed-loop at this time.[5] Further work will be required to better understand how thalamic activity may be used as a biomarker of seizure activity and how it may correlate with clinical response.

CLINICS CARE POINTS

- There is currently no clear set of monitoring parameters that allow for tracking of clinical response, and prior research has included parameters that are currently not supported by the clinical device.
- Tracked local field potential power may not necessarily correlate with a patient's clinical response.

- Offline analysis of a patient's interictal and ictal local field potentials may be required to optimally identify features that correlate with ictal activity.

DISCLOSURE

Dr R.E. Gross serves as a consultant to Medtronic, which manufactures products related to the research described in this article, and receives compensation for these services. Additionally, Dr R.E. Gross receives research support for clinical trials from Medtronic. The terms of these arrangements have been reviewed and approved by Emory University in accordance with conflict-of-interest policies. The other authors declare no conflicts of interested related to this article.

REFERENCES

1. Fisher R, Salanova V, Witt T, et al. Electrical stimulation of the anterior nucleus of thalamus for treatment of refractory epilepsy. Epilepsia 2010;51(5): 899–908.
2. Peltola J, Colon AJ, Pimentel J, et al. Deep Brain Stimulation of the Anterior Nucleus of the Thalamus in Drug Resistant Epilepsy in the MORE Multicenter Patient Registry. Neurology 2023. https://doi.org/10.1212/WNL.0000000000206887.
3. Salanova V, Witt T, Worth R, et al. Long-term efficacy and safety of thalamic stimulation for drug-resistant partial epilepsy. Neurology 2015;84(10):1017–25.
4. Fasano A, Eliashiv D, Herman ST, et al. Experience and consensus on stimulation of the anterior nucleus of thalamus for epilepsy. Epilepsia 2021;62(12): 2883–98.
5. Simpson HD, Schulze-Bonhage A, Cascino GD, et al. Practical considerations in epilepsy neurostimulation. Epilepsia 2022;63(10):2445–60.
6. Salanova V, Sperling MR, Gross RE, et al. The SANTÉ study at 10 years of follow-up: Effectiveness, safety, and sudden unexpected death in epilepsy. Epilepsia 2021;62(6):1306–17.
7. Child ND, Benarroch EE. Anterior nucleus of the thalamus. Neurology 2013;81(21):1869–76.
8. Takebayashi S, Hashizume K, Tanaka T, et al. The Effect of Electrical Stimulation and Lesioning of the Anterior Thalamic Nucleus on Kainic Acid–Induced Focal Cortical Seizure Status in Rats. Epilepsia 2007;48(2):348–58.
9. van der Vlis TAMB, Schijns OEMG, Schaper FLWVJ, et al. Deep brain stimulation of the anterior nucleus of the thalamus for drug-resistant epilepsy. Neurosurg Rev 2019;42(2):287–96.
10. Bertram EH, Zhang DX, Mangan P, et al. Functional anatomy of limbic epilepsy: a proposal for central

synchronization of a diffusely hyperexcitable network. Epilepsy Res 1998;32(1–2):194–205.

11. Bertram EH, Mangan PS, Zhang D, et al. The Midline Thalamus: Alterations and a Potential Role in Limbic Epilepsy. Epilepsia 2001;42(8):967–78.

12. Yu T, Wang X, Li Y, et al. High-frequency stimulation of anterior nucleus of thalamus desynchronizes epileptic network in humans. Brain 2018;141(9): 2631–43.

13. Yan H, Wang X, Yu T, et al. The anterior nucleus of the thalamus plays a role in the epileptic network. Ann Clin Transl Neur 2022;9(12):2010–24.

14. Pizarro D, Ilyas A, Chaitanya G, et al. Spectral organization of focal seizures within the thalamotemporal network. Ann Clin Transl Neur 2019;6(9):1836–48.

15. Ilyas A, Toth E, Chaitanya G, et al. Ictal high-frequency activity in limbic thalamic nuclei varies with electrographic seizure-onset patterns in temporal lobe epilepsy. Clin Neurophysiol 2022;137: 183–92.

16. Hodaie M, Wennberg RA, Dostrovsky JO, et al. Chronic Anterior Thalamus Stimulation for Intractable Epilepsy. Epilepsia 2002;43(6):603–8.

17. Zumsteg D, Lozano AM, Wennberg RA. Rhythmic cortical EEG synchronization with low frequency stimulation of the anterior and medial thalamus for epilepsy. Clin Neurophysiol 2006;117(10):2272–8.

18. Jimenez-Shahed J. Device profile of the percept PC deep brain stimulation system for the treatment of Parkinson's disease and related disorders. Expert Rev Med Devic 2021;18(4):319–32.

19. Stanslaski S, Afshar P, Cong P, et al. Design and Validation of a Fully Implantable, Chronic, Closed-Loop Neuromodulation Device with Concurrent Sensing and Stimulation. Ieee T Neur Sys Reh 2012;20(4):410–21.

20. Gregg NM, Marks VS, Sladky V, et al. Anterior nucleus of the thalamus seizure detection in ambulatory humans. Epilepsia 2021;62(10):e158–64.

21. Frey J, Cagle J, Johnson KA, et al. Past, Present, and Future of Deep Brain Stimulation: Hardware, Software, Imaging, Physiology and Novel Approaches. Front Neurol 2022;13:825178.

22. Worrell GA, Kremen V. Neurostimulation for Epilepsy, 2023, 215-227. doi: 10.1016/b978-0-323-91702-5.00 009-8.

23. Fisher R. Neurostimulation for Epilepsy. 2023;133–159.

24. Elder C, Friedman D, Devinsky O, et al. Responsive neurostimulation targeting the anterior nucleus of the thalamus in 3 patients with treatment-resistant multifocal epilepsy. Epilepsia Open 2019;4(1):187–92.

25. Fasano A, Gorodetsky C, Paul D, et al. Local Field Potential-Based Programming: A Proof-of-Concept Pilot Study. Neuromodulation Technology Neural Interface 2021;25(2):271–5.

26. Lopes EM, Rego R, Rito M, et al. Estimation of ANT-DBS Electrodes on Target Positioning Based on a New PerceptTM PC LFP Signal Analysis. Sensors Basel Switz 2022;22(17):6601.

27. Stypulkowski PH, Stanslaski SR, Jensen RM, et al. Brain Stimulation for Epilepsy – Local and Remote Modulation of Network Excitability. Brain Stimul 2014;7(3):350–8.

28. Grinenko O, Li J, Mosher JC, et al. A fingerprint of the epileptogenic zone in human epilepsies. Brain 2017;141(1):117–31.

29. Afshar P, Khambhati A, Stanslaski S, et al. A translational platform for prototyping closed-loop neuromodulation systems. Front Neural Circuits 2013;6:117.

30. Stypulkowski PH, Stanslaski SR, Giftakis JE. Modulation of hippocampal activity with fornix Deep Brain Stimulation. Brain Stimul 2017;10(6):1125–32.

Utility of Chronic Intracranial Electroencephalography in Responsive Neurostimulation Therapy

Ankit N. Khambhati, PhD

KEYWORDS

- Responsive neurostimulation • Direct electrical stimulation • Closed loop stimulation
- Intracranial EEG • Electrocorticography • Chronic neural recordings • Focal seizures

KEY POINTS

- Responsive neurostimulation (RNS) therapy utilizes a closed loop design to continuously sense intracranial electroencephalography (iEEG) signals and deliver electrical stimulation to the brain.
- Algorithms integrated in the RNS System are programmed to detect seizure onset patterns and to trigger responsive stimulation and abort the seizure.
- Storage of iEEG recordings and hourly counts of detection and stimulation events by the RNS system yields a chronic dataset that can help configure device parameters.
- Offline quantitative analyses of stored data are beginning to reveal insights into acute and chronic mechanisms of RNS therapy.
- Chronic datasets from the RNS System can enable exploratory research of novel biomarkers to prognosticate clinical outcome and rapidly optimize device algorithms.

INTRODUCTION

Nearly 20 million people with epilepsy suffer from seizures that are poorly controlled by medication.[1] For many of these individuals, seizures originate from 1 or more focal areas within the brain and will often spread to surrounding tissue, momentarily impacting function in otherwise normal brain regions.[2] Surgical treatments that destroy brain tissue underlying seizures, such as resection[3] or ablation,[4] can be highly effective but are irreversible and carry risk of neurologic deficits. In patients for whom removal of brain tissue is not an option, a reversible alternative for seizure control has emerged in medical devices that are implanted chronically and deliver therapeutic electrical stimulation pulses to discrete anatomic structures within a patient's epileptic brain network.

To best target the seizure network and tailor stimulation therapy for an individual,[5] many options exist—Food and Drug Administration–approved devices range from either open-loop systems,[6] such as in vagus nerve stimulation (VNS) and deep brain stimulation (DBS), where stimulation is applied at fixed intervals, or closed loop systems,[6,7] such as in the Responsive Neurostimulation System (NeuroPace Inc. RNS System; hereafter "RNS System"), where stimulation is triggered based on the presence of a detected biomarker. Stimulation therapies can be highly effective in some patients, with seizure frequency

Department of Neurosurgery, Weill Institute for Neurosciences, University of California, San Francisco, Joan and Sanford I. Weill Neurosciences Building, 1651 4th Street, 671C, San Francisco, CA 94158, USA
E-mail address: ankit.khambhati@ucsf.edu
Twitter: ankhambhati (A.N.K.)

Neurosurg Clin N Am 35 (2024) 125–133
https://doi.org/10.1016/j.nec.2023.09.004
1042-3680/24/© 2023 Elsevier Inc. All rights reserved.

reductions up to 63% for VNS[8] and up to 75% for DBS[9–11] and RNS[12–14] over long-term treatment. Yet, for most patients, treatments are palliative— patients rarely experience continuous seizure freedom for periods longer than 1 year[8,11,13] and clinical responses are often slow, highly variable, and difficult to predict.[14] A critical barrier toward improved outcomes is that rational mechanisms of effective stimulation therapy and biomarkers indicative of treatment response are elusive.

Tracking of chronic brain network physiology alongside neurostimulation therapy may help optimize treatment for individual patients. Advancements in neurotechnology have made possible the additional capability to read-out brain activity signals chronically using the same devices used to deliver stimulation treatment.[15] Read-out of chronic intracranial electroencephalography (iEEG) is rapidly emerging as an important tool in the practitioner's arsenal. Presently, the RNS System is one of only 2 approved devices for epilepsy that stores iEEG recordings.[16] In this review, the authors focus on the utility of chronic iEEG recordings in optimizing responsive neurostimulation (RNS) therapy.

DESIGN OF THE RESPONSIVE NEUROSTIMULATION SYSTEM

The RNS System was conceptualized on the premise that a seizure can be aborted early by delivering responsive electrical stimulation directly to the epileptic focus.[17] To achieve this goal, the RNS System (**Fig. 1**A) utilizes a bidirectional neural sensing and stimulation interface spanning a cranially implanted neurostimulator and 2 four-contact leads (depth and/or subdural strip electrodes).[18] The neurostimulator continuously senses a total of 4 channels of bipolar-referenced iEEG from the leads and monitors the iEEG signal for patterns, or biomarker, of epileptic activity. If a signal pattern satisfies clinician-defined threshold criteria, the neurostimulator delivers electrical stimulation pulses to the brain via the leads. Device parameters that specify how the implanted neurostimulator should sense biomarkers and deliver stimulation are configured using an external RNS Tablet programmer and telemetry wand. The RNS System allows the clinician-user to configure signal pattern detectors,[18] including line length, area, and bandpass, that reflect the biomarker of epileptic activity used to trigger stimulation. Stimulation parameters, including amplitude, pulse width, frequency, charge density, and any configuration of electrode contacts (monopolar or bipolar), may also be defined.

CHRONIC RECORDING AND STORAGE OF NEUROSTIMULATOR DATA

Ongoing patient and therapy performance data are tracked and temporarily stored on the implanted neurostimulator and must be periodically downloaded to the Patient Data Management System (PDMS) by the patient using a remote monitor and wand.[18] The RNS System continuously senses up to 4 channels of the iEEG signal at 250 Hz and can store the following types of data (**Fig. 1**B): (1) raw, time-limited recordings of iEEG signals and (2) timings of detected events.

Raw Intracranial Electroencephalography Recordings

Storage of an iEEG recording is not continuous and must be triggered by 1 of the following events: (i) a swipe of the telemetry wand near the neurostimulator by the patient, (ii) saturation of the recording amplifier on the neurostimulator due to a high-amplitude event, (iii) detection of a clinician-defined signal pattern (typically an electrographic signature signifying the start of a seizure[19]), or (iv) pre-defined, or "scheduled", times of the day. A qualifying event trigger will result in storage of the recorded iEEG for a user-defined length of time before the trigger and a user-defined length of time after the trigger. Devices may be configured to trigger iEEG recordings during detected epileptiform events to sample the seizure state[20,21] and during scheduled times of day to sample the non-seizure, or "interictal", state.[22–24]

Memory limitations must be considered when configuring the RNS System to store raw iEEG recordings.[24] First, the maximum duration of a single iEEG recording spanning the pre-trigger and post-trigger period is typically 90 seconds. Second, limited memory slots onboard the neurostimulator device constrain the number of individual iEEG recordings that may be stored between each data download period. Third, the clinician may configure a priority list for storing each type of iEEG recording trigger; and events containing detected epileptiform activity typically receive greater priority than other event types. Thus, the sampling of interictal iEEG recordings over time may be impacted by the amount of epileptiform activity detected or by the frequency of data downloading.[24] These sampling biases should be considered during post-hoc analysis and interpretation of chronic iEEG data stored by the RNS System.

Detection Events

Through its continuous sensing and monitoring capabilities, the RNS System also detects, tabulates,

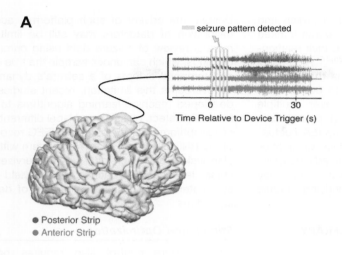

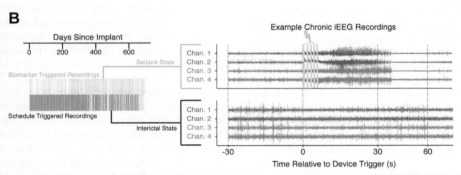

Fig. 1. Chronicity of neural recordings stored by the RNS System. (*A*) (*left*) Schematic of the RNS System comprised of a cranially implanted neurostimulator (*gray*) and 2 intracranial leads consisting of 8 electrodes contacts designed to record iEEG activity and deliver electrical stimulation. (*right*) Example of a raw iEEG signal recording (4 bipolar channels) and accompanying stimulation triggered by the device after a detected seizure onset pattern (*yellow*). (*B*) (*left*) Distribution of chronic data collected in an individual implanted with the RNS System over 600 days; each vertical line reflects an individual iEEG recording triggered either by the detection of a seizure onset biomarker (*orange*) or by scheduled time of day (*black*). (*right*) Each event triggered by the RNS System resulted in the storage of a brief iEEG recording. Recordings triggered by a biomarker detection tend to reflect the seizure state (*top*) and those triggered according to a schedule tend to reflect the interictal state (*bottom*). iEEG, intracranial electroencephalography; RNS, responsive neurostimulation. (*From* Khambhati AN, Shafi A, Rao VR, Chang EF. Long-term brain network reorganization predicts responsive neurostimulation outcomes for focal epilepsy. Sci Transl Med. 2021;13(608):eabf6588. Reprinted with permission from AAAS.)

and tracks the occurrence of clinician-defined events in the iEEG signal. An event occurs when the iEEG signal exhibits a pattern that passes amplitude and duration criteria configured by the clinician. Tabulation of the detected event by the neurostimulator entails storage of the following data: (i) which of the user-defined patterns were detected, (ii) whether the event was accompanied by responsive stimulation, and (iii) whether the detected signal pattern is sustained beyond a user-defined duration, termed a 'long episode'. A common practice is to use the long episode as a surrogate marker for electrographic seizures by defining the duration threshold as the minimum duration of the patient's seizures.[19,25,26] Detection

events that are not prolonged and fail to meet the duration criteria are typically considered to be discharges that reflect interictal epileptiform activity (IEA).[25] Event occurrences are aggregated and stored by the neurostimulator on an hourly basis. If data are downloaded frequently, then the hourly event counts can provide a continuous read-out of the fluctuating rate of detected epileptiform activity.[25] Indeed, the rate of detected events will depend on sensitivity and specificity of the signal pattern detector thresholds configured by the programmer. Thus, a key step in post-hoc analysis of detection event count data is to treat and process data collected during each period of constant detector settings separately.[25]

Recent studies have examined circadian and multiday fluctuations in IEA event counts tracked chronically by the RNS System and their relationship to electrographic seizures.[25,27] A seminal finding from that body of work is that electrographic seizures are more likely to occur when IEA fluctuates more frequently over multiple days.[25] Subsequent studies using probabilistic models demonstrated that multiday IEA fluctuations could reliably forecast the risk of electrographic seizures up to 5 days in advance.[28,29] Thus, an additional clinically relevant signal may be harnessed in count data underlying chronic biomarker detection events.

ROLE OF CHRONIC DATA IN THERAPY OPTIMIZATION

Despite nearly 2 decades of real-world experience with implantable devices, the mechanism of effective RNS therapy is a 'black box'. Rational tuning of the closed loop strategy (**Fig. 2**A) often requires that the clinician participate in an outer optimization loop to tune device parameters manually and periodically—much like the dosing of antiepileptic medication. Patient electrophysiology, biomarker, and stimulation data derived from PDMS may provide critical feedback to the practitioner and help guide parameter selection.

Biomarker Identification

Identification of a biomarker for closed loop seizure control is a critical first step in optimizing therapy. The current theoretic model underlying RNS therapy suggests that stimulation should be delivered during early detection of the patient's electrographic seizures[19] (**Fig. 2**B). Detectors with high sensitivity or low specificity may reduce the ability to accurately distinguish electrographic seizures from background activity or IEA.[25] In the context of the closed loop model, poorly timed or imprecise stimulation delivery may reduce the effectiveness of stimulation for optimal seizure control.[30] Chronic iEEG recordings stored during detected events may be manually reviewed offline within PDMS to evaluate the performance of the programmed detector. Signal processing algorithms that process the raw iEEG recordings and extract frequency spectrum characteristics of the signal may enhance a patient's electrographic seizure fingerprint and inform initial tuning or periodic retuning of the detector settings.[20,31] Visualization and simulation platforms[30,32] for tuning signal pattern detectors and detector thresholds using the existing repository of a patient's iEEG recordings could improve accuracy and timing of detectors that trigger responsive stimulation.

Despite the advent of such platforms, accurate calibration of detectors may still be limited by manual review of seizure data using chronic recordings, which can under-sample the true spatial and temporal extents of a seizure's dynamics.[33] To overcome this limitation, recent studies have developed machine learning algorithms to automatically detect, classify, and label different types of epileptiform activity in chronic iEEG recordings of the RNS System.[21,31,34,35] In tandem with clinician insight and oversight, semi-supervised machine learning approaches could yield more automated and objective calibration of detector algorithms.

Stimulation Optimization

Acute seizure control also requires periodic adjustment of electrical stimulation parameters. Best practices and recommended strategies for manual tuning of stimulation parameters are currently based on generalized, population-level data from pivotal trial and real-world outcome studies,[13,14] acute experimental studies,[36–38] and anecdotal experience.[32] Stimulation parameters are typically adjusted based on outcomes reported by the patient in their seizure diary,[39] and more recently their electrographic seizures[40] over prolonged clinic visit intervals.[13] This infrequent read-out of clinical outcome impedes more rapid parameter optimization and may contribute to the delay in maximal therapeutic benefit reported in the clinical trial.[13,14] Unfortunately, methods for automated, objective, and personalized optimization of responsive stimulation parameters do not currently exist. Limited understanding of the effects of stimulation on epileptiform activity hinders rational parameter selection based on neural mechanisms. A biomarker-driven approach to calibrate devices and track outcomes could help accelerate the efficacy of RNS therapy.

Biomarkers of therapy effectiveness

An emerging research trend involves reverse engineering the current RNS approach to understand the physiologic basis behind effective therapy. Chronic iEEG recordings provide a rare opportunity to trace biomarkers of treatment response alongside stimulation therapy and seizure relief. This framework has already yielded key insights of the effects of RNS on the brain. First, a restructuring of iEEG signal patterns during seizures was found to be a strong indicator of favorable clinical outcome.[20,21] Second, changes in brain network activity and connectivity may predict therapy effectiveness.[22–24,41,42] Separately, recent studies have also identified utility of mapping brain network

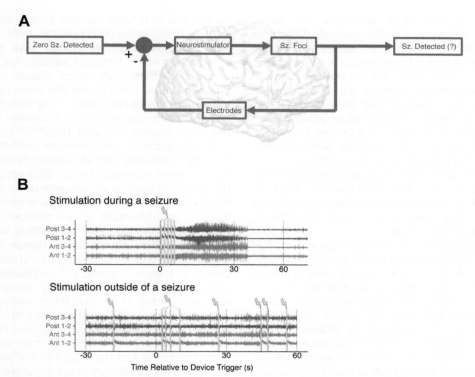

Fig. 2. Optimizing closed loop algorithms for responsive seizure control. (*A*) Conceptual and simplified diagram of the closed loop design employed by the RNS System. First, the desired state of zero electrographic seizures is defined by the practitioner. Second, the desired state is compared against the output of a seizure pattern detector. Third, discrepancy between the measured state and desired state is fed to the neurostimulator. Fourth, the neurostimulator delivers responsive electrical stimulation to seizure foci in the brain. Fifth, the system continues to evaluate whether the desired state has been achieved and the therapy loop is closed. (*B*) Therapy performance may be evaluated based on chronic iEEG recordings stored by the RNS System. (*top*) Pattern detectors correctly trigger stimulation during the start of a seizure. However, stimulation may have been ineffective at abating the seizure. (*bottom*) Pattern detectors with high sensitivity and poor specificity for seizures deliver several rounds of stimulation in response to presumed seizure activity. Detection and stimulation parameters may be adjusted empirically based on the iEEG recordings. iEEG, intracranial electroencephalography; RNS, responsive neurostimulation.

connectivity prior to implantation of the RNS System to predict eventual clinical response.[43,44] Third, actively measuring acute changes in brain activity following individual RNS events may help guide parameter selection.[45,46] Together, the current research evaluating biomarkers of therapy effectiveness suggests that clinically meaningful effects of RNS carry over across seizures and into the interictal period, which is free from stimulation. Features of the iEEG signal measured in these studies were computed using brief recordings less than 2 minutes in duration, which may be measured more quickly and frequently than the conventional seizure tracking approach to therapy optimization. Indeed, existing studies in this area have only evaluated these biomarkers in the context of clinical outcomes. Future studies will need to evaluate the sensitivity and dynamics of

seizure and interictal biomarkers in response to different stimulation parameters.

Alternate paradigms of the closed loop approach

Discovery of novel biomarkers of clinical response to neurostimulation therapy has spurred new mechanistic models that explain how RNS controls seizures. One theory holds that chronic RNS during seizure and interictal brain states drives brain network plasticity that gradually impedes seizure generation and seizure frequency.[20,24,32] While it has been proposed that plasticity is an essential component of effective RNS therapy,[32] the mechanistic driver of this plasticity remains elusive. One potential model may posit that repeated abatement of seizures through responsive stimulation remodels the brain network. Yet, another model contends that abundant stimulation outside of seizures and during the interictal period is responsible for therapeutic plasticity.[24] At present, it is not possible to evaluate and directly compare the 2 hypotheses because the detectors that trigger stimulation are conventionally programmed to maximize discriminability of the onset of a seizure over other interictal activity. A future study evaluating the clinical effectiveness of tuning device detectors to seizures in comparison to biomarkers of plasticity could answer this open question and provide further insight into the interaction effects between biomarkers, responsive stimulation, and network physiology.

A separate mechanistic theory supports the hypothesis that stimulation modulates rhythmic fluctuations of IEA[27] and, consequently, impacts seizure risk.[47] Indeed, a closed loop biomarker of seizure risk may be of significant value for RNS. A recent study examined the impact of RNS on seizure risk and found that the effectiveness of different stimulation parameters is dependent, in part, on whether stimulation is delivered while the patient is in a state of high seizure risk or low seizure risk.[48] This finding defies the assumption that a single stimulation parameter is sufficient for optimal seizure control and demonstrates the potential utility for multiple biomarker detectors—one that relays seizure risk and another that relays brain state—that operate concurrently. Unlike current approaches that rely on infrequent assessment of seizure counts, seizure risk forecasts provide a continuous estimate of seizure likelihood[49] that may be used to rapidly titrate stimulation parameters across the high-dimensional search space.[50]

Mechanistic theories that posit a relationship between effectiveness of RNS therapy and neuroplasticity or seizure risk modulation are still in their infancy. However, it is tempting to speculate a possible relationship between these 2 physiologic processes. Chronic iEEG recordings may be synchronized with IEA count data to study potential interaction effects between brain network plasticity and seizure risk.[51,52] Nonetheless, using either data modality to inform a biomarker for RNS would be a significant departure from the contemporary approach of optimizing therapy based on sparse measures of seizure occurrence.

ADJUNCTIVE APPLICATIONS OF CHRONIC DATA

Outside of its utility as a monitoring tool for seizure control, data from the RNS System have contributed to research across several domains of clinical and basic neuroscience. In focal epilepsy, chronic iEEG recordings have helped localize seizures,[53] lateralize seizures for resective surgery,[54] quantify neural effects of antiepileptic drugs,[55] and model the time-course of the device implantation effect.[22] The RNS System has also been used implanted in tandem (off-label) with anterior thalamic DBS[56,57] and with VNS in 2 novel multi-device setups for distributed network monitoring and stimulation in epilepsy. Beyond focal epilepsy, chronic iEEG recordings from the RNS System are also now being studied in clinical trials for idiopathic generalized epilepsy,[58] post-traumatic stress disorder,[59] and major depressive disorder.[60,61] Multiple areas of human cognitive neuroscience research have leveraged chronic iEEG to study neural representations of speech,[62] memory,[63] and spatial navigation.[64] RNS enables more longitudinal research studies in an ambulatory setting than was previously possible with human intracranial studies in the epilepsy monitoring unit. The unified ecosystem of the RNS System may help promote integration and translation of methods and findings between different areas of human neuroscience and inspire new research directions and approaches in epilepsy.

SUMMARY

RNS is a powerful tool for delivering personalized, chronic treatment to individuals with drug-resistant, focal epilepsy. Despite the "black box" nature of neurostimulation, RNS is highly effective at reducing seizures. Chronic electrophysiology and therapy data stored by the RNS System can help refine device parameters. Emerging research avenues may disentangle complex relationships between stimulation, brain network physiology, and clinical outcomes to maximize benefits and accelerate efficacy to the broader patient population with focal epilepsy.

CLINICS CARE POINTS

- Responsive neurostimulation therapy may reduce seizure frequency by up to 75%.
- Therapy effectiveness improves over time.
- Chronic neural recordings can help manually tune device parameters.
- Devices are programmed to discriminate seizures from background brain activity.

DISCLOSURE

The authors have nothing to disclose.

REFERENCES

1. French JA. Refractory epilepsy: Clinical overview. Epilepsia 2007;48:3–7.
2. Rosenow F, Lüders H. Presurgical evaluation of epilepsy. Brain 2001;124(9):1683–700.
3. Kwan P, Schachter SC, Brodie MJ. Drug-resistant epilepsy. N Engl J Med 2011;365(10):919–26.
4. Medvid R, Ruiz A, Komotar RJ, et al. Current applications of MRI-guided laser interstitial thermal therapy in the treatment of brain neoplasms and epilepsy: a radiologic and neurosurgical overview. Am J Neuroradiol 2015;36(11):1998–2006.
5. Piper RJ, Richardson RM, Worrell G, et al. Towards network-guided neuromodulation for epilepsy. Brain 2022;145(10):3347–62.
6. Markert MS, Fisher RS. Neuromodulation-science and practice in epilepsy: vagus nerve stimulation, thalamic deep brain stimulation, and responsive neurostimulation. Expert Rev Neurother 2019;19(1):17–29.
7. Foutz TJ, Wong M. Brain stimulation treatments in epilepsy: Basic mechanisms and clinical advances. Biomed J 2022;45(1):27–37.
8. Englot DJ, Rolston JD, Wright CW, et al. Rates and predictors of seizure freedom with vagus nerve stimulation for intractable epilepsy. Neurosurgery 2016;79(3):345–53.
9. Fisher R, Salanova V, Witt T, et al, SANTE Study Group. Electrical stimulation of the anterior nucleus of thalamus for treatment of refractory epilepsy. Epilepsia 2010;51:899–908.
10. Salanova V, Witt T, Worth R, et al, SANTE Study Group. Long-term efficacy and safety of thalamic stimulation for drug-resistant partial epilepsy. Neurology 2015;84(10):1017–25.
11. Salanova V, Sperling MR, Gross RE, et al, SANTÉ Study Group. The SANTÉ study at 10 years of follow-up: effectiveness, safety, and sudden unexpected death in epilepsy. Epilepsia 2021;62(6):1306–17.
12. Bergey GK, Morrell MJ, Mizrahi EM, et al. Long-term treatment with responsive brain stimulation in adults with refractory partial seizures. Neurology 2015;55(3):1–2.
13. Nair DR, Laxer KD, Weber PB, et al. on behalf of the RNS System LTT Study. Nine-year prospective efficacy and safety of brain-responsive neurostimulation for focal epilepsy. Neurology 2020;95(9):1244–56.
14. Razavi B, Rao VR, Lin C, et al. Real-world experience with direct brain-responsive neurostimulation for focal onset seizures. Epilepsia 2020;61(8):1749–57.
15. Stacey WC, Litt B. Technology insight: Neuroengineering and epilepsy-designing devices for seizure control. Nat Clin Pract Neurol 2008;4(4):190–201.
16. Duun-Henriksen J, Baud M, Richardson MP, et al. A new era in electroencephalographic monitoring? Subscalp devices for ultra-long-term recordings. Epilepsia 2020;61(9):1805–17.
17. Kossoff EH, Ritzl EK, Politsky JM, et al. Effect of an External Responsive Neurostimulator on Seizures and Electrographic Discharges during Subdural Electrode Monitoring. Epilepsia 2004;45(12):1560–7.
18. NeuroPace RNS System Physician Manual website. http://www.neuropace.com/manuals/RNS_System_Physician_Manual.pdf. Accessed August 1, 2023.
19. Sun FT, Morrell MJ. The RNS system: responsive cortical stimulation for the treatment of refractory partial epilepsy. Expert. Rev Med Devices 2014;11:563–72.
20. Kokkinos V, Sisterson ND, Wozny TA, et al. Association of Closed-Loop Brain Stimulation Neurophysiological Features with Seizure Control among Patients with Focal Epilepsy. JAMA Neurol 2019;15213:1–5.
21. Constantino AC, Sisterson ND, Zaher N, et al. Expert-Level Intracranial Electroencephalogram Ictal Pattern Detection by a Deep Learning Neural Network. Front Neurol 2021;12:603868.
22. Sun FT, Arcot Desai S, Tcheng TK, et al. Changes in the electrocorticogram after implantation of intracranial electrodes in humans: The implant effect. Clin Neurophysiol 2018;129(3):676–86.
23. Arcot Desai S, Tcheng TK, Morrell MJ. Quantitative electrocorticographic biomarkers of clinical outcomes in mesial temporal lobe epileptic patients treated with the RNS® system. Clin Neurophysiol 2019;130(8):1364–74.
24. Khambhati AN, Shafi A, Rao VR, et al. Long-term brain network reorganization predicts responsive neurostimulation outcomes for focal epilepsy. Sci Transl Med 2021;13(608):eabf6588.
25. Baud MO, Kleen JK, Mirro EA, et al. Multi-day rhythms modulate seizure risk in epilepsy. Nat Commun 2018;9(1):88.
26. Spencer DC, Sun FT, Brown SN, et al. Circadian and ultradian patterns of epileptiform discharges differ by seizure-onset location during long-term ambulatory intracranial monitoring. Epilepsia 2016;57:1495–502.
27. Karoly PJ, Rao VR, Gregg NM, et al. Cycles in epilepsy. Nat Rev Neurol 2021;17(5):267–84.
28. Proix T, Truccolo W, Leguia MG, et al. Forecasting seizure risk in adults with focal epilepsy: a development and validation study. Lancet Neurol 2021;20(2):127–35.
29. Leguia MG, Rao VR, Tcheng TK, et al. Learning to generalize seizure forecasts. Epilepsia 2022.

30. Sisterson ND, Wozny TA, Kokkinos V, et al. A rational approach to understanding and evaluating responsive neurostimulation. Neuroinformatics 2020;18: 365–75.

31. Venkatesh P, Sneider D, Danish M, et al. Quantifying a frequency modulation response biomarker in responsive neurostimulation, *J Neural Eng*, 18 (4), 2021, 1-12.

32. Sisterson ND, Wozny TA, Kokkinos V, et al. Closed-Loop Brain Stimulation for Drug-Resistant Epilepsy: Towards an Evidence-Based Approach to Personalized Medicine. Neurotherapeutics 2019;16(1): 119–27.

33. Quigg M, Sun F, Fountain NB, et al. Interrater reliability in interpretation of electrocorticographic seizure detections of the responsive neurostimulator. Epilepsia 2015;56(6):968–71.

34. Arcot Desai S, Tcheng T, Morrell M. Non-linear Embedding Methods for Identifying Similar Brain Activity in 1 Million iEEG Records Captured From 256 RNS System Patients. Frontiers in big Data 2022;5:840508.

35. Peterson V, Kokkinos V, Ferrante E, et al. Deep net detection and onset prediction of electrographic seizure patterns in responsive neurostimulation. Epilepsia 2023;64(8):2056–69.

36. Motamedi GK, Lesser RP, Miglioretti DL, et al. Optimizing parameters for terminating cortical afterdischarges with pulse stimulation [published correction appears in Epilepsia 2002 Nov;43(11): 1441]. Epilepsia 2002;43(8):836–46.

37. Rolston JD, Desai SA, Laxpati NG, et al. Electrical stimulation for epilepsy: experimental approaches. Neurosurg Clin N Am 2011;22(4):425–v.

38. Osorio I, Frei MG, Sunderam S, et al. Automated seizure abatement in humans using electrical stimulation. Ann Neurol 2005;57(2):258–68.

39. Fisher RS, Blum DE, DiVentura B, et al. Seizure diaries for clinical research and practice: Limitations and future prospects. Epilepsy Behav 2012;24: 304–10.

40. Quigg M, Skarpaas TL, Spencer DC, et al. Electrocorticographic events from long-term ambulatory brain recordings can potentially supplement seizure diaries, *Epilepsy Res*, 161, 2020, 1-7.

41. Geller AS, Friedman D, Fang M, et al. Running-down phenomenon captured with chronic electrocorticography. Epilepsia open 2018;3(4):528–34.

42. Kundu B, Charlebois CM, Anderson DN, et al. Chronic intracranial recordings after resection for epilepsy reveal a 'running down' of epileptiform activity. Epilepsia 2023;64(7):e135–42.

43. Scheid BH, Bernabei JM, Khambhati AN, et al. Intracranial electroencephalographic biomarker predicts effective responsive neurostimulation for epilepsy prior to treatment. Epilepsia 2022;63(3): 652–62.

44. Fan JM, Lee AT, Kudo K, et al. Network connectivity predicts effectiveness of responsive neurostimulation in focal epilepsy. Brain communications 2022; 4(3):fcac104.

45. Rønborg SN, Esteller R, Tcheng TK, et al. Acute effects of brain-responsive neurostimulation in drug-resistant partial onset epilepsy. Clin Neurophysiol 2021;132(6):1209–20.

46. Sohal VS, Sun FT. Responsive neurostimulation suppresses synchronized cortical rhythms in patients with epilepsy. Neurosurg Clin 2011;22(4):481.

47. Gregg NM, Sladky V, Nejedly P, et al. Thalamic deep brain stimulation modulates cycles of seizure risk in epilepsy. Sci Rep 2021;11(1).

48. Chiang S, Khambhati AN, Wang ET, et al. Evidence of state-dependence in the effectiveness of responsive neurostimulation for seizure modulation. Brain stimulation 2021;14(2):366–75.

49. Baud MO, Proix T, Gregg NM, et al. Seizure forecasting: Bifurcations in the long and winding road. Epilepsia 2022;1–21.

50. Dabiri S, Cole ER, Gross RE. Adaptive bayesian optimization for state-dependent brain stimulation. Baltimore, MD, USA: 11th International IEEE/EMBS Conference on Neural Engineering (NER); 2023. p. 1–4.

51. Saboo KV, Cao Y, Kremen V, et al. Individualized seizure cluster prediction using machine learning and chronic ambulatory intracranial EEG. IEEE Trans NanoBioscience 2023;1–10.

52. Ojemann WK, Scheid BH, Mouchtaris S, et al. Resting-state background features demonstrate multidien cycles in long-term EEG device recordings. medRxiv 2023;1–21.

53. Chan AY, Knowlton RC, Chang EF, et al. Seizure localization by chronic ambulatory electrocorticography. Clinical Neurophysiology Practice 2018;3: 174–6.

54. Hirsch LJ, Mirro EA, Salanova V, et al. Mesial temporal resection following long-term ambulatory intracranial EEG monitoring with a direct brain-responsive neurostimulation system. Epilepsia 2020;61(3): 408–20.

55. Skarpaas TL, Tcheng TK, Morrell MJ. Clinical and electrocorticographic response to antiepileptic drugs in patients treated with responsive stimulation. Epilepsy Behav 2018;83:192–200.

56. Silva AB, Khambhati AN, Speidel BA, et al. Effects of anterior thalamic nuclei stimulation on hippocampal activity: Chronic recording in a patient with drug-resistant focal epilepsy. Epilepsy & behavior reports 2021;16:100467.

57. Ernst LD, Steffan PJ, Srikanth P, et al. Electrocorticography Analysis in Patients With Dual Neurostimulators Supports Desynchronization as a Mechanism of Action for Acute Vagal Nerve Stimulator Stimulation. J Clin Neurophysiol 2023;40(1):37–44.

58. Sisterson ND, Kokkinos V, Urban A, et al. Responsive neurostimulation of the thalamus improves seizure control in idiopathic generalised epilepsy: initial case series. J Neurol Neurosurg Psychiatry 2022;93(5):491–8.

59. Gill JL, Schneiders JA, Stangl M, et al. A pilot study of closed-loop neuromodulation for treatment-resistant post-traumatic stress disorder. Nat Commun 2023;14(1):2997.

60. Sellers KK, Khambhati AN, Stapper N, et al. Closed-Loop Neurostimulation for Biomarker-Driven, Personalized Treatment of Major Depressive Disorder. J Vis Exp 2023;197:1–15.

61. Sellers KK, Stapper N, Astudillo Maya DA, et al. sChanges in intracranial neurophysiology associated with acute COVID-19 infection. Clin Neurophysiol 2023;148:29–31.

62. Rao VR, Leonard MK, Kleen JK, et al. Chronic ambulatory electrocorticography from human speech cortex. Neuroimage 2017;153:273–82.

63. Henin S, Shankar A, Hasulak N, et al. Hippocampal gamma predicts associative memory performance as measured by acute and chronic intracranial EEG. Sci Rep 2019;9(1):593.

64. Topalovic U, Aghajan ZM, Villaroman D, et al. Wireless programmable recording and stimulation of deep brain activity in freely moving humans. Neuron 2020;108(2):322–34.

Electrode Development for Epilepsy Diagnosis and Treatment

Angelique C. Paulk, PhD*, Pariya Salami, PhD, Rina Zelmann, PhD,
Sydney S. Cash, MD, PhD

KEYWORDS

• sEEG • Grids • Microelectrodes • Intracortical • Strips • ECoG

KEY POINTS

- A wide range and substantial diversity of novel recording systems are in research use and becoming available for clinic use in the care of patients with epilepsy.
- These devices focus on increasing spatial resolution as well as increased the capability of recording single-unit neuronal activity.
- Systems which record from the cortical surface as well as devices made for recording from the gray matter and deep structures in the brain are available.
- Challenges remain in designing and fabricating these systems and in making optimal use of the large quantity and complexity of the resulting data.
- In the near future, it is expected that some of these approaches will become part of routine clinical care in the treatment of patients with epilepsy and other neurologic diseases.

HISTORY

Intracranial recording of human neural activity has been a clinical staple for over 50 years for a wide range of neuropsychiatric disorders and pathologies. The first intracranial recordings, by Förster and Altenburger, were made within 5 years after Hans Berger's 1929 introduction of electroencephalography (EEG) for humans.[1,2] Toward the end of the 1930s, Wilder Penfield and Herbert Jasper achieved major milestones in the use of intracranial recordings and stimulation in understanding and treating epilepsy.[3,4] Their combined neurologic and neurosurgical approaches inspired a new interdisciplinary model toward understanding and utilizing brain physiology for both diagnosis and treatment. During this same period, Penfield characterized functions of several brain areas through recording and stimulation of different brain regions during neurosurgical procedures and developed the concept of the "homunculus."[3] It is also in this period that longer term intracranial epidural recordings first succeeded. In 1949, Hayne and Meyers published the first report showing the utility of stereotactically placed electrodes (stereoelectroencephalography or sEEG),[5] but it was Talairach and Bancaud who developed stereotactic methods for the implantation of intraparenchymal arrays of electrodes.[6–9] The Talairach stereotaxic frame used proportional grids with imaging to map the individual's brain to a common coordinate space. Before the advent of sEEG, ictal activities were rarely recorded during short-term acute recording of intraoperative procedures. The use of sEEG semi-chronically implanted for several days to weeks enabled capturing ictal and interictal activity during day and night, improving the course of epilepsy monitoring.

Over the next 50 years, improved imaging, continued refinement of stereotactic techniques,

Department of Neurology, Center for Neurotechnology and Neurorecovery, Massachusetts General Hospital and Harvard Medical School, 55 Fruit Street, Boston, MA 02114, USA
* Corresponding author.
E-mail address: apaulk@mgh.harvard.edu

Neurosurg Clin N Am 35 (2024) 135–149
https://doi.org/10.1016/j.nec.2023.09.003
1042-3680/24/© 2023 Elsevier Inc. All rights reserved.

and the widespread adaptation of digital EEG systems, all led to changes in practice patterns and utilization of intracranial investigations in both the acute (intraoperative, occurring only in the operating room or OR) and semi-chronic (eg, epilepsy monitoring unit or EMU, for neurophysiological monitoring for up to 29 days in the hospital) environments.[10,11] Subdural grids were introduced in the late 1960s and became more common in the United States in the 1980s and onward, while stereotactic (depth) electrodes remained the approach of choice in Europe and Canada (**Fig. 1**).[10–12] Frameless implantation was introduced in the 1970s.[13,14] MRI, commercially available since the 1980s, changed the way epilepsy was approached for presurgical planning and localization of pathologic tissue. Still, the essential technologies for recording neuronal activity from inside the brain remained relatively unchanged in their major features until the turn of the century. This included the use of platinum contacts using biocompatible materials on the scale of millimeters (see **Fig. 1**A).[15,16]

The first microelectrode recordings in humans date from the 1970s.[17] In-vivo single-unit recordings in humans were regularly obtained since the end of the 1990s using sEEG with microwires at the tip of the electrode shaft.[15,18–22] These microelectrodes also allowed the first recordings of high-frequency oscillations in the human hippocampus, which previously were only observed in animals.[15]

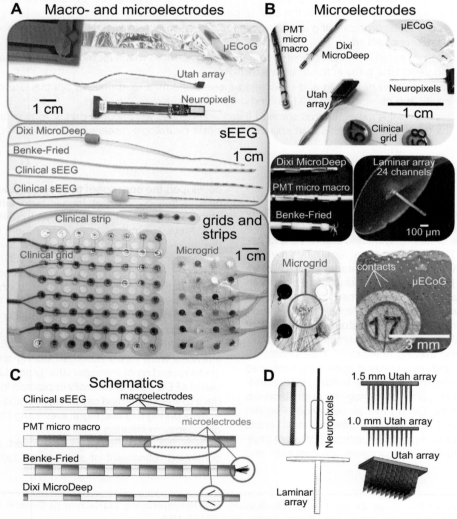

Fig. 1. Electrodes to record human neural activity. (*A*) Macro and microelectrodes used for recording human brain activity at different scales. (*B*) Array of devices used acutely and semi-chronically with channel count ranges included in **Table 1**. (*C*, *D*) Schematic representations of the devices with an inset photo closeup of the Neuropixels array (*upper left*).

In recent years major advances in materials sciences, manufacturing techniques, and digital and computational approaches have led to a wide and evergrowing range of systems for recording intracranial information across multiple scales and in multiple environments.[23–42] Only 5 years ago, clinically, it was common to record from only 100 to 150 macroelectrodes in patients with epilepsy with possible limited access to a small number of microelectrode contacts in the OR.[10] We now can routinely record from more than 250 clinical electrodes over several days in patients with intractable epilepsy[10,43–45] and have begun using microelectrode grids with 1024 channels in the OR.[31] We now focus on the most prevalent systems now in use in the OR or in the semi-chronic recording environment.

DISCUSSION: CHANGING MATERIALS AND METHODS FOR RECORDINGS

Since ~2000, there has been an increased interest in intracranial recordings for both clinical and research purposes.[10,46] Updated materials with higher spatial and temporal resolution can answer fundamental questions regarding how the human brain works on the cellular, and possibly synaptic, level and why specific pathologies, such as epilepsy and tumors, can affect function (see **Fig. 1**; **Fig. 2**). Going from sampling the population activity of a few neurons to hundreds and then to thousands of neurons at high-resolution micrometer-level spatial resolution could help us get that much closer to the mechanisms underlying brain function, behavior, and neuropsychological pathologies.[23,24,31,47,48] These advances have enabled the concomitant use of macroelectrodes (contacts with exposed surface area usually > 4 mm^2) as well as microelectrodes (via electrical contacts on the order of 0.002 mm^2).

New electrodes could help improve the clinical care of our patients with epilepsy and provide, at the same time, research opportunities to directly record from the human brain, delineate the function of different brain regions, and evaluate how their interactions may define normal and pathologic behavior. Three major situations provide a unique opportunity to record with microelectrodes: (i) semi-chronic recording in the EMU, (ii) intraoperative recordings during resective surgery, and (iii) intraoperative recording during placement of neurostimulation devices for the treatment of movement disorders or, more recently, of epilepsy. In cases where the clinical team finds it suitable, the patient, following consent to participating in an institutional review board (IRB) research

protocol, might be considered for possible placement of microelectrodes (see **Fig. 1**).

In the semi-chronic setting, neural activities are recorded from patients with medically refractory epilepsy whose epileptogenic areas were otherwise unidentified via noninvasive techniques (PET, MRI, functional MRI, video-EEG monitoring, and so forth).[10,49] Based on preliminary data obtained through noninvasive approaches, a team of clinicians plans the electrode placement procedure to further evaluate the patient's epileptogenic area. This intracranial sampling can be used to examine whether the patient might be a candidate for resective surgery, neurostimulation, or other treatments.[10] The electrode types utilized in this procedure are limited to electrocorticography (EcoG) and sEEG electrodes that vary in length, contact type, width, and other properties (see **Fig. 1**, **Table 1**).

The second opportunity for recording brain activity is in the OR for acute recordings, during resection of brain tissue through an open craniotomy procedure for patients with epilepsy or brain tumors.[31,39,48,50,51] When clinically indicated, direct electrical stimulation may be planned for mapping the eloquent cortex and surgery can be performed awake (particularly with language mapping).[37,38,52] As in the aforementioned case , a combination of macroelectrode and microelectrode systems are available to stimulate and record large-scale, population-level neural activity. The surgeon and team interact with the patient to elicit behaviors (eg, speech) whose disruption with direct cortical stimulation is used to localize the primary eloquent cortex.[37] Direct access to the cortex is inherent to this process and does not compromise patient safety or clinical prerogatives.

Lastly, the third opportunity that gives us direct access to human neurophysiology is during the placement of a deep brain stimulation (DBS) device with acute recordings. Patients with movement disorders (eg, Parkinson's disease) and certain neuropsychiatric disorders (eg, obsessive-compulsive disorder) may be candidates for a DBS implant.[35,53–58] In most cases, this procedure is done with an awake patient, providing another unique opportunity to record directly from the brain while specific cognitive behaviors are tested.[32–34,59,60] In awake DBS surgery, single-unit recordings in subcortical target regions are obtained as part of the clinical procedure.[32,60] However, other electrodes (eg, high-density EcoG, high-density Neuropixels probe, and so forth) may temporarily be placed during research tasks.[27,31,50,61–64]

There is a fourth scenario, which involves chronic recordings used for clinical purposes,

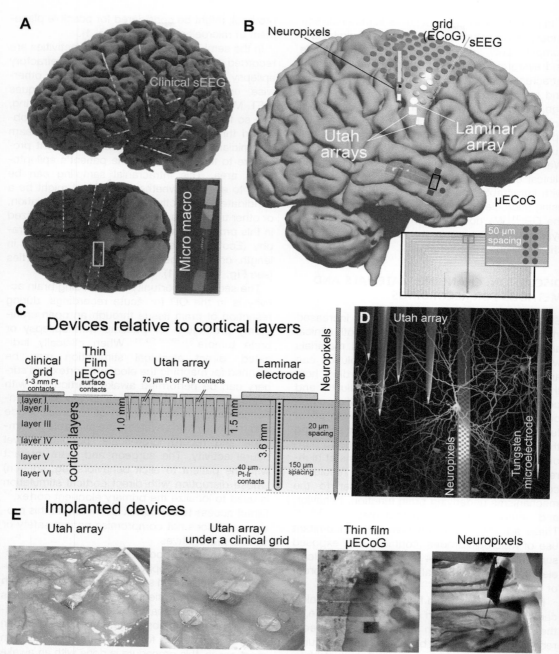

Fig. 2. Size and scale of electrodes relative to the human brain and neurons. (*A*) Example stereoelectroencephalography implant with a micro-macro lead in 1 trajectory, highlighted below. Electrode contacts are light blue. (*B*) Implanted devices and the scale relative to the brain including surface and intraparenchymal (penetrating) devices in the human brain. (*C*) The relative scale of the devices to cortical layers. (*D*) Reconstructions of human pyramidal cells and inhibitory interneurons with cells from NeuroMorpho.Org [68–71] relative to the Neuropixels array, 1.5-mm Utah array and a single sharpened tungsten lead. (*E*) Microelectrode devices implanted into the brain or on the surface, including the Utah array, thin film surface electrode, and Neuropixels examples, all intraoperatively captured.[48,50]

Table 1
Common channel counts, dimensions, uses, and Food and Drug Administration approvals for different types of devices used in the acute and semi-chronic recording setting

Device	Dimension Range of Implanted Portion of Electrode	Common Implantation Locations	Implantation Duration	Common Active Contact Count Ranges per Device	Current FDA Approval
Platinum macro contacts in a grid (n x n channels) in a silastic sheet	10 × 10 × 1 mm to 60 × 60 × 1 cm	Subdural or epidural	Semi-chronic, chronic, or acute	4–64 contacts	Yes
Platinum macro contacts strip (1 x n channels) in a silastic sheet	10 × 1 × 1 mm to 60 × 1 × 1 mm	Subdural or epidural	Semi-chronic, chronic, or acute	1–12 contacts	Yes
Microgrid with platinum wires in a silastic sheet (can be with or without macro-contacts)	10 × 10 × 1 mm to 60 × 60 × 1 cm	Subdural or epidural	Semi-chronic or acute	4–64 contacts	Yes
sEEG depth electrode	20 (length) x 0.8–1.3 (diameter) mm to 60 (length) x 0.8–1.3 (diameter) mm	Intraparenchymal (inside brain)	Semi-chronic or acute	2–18 contacts	Yes
Deep brain stimulation electrode	60 (length) x 0.8–1.3 (diameter) mm	Intraparenchymal (inside brain)	Semi-chronic, chronic, or acute	2–10 contacts	Yes
sEEG Behnke-Fried, Dixi MicroDeep, PMT micro-macro depth electrodes with both macro and micro electrode contacts	20 (length) x 0.8–1.3 (diameter) mm to 60 (length) x 0.8–1.3 (diameter) mm	Intraparenchymal (inside brain)	Semi-chronic or acute	2–18 contacts	Yes
Utah array	4 × 4 x 1–1.5 mm	Intraparenchymal (inside brain)	Semi-chronic, chronic, or acute	100 contacts	Yes
Thin film μECoG arrays with micro or macro contacts	Wide range	Subdural or epidural	Acute	2–2048 contacts	Some devices (NeuroOne)
Laminar arrays	1.2 × 4 mm	Intraparenchymal (inside brain)	Semi-chronic or acute	16–24 contacts	No
Neuropixels probe	100 μm × 70 μm x 10 mm	Intraparenchymal (inside brain)	Acute	384 contacts (out of 966 total)	No

Abbreviations: FDA, Food and Drug Administration; μECoG, micro-electrocorticography; sEEG, stereoelectroencephalography.

including the use of closed loop neurostimulation as in the responsive neurostimulator system (from NeuroPace).[65,66] We envision that chronically implanted microelectrode recordings could also be feasible in the future but this approach has not been implemented in any way for epilepsy yet.

The type of electrodes used in any of these settings may vary. Generally, the electrodes can be divided into 2 categories based on their level of penetration: surface electrodes and penetrating (intraparenchymal) electrodes (see **Fig. 2**, **Table 1**). Surface electrodes are intended for use on the epidural or subdural surface of the exposed brain. These are non-penetrating electrode arrays which are akin to a clinical grid. In contrast, the penetrating electrodes are designed to record directly from the gray matter and/or deeper, subcortical structures (see **Fig. 2**).

Recording with macroelectrodes as done as part of standard clinical care combined with microelectrodes could provide a more directed, targeted control point. More specifically, this combination of macroelectrode and microelectrode recordings could enable an improved understanding of neural activity from individual neurons to brain networks. Indeed, combining these microelectrodes and macroelectrodes either on the surface or placed in the brain will improve 2 interrelated aspects. The first is the desire to use smaller electrodes that are capable of greater sensitivity to high-frequency activity and, ultimately, extracellularly recorded action potential activity. The second is to enable increasingly higher channel counts for greater spatial coverage and higher resolution (see **Table 1**). Ideally, the acquisition systems should satisfy both needs while also permitting relatively broad coverage.[23] Further altering via direct electrical stimulation would help understand the causal intrinsic and network characteristics of the human brain with unprecedent detail.[67]

ADVANCES IN BRAIN SURFACE TECHNOLOGIES
Microgrids/Micro-electrocorticography

One of the earliest developments toward increasing the density and spatial resolution of recording electrodes while decreasing the size of the contact was the development of microgrid systems. The microgrid systems involved smaller contacts interspersed between more common and clinically used contacts on a typical silastic grid sheet.[72] This is often done using the cut end of an embedded, isolated platinum wire (see **Fig. 1**D).[72] There are various versions—some with the wire

cut flush to the silastic, while others had the wires extended 100 um or so. These systems have proven useful in identifying microphysiologic events such as microseizures[72] but do not appear to consistently produce evidence of single-unit activity. They are 510K approved and available from both Ad-tech and PMT (see **Figs. 1** and **2**). Impedances of these electrodes are in the 100 kOhm range. These devices can be used in both the acute setting and in the semi-chronic setting (see **Table 1**). Although these electrodes provide higher spatial resolution compared to the typical clinical grid, the manufacturing process relying on cut wires entails significant limitations on the total density and number of channels that can be incorporated.

Thin-Film Arrays

To move to even higher density of electrodes, there were 2 major issues to overcome. First, the contacts of small, high-resolution electrodes will inherently have extremely high impedance (and therefore high noise). Second, with the relatively thick silastic membrane used for typical clinical grids and strips, an increase in spatial density is difficult to achieve (see **Fig. 1**).

In the face of these obstacles, multiple groups began working with organic polymers deposited on contacts embedded in a parylene C or polyimide sheet (see **Figs. 1** and **2**; **Fig. 3**).[26,39,41,73] The parylene C or polyimide provides a biocompatible, highly flexible layer which is relatively easy to work with. The organic polymers, particularly high-density poly (3,4-ethylenedioxythiophene) polystyrene sulfonate (PEDOT:PSS) microelectrodes, which provide excellent impedance characteristics, have been used to detect microscale neural activity from large areas of the cortical surface in humans, rodents, and nonhuman primates[39,48,50,51,73–78] (see **Fig. 3**).

One of the first of these systems to be used in humans was the NeuroGrid, which was shown to detect high-frequency events similar to the single-unit activity seen in intraparenchymal recordings with penetrating metal electrodes.[39,51,77] More recent work has involved the use of thin-film electrodes recording activity on the surface of the brain via PEDOT:PSS, as well as the development of platinum nanorod electrodes with more than 1000 channels per device to detect single-cell and local neural activity intraoperatively[31,48,50,51] (see **Figs. 2** and **3**). The high-resolution sampling achieved by the high channel counts of these devices proved to be essential in studying neural mechanisms of movement, epileptiform activity, and direct electrical stimulation, both in the clinic

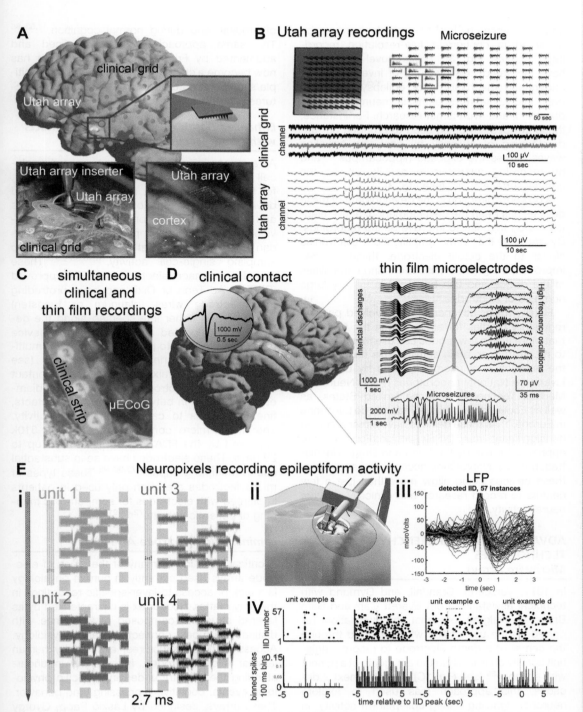

Fig. 3. Types of neural signals captured with the various microelectrodes. (*A*) Utah array recording in the lateral temporal lobe including images of the implanted device and the end of the pneumatic inserter (metal post). (*B*) Evidence of a microseizure localized to a few contacts on the array in the microelectrode local field potential (LFP) recording. Note that the nearby clinical contacts (the contact highlighted in red) did not show a seizure. (*C*) Example of a simultaneous thin film recording with a clinical strip in an intraoperative case. (*D*) Array of different types of signals which can be captured by a clinical lead (*left*) and a thin film micro-electrocorticography (µECoG) array of similar length (right). Where the clinical lead can capture a single interictal discharge (IID), the thin film electrode can record high-frequency oscillations, traveling IIDs, and microseizures at high spatial resolution (50 µm to 1 mm inter-contact spacing).[48] (*E*) (*i*) Example unit waveforms (each color is a separate unit). On the left, original waveforms

and in research,[31,48,50,51] which cannot be observed in concurrent low-resolution recordings[48,50] (see **Fig. 3**). These novel techniques have facilitated new avenues of investigation to understand mechanisms of epilepsy, traumatic brain injury, stroke, anesthesia, neuropsychiatric disorders, and even tumor research. For instance, these devices are being used to broaden our understanding of epilepsy by analyzing traveling waves across the exposed hippocampus,[79] and by recording microseizure activity across the cortical surface[42,48,80] (see **Fig. 3**).

A powerful direction in the development of these devices has been the development of active electronics on thin film to improve neural recordings. By moving the early amplification electronics closer to the actual electrode, these devices improve the signal-to-noise recording capabilities of the device and can be scalable to very large numbers of electrodes.[41,42,81]

Finally, major advances have involved passing regulatory hurdles for acute use in the OR such that more than a few groups can use these devices to record human brain activity. This has involved the production of microelectrodes by Lawrence Livermore National Laboratories[79] and NeuroOne Medical Technologies in the United States, as well as École Polytechnique Fédérale de Lausanne in Europe.[82] As these devices have either received nonsignificant risk (NSR) designations or are approved for use by the Food and Drug Administration (FDA) (NeuroOne), accessibility and use of these devices could allow more than just a few centers to record research and clinically relevant neural activity.

ADVANCES IN INTRAPARENCHYMAL TECHNOLOGIES
Microwire Arrays

In 1971, Verzeano, Crandall, and Dymond with technical assistance from Everett Carr and Sam Brakel (E. Halgren, personal communication) reported on the use of fine wires inserted through the center of a depth electrode to record single-unit activity chronically in the amygdala of a patient with epilepsy[20] (see **Fig. 1**C). Over the next 2 decades, this approach was used to explore neuronal signaling during epileptiform activity, in response to changes in metabolic state or level of arousal, and during normal cognition.[17,83–85] The same approach was later refined and augmented by Fried and Behnke in what has now become a standard approach to obtain multiple single-unit recordings from deep brain structures in humans.[16]

Enhanced Depth Electrodes—Microcontacts with Depth Electrodes

As a way to improve our ability to record single-cell activity while not disrupting clinical workflow, for the past 2 decades, researchers have used devices with combinations of microelectrodes and macroelectrodes along the same depth devices.[16,46,86–89] Once implanted, these devices can be used for clinical recordings while also sampling single-cell activity.[16,46,86–89] These mixed micro-macro electrodes are FDA approved (PMT or Ad-Tech or Dixi) and have protruding microelectrode wires (platinum or tungsten) which can be either interspersed along the devices or are located at the end of the device (see **Figs. 1** and **2**) to permit single-unit or multiunit acquisition during sEEG recordings (see **Fig. 1**).[90–92] The mixed macro-micro contact array is a depth electrode 0.8 to 1.27 mm in diameter which has, in between the macro-contacts, fine microwires to capture single-cell activity. The macro-micro contacts are currently 510k approved by the FDA for use in humans up to 29 days. These electrodes have seen substantial use in multiple groups.[23,72,90–93] These types of microelectrodes are often only used in patients implanted with electrodes for semi-chronic mapping of epileptic activity.[72,88,91,92]

Laminar Microelectrode Arrays

A critical limitation of many of the types of electrode arrays used currently in human physiology is a lack of access to layer-specific recordings in the gray matter. Neocortex is characterized by its layered structure, composed of 6 laminae with distinct cell types, connectivity, and physiology. Access to these structures, enabled by human laminar microelectrodes, is essential in understanding the circuitry underlying specific physiologic events, cognitive processing, and behavior. These arrays, designed by László Papp, György Karmos, and István Ulbert in the late 1990s consist

---

are overlaid relative to the recorded channels, with the gray bars to the left indicating the location of the units along the probe. (*ii-iii*). Neuropixels array and recording in lateral temporal lobe (*left, ii*) while detecting interictal discharges (IIDs) in the local field potential (*right, iii*). (*iv*). Individual unit example spike timing relative to the peak of the interictal discharges (IIDs) as both a raster plot and a peristimulus time histogram.[27]

of a linear array of 24 contacts with 150 μm spacing.[94,95] The contacts are cut ends of platinum-iridium which provides biocompatibility as well as relatively low impedances (500 kΩ–1 MΩ) to provide quality recording characteristics. The entire array is 3.6 mm, allowing it to span the cortical depth while sampling each cortical layer with multiple channels (see **Figs. 1** and **2**). This spatial sampling enables the collection of action potentials as well as their proxies, multiunit activity and high gamma power.[94–97] Perhaps more importantly, net transmembrane currents due to synaptic activity and active channels can be estimated by the current source density within individual laminae which have been informative in identifying layer-specific activity during epileptiform neural activity and seizures.[96–103]

These platinum-iridium laminar electrodes come in 2 designs—one for superficial, neocortical structures and the other for deeper structures which could include the cingulate gyrus or hippocampus and amygdala. These laminar devices are not FDA-approved devices but have been used by multiple groups under local IRB oversight (see **Table 1**). The version designed for the lateral neocortex is anchored to the cortical surface via a thin silicone sheet that sits on the pia. This holds the probe in place and keeps it normal to the cortical surface/perpendicular to cortical layers (see **Figs. 1** and **2**). These arrays are inserted manually under visual guidance.[94]

The second version of the laminar electrode is akin to the microwires and is also used in conjunction with a Behnke-Fried depth electrode which has a hollow core and opening at the distal end. The depth version of the laminar microelectrode protrudes from the end of the clinical depth electrode and therefore can sample deep structures.[94,95] Recordings can be made acutely (within the OR, ~1 hour) and/or semi-chronically within the epilepsy-monitoring-unit.

Utah Arrays

In the early 1990s, Richard Norman and collaborators created an etched silicon array of 100 probes, known as the Utah array.[104] This has now been used extensively in rodent, feline, and nonhuman primate experiments.[28,29,105,106] It has also become a mainstay of human neocortical research particularly in the field of brain-computer interfaces[30,107–109] (see **Figs. 1–3**; currently available through BlackRock microsystems as the Neuro-Port array). The Utah array has also been used extensively in semi-chronic recordings in patients with epilepsy,[110–113] including detecting microseizures not present on the concurrent clinical

electrode recordings (see **Fig. 3**). Versions of the Utah arrays have platinum or platinum-iridium tips and can come in 1-mm and 1.5-mm configurations for human use (see **Fig. 1**, **Table 1**).

Unlike all other systems currently available for human use, insertion of this array of electrodes requires a specialized system consisting of a pneumatic piston which, when triggered, taps the electrode through the pia and into the parenchyma (see **Fig. 3**A, **Table 1**). This system provides reproducible results and overcomes the surface tension resulting from pushing 100 tines through the pial membrane.

Neuropixels Arrays

A more recent set of devices able to record from hundreds of human brain cells at the same time in a small area of the cortex includes Neuropixel arrays (see **Figs. 2** and **3**).[27,40,114] Neuropixels probes (NP v S 1.0, Interuniversity Microelectronics Centre) used in humans include an electrode shank (width: 70 μm, length: 10 mm, thickness: 90 μm) of 966 total possible sites with 384 active sites possible to record from laid-out-in-a-checkerboard or grid pattern of a silicon probe with porous TiN contacts of ~18 μm site-to-site distances.[27,40,114,115] Neuropixels arrays have been used to record neural activity across multiple species, including humans, for which researchers have established a validated sterilization protocol for the arrays with BioSeal Inc (Placentia, CA, USA).[27,40,114,116] These arrays can also detect epileptiform activity in the local field potential (LFP) along with single-unit activity, sometimes capturing up to 200 units in a single recording[27,40] (see **Fig. 3**).

Commercial Systems Not yet in Human Use

Neuralink

While not intended for the investigation of epilepsy per se, and not yet in clinical trials, the Neuralink approach to developing intracortical arrays has received substantial media attention.[117] Press releases from the company suggest that a recording system using thin and flexible 'threads' of electrodes can be inserted using robotic control and achieve recordings from ~3000 channels.[117] Maturity of this system for recording may provide a method for acquiring large numbers of single neurons across a wider area of cortex than current technologies can provide and would likely present novel opportunities for understanding a variety of neurologic diseases including epilepsy.

Paradromics

While also not yet used in patients, Paradromics has developed the Argo system.[118] This is a parallel neural recording system based on platinum-iridium microwire electrode arrays bonded to a complementary metal-oxide semiconductor voltage amplifier array. It currently supports simultaneous recording from 65,536 channels, sampled at 32 kHz and 12-bit resolution.[118] This system, being compatible with both penetrating and surface microelectrodes, was designed for cortical recordings, and was tested on the benchtop and some animal models.[118] It, too, potentially represents a substantial step forward in obtaining a large number of single neuronal and microscale LFPs which can be of importance in epilepsy and other neurologic diseases.

Challenges from data acquisition to widespread adoption

Currently, patients and research participants whose cortical activity is recorded with a single (4 × 4 mm) Utah array can easily generate several terabytes (TB) of data that contain information on 100+ recorded neurons. Indeed, the full bandwidth of neural data when captured from 1 array at current resolutions produces ~500 gigabytes per day. Continuous storage of neural data from 1 individual with 2 implanted arrays would yield 365 TB in 1 year. Even though storage costs for data are declining and our ability to handle that data from a purely logistical perspective is improving for an average laboratory or a clinical setting, this represents a challenge. More importantly, beyond simple storage challenges, data processing of this scale requires specialized techniques for extracting meaningful information. In the clinic, neural data are reviewed visually, which may require spectral analysis or other approaches for a more comprehensive evaluation.

The ability to analyze 100s or 1000s of channels of data spanning a large frequency space (from ~1 Hz–30 kHz) in a clinical setting is essentially nonexistent at this point. In time, advances in point process techniques, dimensionality reduction, data compression techniques, and other approaches are expected to enable these large-scale data analyses[119–123] and their incorporation into the clinical workflow for patients with epilepsy.

A CHANGING LANDSCAPE OF ACADEMIC AND INDUSTRIAL INTEREST AND REGULATORY CONSIDERATIONS

Currently, the number of patients who have been involved in the use of microelectrode systems remains relatively small, but it has been growing and is likely to grow even further as more systems become available and as regulatory processes are worked through. In addition, the indications for use are likely to expand from patients with intractable focal epilepsy or those undergoing resective surgery to patients in neurocritical care settings or even patients with epilepsy in outpatient settings, as well as patients with a wide variety of other neurologic and neuropsychiatric diseases.[10,35,46,55]

However, a key issue of advancing these technologies is that these devices are first used for research purposes under local regulatory (IRB) research approvals. As such, there are ongoing local discussions at each research site regarding whether the use of these electrodes is considered significant risk or NSR and whether their use requires FDA approvals for investigational device exemptions (in the United States) or other regulatory approvals.[124–126] These determinations will also vary with the different types of devices and the level of overall risk. Further, if the work involves local regulatory (IRB) approvals, patient consent should be fully informed with regard to the risks of participating in these studies. For instance, while there is possible increased risk of infection, this risk should be mitigated by using validated sterilization practices in combination with sterile tools in the OR as well as keeping the duration of intraoperative recordings low (as infection risk could relate to the length of the surgery). All of these risks must be communicated clearly to prospective participants in a rigorous informed consent process.[46,127,128] Following these approved local regulatory practices, however, has been crucial to produce the initial demonstrations of the capabilities of these devices, particularly before companies and groups move forward through the regulatory pathway to FDA approval.[28,29,94,105]

SUMMARY

The treatment of epilepsy has relied on recordings of neural activity for almost a century. Only recently, however, have we seen a rapid and accelerating change in the kinds of recordings that are possible in patients. Novel recording systems are now in use which allow for very high spatial resolution recordings as well as capturing single neuronal activities. Use of these systems has shed important light on normal cognitive function, sleep, anesthesia, and, most importantly, the physiology of epilepsy. While these systems are not yet in use for clinical purposes, the authors expect that it will not be too much time before they do become a regular part of clinical management of epilepsy. This is especially true as other challenges with these devices are overcome, including large and complex data sets, regulatory and manufacturing issues, and movement from purely academic interest to commercial interest so that devices are made in a scalable and regulated fashion. Ultimately, the set of tools available to the functional neurosurgeon and clinical care team in epilepsy will be more varied, more powerful, and more capable in ways which are likely to substantially change how we approach and treat epilepsy.

CLINICS CARE POINTS

- Clinicians are going to see an increasing diversity of recording systems for mapping out epileptic foci and understanding epileptic networks and their relationship to eloquent cortex.

- Semi-chronic microelectrode recordings will help to delineate the epileptogenic region and eloquent regions more precisely, improving prognosis.

- Acute recordings with new electrodes in the OR will allow more precise delineation of lesions, the epileptogenic zone, and borders of tumors.

- Combined information at different spatial scales will bridge the gap between current clinical care and basic neuroscience knowledge leading to greater understanding of the mechanisms underlying epilepsy, ultimately facilitating the development of new treatments.

DISCLOSURE

The MGH Translational Research Center has clinical research support agreements with Neuralink, Paradromics, and Synchron, for which S.S. Cash provides consultative input. The remaining authors declare no competing interests.

REFERENCES

1. Berger H. Über das Elektrenkephalogramm des Menschen. Archiv für Psychiatrie und Nervenkrankheiten 1929;87(1):527–70.

2. Foerster O, Altenburger H. Elektrobiologische Vorgänge an der menschlichen Hirnrinde. Dtsch Z für Nervenheilkd 1935;135:277–88.

3. Penfield W, Boldrey E. Somatic motor and sensory representation in the cerebral cortex of man as studied by electrical stimulation1. Brain 1937;60(4):389–443.

4. Penfield W, Jasper H. Epilepsy and the functional anatomy of the human brain. Boston: Little, Brown & Co; 1954. p. xv, 896.

5. Hayne R, Meyers R. An Improved Model of a Human Stereotaxic Instrument. J Neurosurg 1950;7(5):463–6.

6. Reif PS, Strzelczyk A, Rosenow F. The history of invasive EEG evaluation in epilepsy patients. Seizure 2016;41:191–5.

7. Bourdillon P, Apra C, Lévêque M, et al. Neuroplasticity and the brain connectome: what can Jean Talairach's reflections bring to modern psychosurgery? Neurosurg Focus 2017;43(3):E11.

8. Talairach J, Bancaud J, Bonis A, et al. Functional stereotaxic exploration of epilepsy. Confin Neurol 1962;22:328–31.

9. Harary M, Cosgrove GR. Jean Talairach: a cerebral cartographer. Neurosurg Focus 2019;47(3):E12.

10. Mercier MR, Dubarry AS, Tadel F, et al. Advances in human intracranial electroencephalography research, guidelines and good practices. Neuroimage 2022;119438. https://doi.org/10.1016/j.neuroimage.2022.119438.

11. Branco MP, Geukes SH, Aarnoutse EJ, et al. Nine decades of electrocorticography: A comparison between epidural and subdural recordings. Eur J Neurosci 2023;(September 2022). https://doi.org/10.1111/ejn.15941.

12. Tandon N, Tong BA, Friedman ER, et al. Analysis of Morbidity and Outcomes Associated with Use of Subdural Grids vs Stereoelectroencephalography in Patients with Intractable Epilepsy. JAMA Neurol 2019;76(6):672–81.

13. Olivier A, Germano IM, Cukiert A, et al. Frameless stereotaxy for surgery of the epilepsies: preliminary experience. Technical note. J Neurosurg 1994;81(4):629–33.

14. Otsubo H, Hwang PA, Hunjan A, et al. Use of frameless stereotaxy with location of electroencephalographic electrodes on three-dimensional computed tomographic images in epilepsy surgery. J Clin Neurophysiol 1995;12(4):363–71.

15. Bragin A, Engel JJ, Wilson CL, et al. High-frequency oscillations in human brain. Hippocampus 1999;9(2):137–42.

16. Fried I, Wilson CL, Maidment NT, et al. Cerebral microdialysis combined with single-neuron and electroencephalographic recording in neurosurgical patients: Technical note. J Neurosurg 1999;91(4):697–705.

17. Halgren E, Babb TL, Rausch R, et al. Neurons in the human basolateral amygdala and hippocampal formation do not respond to odors. Neurosci Lett 1977;4(6):331–5.

18. Babb TL, Wilson CL, Isokawa-Akesson M. Firing patterns of human limbic neurons during stereoencephalography (SEEG) and clinical temporal lobe seizures. Electroencephalogr Clin Neurophysiol 1987;66(6):467–82.

19. Babb TL, Crandall PH. Epileptogenesis of human limbic neurons in psychomotor epileptics.

Electroencephalogr Clin Neurophysiol 1976;40(3): 225–43.

20. Verzeano M, Crandall PH, Dymond A. Neuronal activity of the amygdala in patients with psychomotor epilepsy. Neuropsychologia 1971;9(3):331–44.

21. Kawasaki H, Adolphs R, Kaufman O, et al. Single-neuron responses to emotional visual stimuli recorded in human ventral prefrontal cortex. Nat Neurosci 2001;4(1):15–6.

22. Rutishauser U, Schuman EM, Mamelak AN. Online detection and sorting of extracellularly recorded action potentials in human medial temporal lobe recordings, in vivo. J Neurosci Methods 2006;154(1–2):204–24.

23. Chari A, Thornton RC, Tisdall MM, et al. Microelectrode recordings in human epilepsy: a case for clinical translation. Brain Communications 2020;2(2). https://doi.org/10.1093/braincomms/fcaa082.

24. Cash SS, Hochberg LR. The emergence of single neurons in clinical neurology. Neuron 2015;86(1): 79–91.

25. Hermiz J, Rogers N, Kaestner E, et al. A clinic compatible, open source electrophysiology system. Annu Int Conf IEEE Eng Med Biol Soc 2016;4511–4. https://doi.org/10.1109/EMBC.2016.7591730.

26. Ganji M, Kaestner E, John H, et al. Development and Translation of PEDOT:PSS Microelectrodes for Intraoperative Monitoring. Adv Funct Mater 2017;28(12):1700232.

27. Paulk AC, Kfir Y, Khanna AR, et al. Large-scale neural recordings with single neuron resolution using Neuropixels probes in human cortex. Nat Neurosci 2022;25:252–63.

28. Maynard EM, Nordhausen CT, Normann RA. The Utah Intracortical Electrode Array: A recording structure for potential brain-computer interfaces. Electroencephalogr Clin Neurophysiol 1997; 102(3):228–39.

29. Nordhausen CT, Rousche PJ, Normann RA. Optimizing recording capabilities of the Utah Intracortical Electrode Array. Brain Res 1994;637(1–2): 27–36.

30. Hochberg LR, Serruya MD, Friehs GM, et al. Neuronal ensemble control of prosthetic devices by a human with tetraplegia. Nature 2006;442(7099): 164–71.

31. Tchoe Y, Bourhis AM, Cleary DR, et al. Human Brain Mapping with Multi-Thousand Channel PtNRGrids Resolves Novel Spatiotemporal Dynamics. Sci Transl Med 2022;14:eabj1441.

32. Amirnovin R, Williams ZM, Cosgrove GR, et al. Experience with microelectrode guided subthalamic nucleus deep brain stimulation. Neurosurgery 2006;58:ONS96–102.

33. Jamali M, Grannan B, Fedorenko E, et al. Single-neuronal predictions of others' beliefs in humans. Nature 2021;591:610–4.

34. Sheth SA, Mian MK, Patel SR, et al. Human dorsal anterior cingulate cortex neurons mediate ongoing behavioural adaptation. Nature 2012;488(7410): 218–21.

35. Sheth SA, Bijanki KR, Metzger B, et al. Deep Brain Stimulation for Depression Informed by Intracranial Recordings. Biol Psychiatr 2021;1–6. https://doi.org/10.1016/j.biopsych.2021.11.007.

36. Krishna S, Choudhury A, Keough MB, et al. Glioblastoma remodelling of human neural circuits decreases survival. Nature 2023. https://doi.org/10.1038/s41586-023-06036-1.

37. Berger MS, Ojemann GA. Intraoperative brain mapping techniques in neuro-oncology. Stereotact Funct Neurosurg 1992;58:153–61.

38. Borchers S, Himmelbach M, Logothetis N, et al. Direct electrical stimulation of human cortex — the gold standard for mapping brain functions? Nat Rev Neurosci 2012;13(January 2012):63–70.

39. Khodagholy D, Gelinas JN, Thesen T, et al. NeuroGrid: recording action potentials from the surface of the brain. Nat Neurosci 2015;18(2):310–5.

40. Chung JE, Sellers KK, Leonard MK, et al. High-density single-unit human cortical recordings using the Neuropixels probe. Neuron 2022;1–13. https://doi.org/10.1016/j.neuron.2022.05.007.

41. Chiang CH, Wang C, Barth K, et al. Flexible, high-resolution thin-film electrodes for human and animal neural research. J Neural Eng 2021;18(4). https://doi.org/10.1088/1741-2552/ac02dc.

42. Barth KJ, Sun J, Chiang CH, et al. Flexible, high-resolution cortical arrays with large coverage capture microscale high-frequency oscillations in patients with epilepsy. Epilepsia 2023. https://doi.org/10.1111/epi.17642.

43. Salami P, Borzello M, Kramer MA, et al. Quantifying seizure termination patterns reveals limited pathways to seizure end. Neurobiol Dis 2022;165:105645.

44. Salami P, Peled N, Nadalin JK, et al. Seizure onset location shapes dynamics of initiation. Clin Neurophysiol 2020. https://doi.org/10.1016/j.clinph.2020.04.168.

45. Paulk AC, Zelmann R, Crocker B, et al. Local and distant cortical responses to single pulse intracranial stimulation in the human brain are differentially modulated by specific stimulation parameters. Brain Stimul 2022;15(2):491–508.

46. Feinsinger A, Pouratian N, Ebadi H, et al. Ethical commitments , principles , and practices guiding intracranial neuroscientific research in humans. Neuron 2022;110(2):188–94.

47. Chan AM, Dykstra AR, Jayaram V, et al. Speech-specific tuning of neurons in human superior temporal gyrus. Cerebr Cortex 2014;24(10):2679–93.

48. Yang JC, Paulk AC, Salami P, et al. Microscale dynamics of electrophysiological markers of epilepsy. Clin Neurophysiol 2021;32:2916–31.

49. Anand A, Magnotti JF, Smith DN, et al. Predictive value of magnetoencephalography in guiding the intracranial implant strategy for intractable epilepsy. J Neurosurg 2022;1–11. https://doi.org/10.3171/2022.1.JNS212943.

50. Paulk AC, Yang JC, Cleary DR, et al. Microscale Physiological Events on the Human Cortical Surface. Cerebr Cortex 2021;31(8):3678–700.

51. Hassan AR, Zhao Z, Ferrero JJ, et al. Translational Organic Neural Interface Devices at Single Neuron Resolution. Adv Sci 2022;2202306:1–11.

52. Formaggio E, Storti SF, Tramontano V, et al. Frequency and time-frequency analysis of intraoperative ECoG during awake brain stimulation. Front Neuroeng 2013;6(FEB):1–8.

53. Bahramisharif A, Mazaheri A, Levar N, et al. Deep Brain Stimulation Diminishes Cross-Frequency Coupling in Obsessive-Compulsive Disorder. Biol Psychiatr 2016;80(7):e57–8.

54. Bourne SK, Eckhardt CA, Sheth SA, et al. Mechanisms of deep brain stimulation for obsessive compulsive disorder: effects upon cells and circuits. Front Integr Neurosci 2012;6:29.

55. Provenza NR, Sheth SA, Rijn EMD van, et al. Long-term ecological assessment of intracranial electrophysiology synchronized to behavioral markers in obsessive-compulsive disorder. Nat Med 2021. https://doi.org/10.1038/s41591-021-01550-z.

56. Bronstein JM, Tagliati M, Alterman RL, et al. Deep brain stimulation for parkinson disease: An expert consensus and review of key issues. Arch Neurol 2011;68(2):165–71.

57. Deng J, Luan G. Mechanisms of Deep Brain Stimulation for Epilepsy and Associated Comorbidities. Neuropsychiatry 2017;S(1):31–7.

58. Herrington TM, Cheng JJ, Eskandar EN. Mechanisms of deep brain stimulation. J Neurophysiol 2016;115(1):19–38.

59. Mian MK, Sheth SA, Patel SR, et al. Encoding of rules by neurons in the human dorsolateral prefrontal cortex. Cerebr Cortex 2014;24(3):807–16.

60. Eden UT, Gale JT, Amirnovin R, et al. Characterizing the spiking dynamics of subthalamic nucleus neurons in Parkinson's disease using generalized linear models. Front Integr Neurosci 2012;6(June):1–10.

61. Hermiz J, Rogers N, Kaestner E, et al. Sub-millimeter ECoG pitch in human enables higher fidelity cognitive neural state estimation. Neuroimage 2018;176:454–64.

62. Bush A, Chrabaszcz A, Peterson V, et al. Differentiation of speech-induced artifacts from physiological high gamma activity in intracranial recordings. Neuroimage 2022;250(October 2021):118962.

63. Chrabaszcz A, Neumann WJ, Stretcu O, et al. Subthalamic Nucleus and Sensorimotor Cortex Activity During Speech Production. J Neurosci 2019; 39(14):2698–708.

64. Peterson V, Merk T, Bush A, et al. Movement decoding using spatio-spectral features of cortical and subcortical local field potentials. Exp Neurol 2022;359(October 2022):114261.

65. Lee B, Zubair MN, Marquez YD, et al. A Single-Center Experience with the NeuroPace RNS System: A Review of Techniques and Potential Problems. World Neurosurgery 2015;84(3):719–26.

66. Nair DR, Laxer KD, Weber PB, et al. Nine-year prospective efficacy and safety of brain-responsive neurostimulation for focal epilepsy. Neurology 2020;95(9):e1244–56.

67. Titiz AS, Hill MRH, Mankin EA, et al. Theta-burst microstimulation in the human entorhinal area improves memory specificity. Elife 2017;6:1–18.

68. Koch C, Jones A. Big Science, Team Science, and Open Science for Neuroscience. Neuron 2016; 92(3):612–6.

69. Ascoli GA. Mobilizing the base of neuroscience data: the case of neuronal morphologies. Nat Rev Neurosci 2006;7(4):318–24.

70. Ascoli GA, Donohue DE, Halavi M. NeuroMorpho.Org: A central resource for neuronal morphologies. J Neurosci 2007;27(35):9247–51.

71. Tóth K, Hofer KT, Kandrács Á, et al. Hyperexcitability of the network contributes to synchronization processes in the human epileptic neocortex. J Physiol 2018;596(2):317–42.

72. Worrell GA, Gardner AB, Stead SM, et al. High-frequency oscillations in human temporal lobe: Simultaneous microwire and clinical macroelectrode recordings. Brain 2008;131(4):928–37.

73. Cellot G, Lagonegro P, Tarabella G, et al. PEDOT: PSS interfaces support the development of neuronal synaptic networks with reduced neuroglia response in vitro. Front Neurosci 2016;9(JAN): 1–11.

74. Wilks SJ, Woolley AJ, Ouyang L, et al. In vivo polymerization of poly(3,4-ethylenedioxythiophene) (PEDOT) in rodent cerebral cortex. 2011 Annual International Conference of the IEEE Engineering in Medicine and Biology Society; 2011. p. 5412–5. https://doi.org/10.1109/IEMBS.2011.6091338.

75. Hermiz J, Hossain L, Arneodo EM, et al. Stimulus driven single unit activity from micro-electrocorticography. Front Neurosci 2020;14(February):1–10.

76. Sessolo M, Khodagholy D, Rivnay J, et al. Easy-to-fabricate conducting polymer microelectrode arrays. Adv Mater 2013;25(15):2135–9.

77. Khodagholy D, Gelinas JN, Zhao Z, et al. Organic electronics for high-resolution electrocorticography of the human brain. Sci Adv 2016;2(November): e1601027.

78. Khodagholy D, Gelinas JN, Buzsáki G. Learning-enhanced coupling between ripple oscillations in association cortices and hippocampus. Science 2017;372(October):369–72.

79. Kleen JK, Chung JE, Sellers KK, et al. Bidirectional propagation of low frequency oscillations over the human hippocampal surface. Nat Commun 2021; 12(1):2764.

80. Sun J, Barth K, Qiao S, et al. Intraoperative microseizure detection using a high-density micro-electrocorticography electrode array. Brain Communications 2022;4(3):fcac122.

81. Viventi J, Kim DH, Vigeland L, et al. Flexible, foldable, actively multiplexed, high-density electrode array for mapping brain activity in vivo. Nat Neurosci 2011;14(12):1599–605.

82. Tringides CM, Vachicouras N, de Lázaro I, et al. Viscoelastic surface electrode arrays to interface with viscoelastic tissues. Nat Nanotechnol 2021; 16(9):1019–29.

83. Babb TL, Halgren E, Wilson C, et al. Neuronal firing patterns during the spread of an occipital lobe seizure to the temporal lobes in man. Electroencephalogr Clin Neurophysiol 1981;51(1):104–7.

84. Wilson CL, Babb TL, Halgren E, et al. Visual receptive fields and response properties of neurons in human temporal lobe and visual pathways. Brain 1983;106(2):473–502.

85. Ravagnati L, Halgren E, Babb TL, et al. Activity of human hippocampal formation and amygdala neurons during sleep. Sleep 1980;2(2):161–73.

86. Fried I. Neurons as will and representation. Nat Rev Neurosci 2021. https://doi.org/10.1038/s41583-021-00543-8.

87. Fried I, Cameron KA, Yashar S, et al. Inhibitory and excitatory responses of single neurons in the human medial temporal lobe during recognition of faces and objects. Cerebr Cortex 2002;12(6):575–84.

88. Carlson AA, Rutishauser U, Mamelak AN. Safety and utility of hybrid depth electrodes for seizure localization and single-unit neuronal recording. Stereotact Funct Neurosurg 2018;96(5):311–9.

89. Zheng J, Schjetnan AGP, Yebra M, et al. Neurons detect cognitive boundaries to structure episodic memories in humans. Nat Neurosci 2022;25(March): 358–68.

90. Despouy E, Curot J, Reddy L, et al. Recording local field potential and neuronal activity with tetrodes in epileptic patients. J Neurosci Methods 2020;(May): 108759. https://doi.org/10.1016/j.jneumeth.2020. 108759.

91. Despouy E, Curot J, Denuelle M, et al. Neuronal spiking activity highlights a gradient of epileptogenicity in human tuberous sclerosis lesions. Clin Neurophysiol 2019;130(4):537–47.

92. Curot J, Barbeau E, Despouy E, et al. Local neuronal excitation and global inhibition during epileptic fast ripples in humans. Brain : a journal of neurology 2023;146(2):561–75.

93. Manning JR, Jacobs J, Fried I, et al. Broadband shifts in local field potential power spectra are correlated with single-neuron spiking in humans. J Neurosci 2009;29(43):13613–20.

94. Ulbert I, Halgren E, Heit G, et al. Multiple microelectrode-recording system for human intracortical applications. J Neurosci Methods 2001; 106(1):69–79.

95. Ulbert I, Karmos G, Heit G, et al. Early discrimination of coherent versus incoherent motion by multiunit and synaptic activity in human putative MT+. Hum Brain Mapp 2001;13(4):226–38.

96. Cash SS, Halgren E, Dehghani N, et al. The human K-complex represents an isolated cortical downstate. Science 2009;324(5930):1084–7.

97. Entz L, Tóth E, Keller CJ, et al. Evoked effective connectivity of the human neocortex. Hum Brain Mapp 2014;35(12):5736–53.

98. Halgren M, Ulbert I, Bastuji H, et al. The generation and propagation of the human alpha rhythm. Proc Natl Acad Sci U S A 2019;116(47):23772–82.

99. Csercsa R, Dombovári B, Fabó D, et al. Laminar analysis of slow wave activity in humans. Brain 2010;133(9):2814–29.

100. Halgren M, Fabó D, Ulbert I, et al. Superficial slow rhythms integrate cortical processing in humans. Sci Rep 2018;8(1):1–12.

101. Fabó D, Maglóczky Z, Wittner L, et al. Properties of in vivo interictal spike generation in the human subiculum. Brain 2008;131(2):485–99.

102. Ujma PP, Hajnal B, Bódizs R, et al. The laminar profile of sleep spindles in humans. Neuroimage 2021; 226(November 2020). https://doi.org/10.1016/j. neuroimage.2020.117587.

103. Kandrács Á, Hofer KT, Tóth K, et al. Presence of synchrony-generating hubs in the human epileptic neocortex. J Physiol 2019;597(23):5639–70.

104. Campbell PK, Jones KE, Normann RA. A 100 electrode intracortical array: structural variability. Biomed Sci Instrum 1990;26:161–5.

105. Nordhausen CT, Maynard EM, Normann RA. Single unit recording capabilities of a 100 microelectrode array. Brain Res 1996;726(1–2):129–40.

106. Shenoy KV, Meeker D, Cao S, et al. Neural prosthetic control signals from plan activity. Neuroreport 2003;14(4):591–6.

107. Willett FR, Avansino DT, Hochberg LR, et al. High-performance brain-to-text communication via handwriting. Nature 2021;593(7858):249–54.

108. Willett FR, Deo DR, Avansino DT, et al. Hand Knob Area of Premotor Cortex Represents the Whole Body in a Compositional Way. Cell 2020;181: 1–14.

109. Churchland MM, Cunningham JP, Kaufman MT, et al. Neural population dynamics during reaching. Nature 2012;487(7405):51–6.

110. Truccolo W, Ahmed OJ, Harrison MT, et al. Neuronal Ensemble Synchrony during Human Focal Seizures. J Neurosci 2014;34(30):9927–44.

111. Truccolo W, Donoghue JA, Hochberg LR, et al. Single-neuron dynamics in human focal epilepsy. Nat Neurosci 2011;14(5):635–41.

112. Schevon CA, Goodman RR, McKhann G, et al. Propagation of epileptiform activity on a submillimeter scale. J Clin Neurophysiol 2010;27(6):406–11.

113. Schevon CA, Weiss SA, McKhann G, et al. Evidence of an inhibitory restraint of seizure activity in humans. Nat Commun 2012;3:1011–60.

114. Jun JJ, Steinmetz NA, Siegle JH, et al. Fully integrated silicon probes for high-density recording of neural activity. Nature 2017;551(7679):232–6.

115. Dutta B, Andrei A, Harris TD, et al. The Neuropixels probe: a CMOS based integrated microsystems platform for neuroscience and brain-computer interfaces. 2019 IEEE International Electron Devices Meeting (IEDM); 2019. https://doi.org/10.1109/IEDM19573.2019.8993611.

116. Jia X, Siegle JH, Bennett C, et al. High-density extracellular probes reveal dendritic backpropagation and facilitate neuron classification. J Neurophysiol 2019;121(5):1831–47.

117. Musk E, Neuralink. An integrated brain-machine interface platform with thousands of channels. bioRxiv 2019;703801. https://doi.org/10.1101/703801.

118. Sahasrabuddhe K, Khan AA, Singh AP, et al. The Argo: A high channel count recording system for neural recording in vivo. J Neural Eng 2021;18:015002.

119. Shenoy KV, Kao JC. Measurement, manipulation and modeling of brain-wide neural population dynamics. Nat Commun 2021;12:633.

120. Kemere C, Santhanam G, Yu BM, et al. Neural-State Transitions Using Hidden Markov Models for Motor Cortical Prostheses. J Neurophysiol 2008;100:2441–52.

121. Eden UT, Frank LM, Barbieri R, et al. Dynamic Analysis of Neural Encoding by Point Process Adaptive Filtering. Neural Comput 2004;16(5):971–98.

122. Truccolo W. From point process observations to collective neural dynamics: Nonlinear Hawkes process GLMs, low-dimensional dynamics and coarse graining. J Physiol Paris 2016;110(4):336–47.

123. Trautmann EM, Stavisky SD, Lahiri S, et al. Accurate Estimation of Neural Population Dynamics without Spike Sorting. Neuron 2019;103(2):292–308.e4.

124. Investigational Device Exemptions. 21 CFR § 812. Published January 17, 2023. https://www.accessdata.fda.gov/scripts/cdrh/cfdocs/cfCFR/CFRSearch.cfm?CFRPart=812.

125. *Human Services Food and Drug Administration Center for Devices and Radiological Health (CDRH)*. Published onlineInformation sheet guidance for IRBs, clinical Investigators, and sponsors. Significant risk and nonsignificant risk medical device studies. US Department of Health and; 2006. https://www.fda.gov/media/75459/download.

126. Kalb Soma. IDE basics, investigational device exemption (IDE) program office of device evaluation. Center for Devices and Radiological Health U.S. Food and Drug Administration; 2014. https://www.fda.gov/media/127955/download.

127. Greely HT, Grady C, Ramos KM, et al. Neuroethics Guiding Principles for the NIH BRAIN Initiative. J Neurosci 2018;38(50):10586–8.

128. Young MJ, Bernat JL. Emerging Subspecialties in Neurology: Neuroethics: An Emerging Career Path in Neurology. Neurology 2022;98(12):505–8.

Interneuron Transplantation for Drug-Resistant Epilepsy

Derek G. Southwell, MD, PhD*

KEYWORDS

• Epilepsy • Cell therapy • Interneuron transplantation • Neural circuit repair • Regenerative medicine

KEY POINTS

- Diverse populations of cortical interneurons mediate cell type-specific forms of synaptic inhibition, shaping neural circuit activity, network function, and behavior; cell loss and dysfunction of interneurons occurs in epilepsy.
- Immature interneurons have a unique capacity to functionally engraft in the recipient brain when transplanted.
- In rodent models of epilepsy, transplanted interneurons alter recipient synaptic inhibition and improve seizure phenotypes.
- Scientists have advanced in vitro methods for producing donor interneuron populations from allogeneic human pluripotent stem cell lines and autologous induced pluripotent stem cells; these cells have proven therapeutically effective in rodent models of epilepsy.
- A first-in-human study is investigating the safety and efficacy of interneuron transplantation in patients with drug-resistant mesial temporal lobe epilepsy.

INTRODUCTION

Medications are the mainstays of epilepsy treatment, yet they fail to control seizures in 30% to 40% of patients.[1] Epilepsy surgeries, including brain resection, laser ablation, and neurostimulation, are valuable treatment adjuncts for drug-resistant epilepsy. However, these approaches target seizure networks at macroscopic scales, rendering nonspecific and disruptive effects on the physiologic functions of circuits and networks. Current surgical epilepsy treatments are thus limited and underutilized due to their invasiveness, incomplete seizure control outcomes, and neurocognitive impacts. This leaves an unmet need for alternative or supplemental strategies that target the neural underpinnings of seizures in specific and less-disruptive manners.

The pathophysiology of epilepsy involves a variety of molecular and cellular derangements, which together result in the hyperexcitability of circuits and networks.[2,3] Deficiencies of synaptic inhibition are one pathogenetic factor contributing to epileptogenic hyperexcitability. In the cerebral cortex, synaptic inhibition is mediated by local populations of GABAergic interneurons. Various forms of epilepsy, such as Dravet syndrome[4] and mesial temporal lobe epilepsy (MTLE),[5] are marked by the dysfunction and cell loss of interneuron populations.[6,7] Interventions that augment interneuron function may thus be an approach to correcting or compensating for pathologic hyperexcitability in epilepsy.

During the last 20 years, the transplantation of GABAergic cell types has emerged as a targeted, regenerative method for altering recipient neural circuits and networks in epilepsy.[8] When transplanted from the embryonic brain or in vitro cell culture systems, embryonic-stage GABAergic interneuron precursors disperse, survive and

Department of Neurosurgery, Graduate Program in Neurobiology, Duke University, DUMC 3807, 200 Trent Drive, Durham, NC 27710, USA
* Corresponding author.
E-mail address: derek.southwell@duke.edu

Neurosurg Clin N Am 35 (2024) 151–160
https://doi.org/10.1016/j.nec.2023.08.006

differentiate in recipient cortical areas, including the hippocampus. Transplanted interneurons receive synaptic inputs and form functional inhibitory synaptic outputs with recipient neurons, together mediating various forms of cell type-specific synaptic inhibition. Remarkably, interneuron transplantation has been found to improve seizure phenotypes and associated behavioral abnormalities in rodent models of focal and generalized epilepsy. Stem cell engineering techniques have been used to produce clinical-grade human interneuron populations, one of which was recently approved for investigation in epilepsy patients. This article provides a broad update to earlier reviews on interneuron transplantation for epilepsy[9–17] and describes the initiation of a first-in-human clinical trial of interneuron transplantation in patients with MTLE.

DEVELOPMENTAL ORIGIN AND FUNCTION OF CORTICAL INTERNEURONS

Interneurons are highly diverse cell types that together comprise approximately 20% to 30% of the neuronal population of the cerebral cortex.[18] Interneurons have been classified based on their morphologic, electrophysiological, and transcriptional features.[19–22] Neocortical and hippocampal interneurons primarily originate in the embryonic medial ganglionic and caudal ganglionic eminences (MGE and CGE, respectively) and septum of the ventral forebrain (Fig. 1A).[23] Unlike immature cortical excitatory neurons, which are produced locally in the dorsal forebrain, immature interneurons populate the developing cortex primarily through long distance tangential migration. Broadly, the CGE generates vasoactive intestinal peptide (VIP)-expressing interneurons, and the MGE generates parvalbumin (PVALB)-expressing and somatostatin (SST)-expressing interneurons.[24] In the rodent neocortex (where interneuron development and function have been most detailed) CGE-derived interneurons provide inhibitory input onto other interneurons, whereas MGE-derived interneurons primarily inhibit excitatory neurons and CGE-derived interneurons.[25,26] Cortical interneurons typically form local cortical inhibitory projections, although some interneurons make long-distance projections to targets within and outside the cortex.[27] Interneurons project synaptic outputs onto specific subcellular domains of target cells, differentially shaping how their postsynaptic targets integrate synaptic inputs and fire action potentials (Fig. 1B).[28] Interneurons are also highly connected through electrical synapses, and the activity of interneurons contributes to synchronous network oscillatory patterns.[29–31]

Given the critical involvement of interneurons in cortical circuit and network function, interneuron pathologic conditions (ie, "interneuronopathies") contribute to numerous disease phenotypes, including epileptic seizures.[32] Of note, the developmental origins, cellular diversity, and functional roles of human cortical interneurons remain largely uncharacterized.

BASIC STUDIES OF THE FUNCTIONAL INTEGRATION OF TRANSPLANTED INTERNEURONS

The first description of the engraftment (migration, survival, and differentiation) of transplanted cortical interneuron precursors was made in 1999.[33] This initial study and nearly all subsequent experiments have been performed in rodents, with rare exceptions (eg, transplantation has also been performed in a sea lion[34] and in rhesus macaques[35]). These studies have typically used primary cell populations dissected from the mouse embryonic ganglionic eminences, although primary porcine MGE cell transplants have also been tested.[34,36] In the past decade, there has also been increasing study of donor interneuron populations derived from mouse and human pluripotent stem cells (described below).

When transplanted into various structures of the rodent nervous system, such as the neocortex, hippocampus, amygdala, striatum, and spinal cord, rodent MGE and CGE interneuron precursors disperse several millimeters, survive, and develop morphologies characteristic of mature interneurons[12,37–41] (Fig. 2A). Transplanted interneurons express the inhibitory neurotransmitter, gamma-aminobutyric acid (GABA), and they differentiate into histochemically defined subtypes of mature cortical interneurons (eg, PVALB-expressing, SST-expressing, VIP-expressing populations, according to donor site of origin).[37,40–42] Transplanted interneurons receive local and long-distance synaptic inputs from neurons of the recipient brain (Fig. 2B, and C), and they form functional synaptic outputs onto recipient neurons (excitatory vs inhibitory populations of the recipient) in donor site-specific manners (MGE vs CGE; Fig. 2D).[37,43–48] Interneuron transplantation increases synaptic inhibition onto recipient excitatory populations (Fig. 2E, F); transplant outputs onto recipient inhibitory populations have been less characterized.[37,40–42,46,49,50]

In addition to modifying synaptic inhibition, transplanted interneurons also elicit higher order modifications of circuit and network function. For example, interneuron transplantation into the visual cortex induces new periods of local ocular

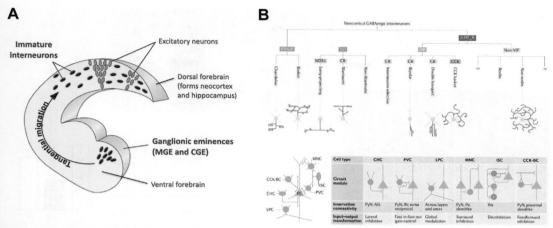

Fig. 1. Embryonic origins and cellular diversity of cortical interneurons. (*A*) Illustration depicting a developing cerebral hemisphere during midgestational stages (coronal plane). Cortical interneurons are generated during embryonic and early postnatal stages. The majority of cortical interneurons (blue) are produced in the MGE and CGE of the ventral forebrain, from which they migrate into the developing cortex, where excitatory neurons (red) are produced by local progenitor cells. (*B*) Basic molecular and morphologic classification of neocortical interneuron types. Cortical interneurons are classified by molecular, morphologic and electrophysiological characteristics. Major molecular/histochemically defined classes include PVALB-expressing, SST-expressing, VIP-expressing populations. Generally, the MGE primarily produces PVALB and SST classes, and the CGE produces VIP classes. Diverse morphologic types of interneurons exhibit varying degrees of specificity in their projections patterns (both with respect to the brain region, cortical layer, subcellular domain and cell type they target; CHC, chandelier cell; CCK-BC, cholecystokinin-basket cell; ISC, interneuron-selective cell; LPC, long-projecting cell; MNC, Martinotti cell; PVC, parvalbumin basket cell). ([*B*] *From* Paul and Huang, 2019.[21])

dominance plasticity, allowing for experience-dependent circuit reorganization.[44,46,51] Transplantation into the amygdala similarly alters plasticity in a manner that facilitates fear memory extinction.[39] Interneuron transplantation also modifies network oscillatory patterns in local and remote brain regions.[52,53]

TRANSPLANTATION OF RODENT INTERNEURONS IN PRECLINICAL EPILEPSY MODELS

During the past 15 years, interneuron transplantation has been evaluated in preclinical rodent models of epilepsy. The first of these studies involved mouse MGE cell transplantation into neonatal mice lacking a voltage-gated potassium channel (Kv1.1), which is mutated in some forms of human epilepsy.[47] In this generalized epilepsy model, MGE cell transplantation reduced recipient spontaneous seizure frequency by approximately 85%. In a second study using a genetic model of epilepsy with absence-like seizures, transplantation into occipital cortex also reduced recipient seizure event frequency and duration.[54] Notably, in both these early studies, transplantation was performed before epilepsy phenotypes manifested in the recipients. Transplants also corrected seizure phenotypes without populating all areas

of the presumed seizure network. In wild type recipients, interneuron transplantation has also been found to increase subsequent thresholds for pharmacologically[55] electrically[56] evoked ictal activity. Thus, in both genetic generalized epilepsy and evoked seizure models, transplantation can yield seizure-protective effects at later stages. Along these lines, transplantation early after traumatic brain injury (before spontaneous seizure onset) also improves posttraumatic seizure phenotypes.[57]

Interneuron transplantation has also been found to improve recipient phenotypes in chronic seizure models. In the pilocarpine model of temporal lobe epilepsy (TLE), hippocampal transplantation of mouse MGE cells has been reduces electrographic seizure frequency and corrects epilepsy-associated behavioral abnormalities (aggression, hyperactivity, and spatial learning deficits).[58] Using this model, another group found that transplantation of MGE interneurons into dentate gyrus, but not entorhinal cortex, improved seizure phenotypes and reduced mossy fiber sprouting in recipient dentate gyrus.[49] Transplants also reversed abnormal patterns of adult neurogenesis in the epileptic recipient hippocampus.[59] The seizure-corrective effects of MGE cell transplantation appear durable in mice, lasting at least 6 to 7 months (the longest period of seizure

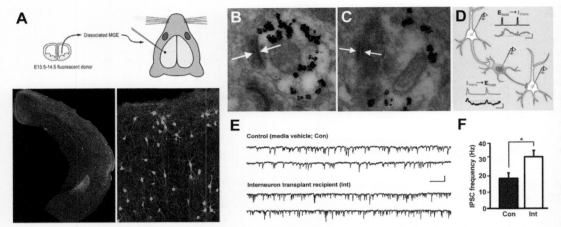

Fig. 2. Transplanted immature interneurons disperse in the recipient brain, synaptically integrate into recipient circuits, and alter synaptic inhibition. (*A*) Transplantation of primary interneuron populations from the embryonic day 13.5 to 14.5 (E13.5–14.5) mouse MGE into mouse recipient cortex (*top*). Immature interneurons can also be generated and transplanted from in vitro culture systems in a similar fashion. Transplanted immature interneurons disperse in the mouse recipient brain (*bottom left*, left cortex in coronal plane) and develop morphologies of mature interneuron subtypes (*bottom right*). (*B*) Electron micrograph of recipient brain tissue following transplantation. Transplanted interneurons, identified by gold particle-conjugated antibodies against a donor-specific marker (*black densities*), receive synaptic inputs (*arrows*) from recipient neurons. (*C*) Transplanted interneurons also form synaptic outputs onto recipient neurons. (*D*) Simultaneous electrode recordings from transplanted interneurons (*red*) and recipient excitatory neurons (*white*). Stimulation of recipient excitatory neurons elicits excitatory postsynaptic potentials in the transplanted interneuron (E_{host} to I_{trans}; *top*), whereas depolarization of the transplanted interneuron elicits inhibitory postsynaptic potentials in the recipient excitatory neuron (I_{trans} to E_{host}; *bottom*). (*E*) Spontaneous inhibitory postsynaptic current traces recorded from excitatory neurons in adult mice following MGE interneuron transplantation (Int.) or control injection (Con.). (*F*) Transplantation increases the frequency of spontaneous inhibitory synaptic events in recipient excitatory neurons. Horizontal bar in E, 200 milliseconds; vertical bar 40 pA. * indicates statistical significance ($p < 0.05$). (*Images adapted from [B–D]* Southwell et al., 2014[12] *and [E, F]* Southwell et al., 2012.[91])

observation reported; 6-7 months is approximately one-quarter the life span of a laboratory mouse).[60] In the same study, CGE interneuron transplantation neither improved nor worsened seizure phenotypes in epileptic recipients.

PRECLINICAL STUDIES OF HUMAN STEM CELL-DERIVED INTERNEURONS

As rodent primary and stem cell-derived interneuron populations proved efficacious in epilepsy models, there has been strong interest in producing human interneurons for preclinical research and clinical endpoints. Several strategies have been devised for generating cortical interneuron-like populations from pluripotent stem cells,[61–66] embryonic stem cells,[67–71] and induced pluripotent stem cells.[70,72] These in vitro methods typically involve the manipulation of signaling pathways engaged during development of the ganglionic eminences, or the induction of interneuron progenitor identities via forced expression of exogenous transcription factors.

Remarkably, in rodent models of TLE, transplanted in vitro-derived human interneurons

have been found to disperse, survive, and synaptically integrate in the recipient hippocampus, durably improving recipient seizure phenotypes and partially correcting epilepsy-associated behavioral abnormalities.[48,61,72,73] In some of these studies, optogenetic activation[48,73] and chemogenetic suppression[72] of transplant activity improved and diminished recipient seizure responses, respectively, indicating that seizure suppression involves transplant recruitment in recipient circuits. Human stem-cell-derived interneurons can also synaptically integrate into live brain tissues collected from human patients with epilepsy.[74]

Some of the challenges and limitations to the successful in vitro derivation, preclinical study, and utilization of human donor interneuron populations include the potential tumorigenicity of residual progenitor populations, the production and selection of specific interneuron that are also developmentally staged to disperse and integrate into the recipient brain, the long timescale of human interneuron differentiation, and the potential immunogenicity of donor cells sourced from allogeneic stem cell lines.[12,61,63,69,70,72,75,76]

Transplant immunogenicity (or requirements for immunosuppression when transplanting allogeneic cells) may be avoided by using autologous transplant populations derived from induced pluripotent stem cells. However, the custom, patient-specific production of good manufacturing practice (GMP)-validated, clinical grade interneuron products is both practically challenging and potentially cost-prohibitive (estimated to be nearly 1M USD for the generation of patient-specific cells).[77]

A FIRST-IN-HUMAN TRIAL OF INTERNEURON TRANSPLANTATION

In 2021, the US Food and Drug Administration (FDA) allowed the initiation of an industry-sponsored, first-in-human trial of GABAergic interneuron transplantation for drug-resistant MTLE (ClinicalTrials.gov Identifier: NCT05135091). This ongoing, multisite, Phase 1/2 study is investigating the safety and efficacy of NRTX-1001, a cryopreserved, off-the-shelf, allogeneic human pluripotent stem cell (hPSC)-derived cortical-type interneuron product developed by Neurona Therapeutics (South San Francisco, CA).

The study sponsor has presented preclinical data evaluating the safety and efficacy of NRTX-1001 in a mouse model of unilateral temporal lobe epilepsy elicited by intrahippocampal kainate injection to immunodeficient recipients.[35,91] These preclinical results indicate that NRTX-1001 cells disperse and persist in the recipient mouse hippocampus to time points at least 7 months from the time of transplantation (transplanted cells did not distribute outside the hippocampus to other brain areas or organs; **Fig. 3**A). Hippocampal transplantation of NRTX-1001 significantly reduced spontaneous focal seizure burden in the mouse model, as measured by recipient video-electroencephalography (**Fig. 3**B). Transplantation also improved the survival of the recipient mice, and it reduced granule cell dispersion in the epileptic hippocampal dentate gyrus (**Fig. 3**C). Summarized preclinical safety data suggest that the NRTX-1001 did not proliferate in the recipient, form teratomas, elicit gross motor, sensory or behavioral changes; or cause other toxicities (eg, weight changes, metabolic derangements on serum chemistry panels, or hematologic abnormalities on blood cytology studies). The sponsor has also presented findings validating the delivery of NRTX-1001 to the nonhuman primate temporal lobe.[78] These data indicated the feasibility of targeting NRTX-1001 to the primate hippocampus, where the cell product dispersed and expressed interneuron histochemical markers (**Fig. 3**D).

The ongoing human study of NRTX-1001 is designed as a 2-stage trial, with stage 1 acting as an open-label, single-arm dose escalation study of the safety of NRTX-1001 administration and stage 2 acting as a masked, randomized, sham-controlled study of NRTX-1001 safety and efficacy. The study is evaluating NRTX-1001 in adult patients with drug-resistant focal onset epilepsy originating from a unilateral mesial temporal lobe (based on clinical semiology, electrographic evaluation, and neuroimaging findings of mesial temporal sclerosis). The patient population is thus one that would typically qualify for standard surgical treatments such as temporal resection, laser ablation, and responsive neurostimulation.

Following administration of the allogeneic cell product, study subjects are receiving immunosuppressive therapy for 1 year, with the option to wean immunosuppression thereafter. The safety and efficacy of NRTX-1001 are being assessed at a 1-year primary endpoint, with long-term follow-up for 15 years from treatment. These evaluations include physical examinations, blood draws, structural imaging, magnetic resonance spectroscopy, electroencephalogram (EEG), neuropsychometric testing, patient seizure diaries, and quality of life surveys. Patients will continue antiepileptic medications (with ongoing medication adjustments per their neurologists), and they may elect to undergo standard of care surgical treatments. Safety of NRTX-1001 administration, the primary outcome measure of the study, will be reported as the frequency of serious or severe adverse events that occur in the first year after treatment. Efficacy, a secondary outcome measure, will involve comparisons of seizure frequency reductions and responder rates between NRTX-1001 recipients and sham-treated subjects. As of May, 2023, the study team described the treatment of 2 sentinel subjects.[80] Following data safety monitoring review, 3 additional patients were then treated in the summer of 2023. As of the time of this publication, patient outcomes data are pending.

KNOWLEDGE GAPS AND BARRIERS TO THE EFFECTIVE CLINICAL APPLICATIONS OF INTERNEURON TRANSPLANTATION

Inhibitory cell therapies for epilepsy will benefit from an improved understanding of how diverse interneuron types contribute to both physiologic and epileptogenic circuit functions. Although recent data suggest that the composition and cellular properties of human interneuron populations may differ significantly from those of mice,[81–83] it is poorly understood how interneuron types function in human inhibitory circuits.

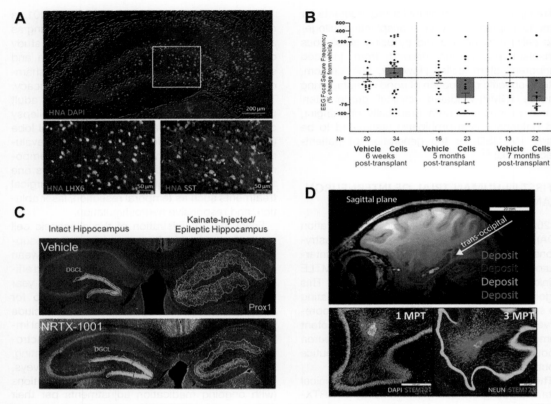

Fig. 3. Preclinical studies of NRTX-1001, a human pluripotent stem-cell derived interneuron product under Phase I/II evaluation in patients with MTLE. (*A*) Seven months posttransplantation (MPT) to mouse hippocampus (sectioned in coronal plane), NRTX-1001 cells (labeled by human nuclear antigen [*red*]) have dispersed and expressed markers of MGE interneurons (eg, Lhx6 and somatostatin). (*B*) By 5 MPT to epileptic mice (unilateral intrahippocampal kainate injection model), hippocampal NRTX-1001 transplantation significantly reduces recipient spontaneous seizure frequency. (*C*) NRTX-1001 transplantation reduces structural changes in the epileptic mouse hippocampus (*right*), decreasing the dispersion of granule cells in the dentate granule cell layer. (*D*) Delivery of NRTX-1001 to the rhesus macaque hippocampus. Top, posttreatment imaging depicts delivery of NRTX-1001 along a transoccipital trajectory, similar to that used for mesial temporal ablation in humans. NRTX-1001 delivery in an MRI contrast dye-containing suspension enables visualization of cell delivery (cells were delivered at 4 points along the trajectory, false-colored here). Bottom, at 1 and 3 MPT, NRTX-1001 cells (labeled by a human marker, STEM121) have dispersed in the hippocampus, where some of them express somatostatin. ** and *** indicate statistical significance. (*Images from* [*A-C*] Priest et al[35] and [*D*] Blum et al.[79])

Additionally, there is much left to be determined as to how specific interneuron types may govern the initiation, propagation, and termination of seizure activity.[84] Speaking to our incomplete understandings of both ictogenesis and the therapeutic mechanisms of interneuron transplantation, some data suggest that interneuron activation drives seizure activity, and, in some circumstances, GABAergic signaling may excite postsynaptic cells in epileptic brain areas.[85] Taken at face value, these findings would indicate that transplanted interneurons might exacerbate seizure phenotypes, an effect that has not been observed in preclinical studies.

Because preclinical studies have primarily investigated and validated transplantation's local effects on inhibitory signaling, interneuron transplantation has been conceptualized as a tool for focally constraining hyperexcitability in the epileptic brain. This has led to applications in which transplants are targeted directly to seizure onset zones. In clinical settings, interneuron transplantation could serve a role (either as an alternative, or augmentative therapy) in treating seizures that originate from eloquent tissues (e.g., operculum and rolandic cortex) or multiple areas (eg, bitemporal epilepsy), scenarios in which resective or laser ablative treatments cannot be safely or effectively used. Network-based applications of interneuron transplantation,[86,87] whereby interneurons may be targeted to sites of ictal organization or propagation outside the seizure onset zone(s), remain relatively unstudied in preclinical settings. This strategy, if effective, could support transplantation for generalized and regional onset epilepsies as well. At a more fundamental level, most transplantation studies have been performed in rodent brain targets, which lack the gross scale and structural complexity of the human brain. As such, the extent of transplant dispersion in the human brain, and the focality of its synaptic inhibitory effects, remain unknown. Both of these phenomena may in turn depend on where transplants are delivered. Additionally, it is unclear how transplantation should be timed with respect to patient disease state and, perhaps, patient seizure cycles; these factors (as well as patient medication regimens) may influence how the immature transplant population differentiates and integrates into the recipient circuitry.[88,89]

Finally, the sourcing of donor cells is another important factor in the clinical implementation of interneuron transplantation. As described above, the use of allogeneic populations requires patient immunosuppression, with its associated medication burdens and potential side-effects. Although the use of autologous cells or cells derived from human leukocyte antigen (HLA)-engineered lines may not require patient immunosuppression, such approaches are highly costly and less flexible than those involving a single and invariant allogeneic cell product.[77] Reprogramming patient brain cell populations into interneurons may be an alternative to exogenous cell transplantation as well.[90]

SUMMARY

Interneuron transplantation is a novel cellular approach to modifying synaptic inhibition in neural circuits. Preclinical studies have demonstrated the seizure-corrective effects of transplantation in rodent models and advanced methods for producing donor human interneuron populations in vitro. A first-in-human study is currently investigating the safety and efficacy of interneuron transplantation in patients with unilateral MTLE. Clinical applications of interneuron transplantation will benefit from a deeper understanding of human interneurons, inhibitory circuit dysfunction in human epilepsy, and the circuit and network effects of interneuron transplants.

CLINICS CARE POINTS

- Interneuron transplantation is a prospective cellular therapy that has been tested in various rodent models of epilepsy. To date, there is no clinical evidence to guide its use in patients.

- A first-in-human Phase I/II study of interneuron transplantation is now evaluating the safety and efficacy of interneuron transplantation for focal onset epilepsy originating from the mesial temporal lobe.

- As a cell-based strategy for modifying epileptogenic neural circuits and networks, interneuron transplantation could prove a minimally invasive, regenerative approach to treating seizures in various forms of epilepsy. Preclinical data thus far best support future applications for focal onset epilepsies originating from one or more onset zones, particularly when resection or laser ablation may have significant influences on patient motor, sensory, or neurocognitive function.

FUNDING

D.G.S. was supported by the NINDS K12 Neurosurgery Research Career Development Program K12 Award, Klingenstein-Simons Foundation, and Duke University Holland-Trice Scholars Program.

DISCLOSURE

The author is a study investigator in the first-in-human clinical trial described in this review. The author has no financial or other conflicts of interest concerning the subjects discussed in this article.

REFERENCES

1. Bialer M, Johannessen SI, Koepp MJ, et al. Progress report on new antiepileptic drugs: A summary of the Fifteenth Eilat Conference on New Antiepileptic Drugs and Devices (EILAT XV). II. Drugs in more advanced clinical development. Epilepsia 2020; 61(11):2365–85.

2. Paz JT, Huguenard JR. Microcircuits and their interactions in epilepsy: is the focus out of focus? Nat Neurosci 2015;18(3):351–9.

3. Pitkänen A, Lukasiuk K, Dudek FE, et al. Epileptogenesis. Cold Spring Harb Perspect Med 2015;5(10). https://doi.org/10.1101/cshperspect.a022822.

4. Bender AC, Morse RP, Scott RC, et al. SCN1A mutations in Dravet syndrome: impact of interneuron dysfunction on neural networks and cognitive outcome. Epilepsy Behav 2012;23(3):177–86.

5. de Lanerolle NC, Kim JH, Williamson A, et al. A retrospective analysis of hippocampal pathology in human temporal lobe epilepsy: evidence for distinctive patient subcategories. Epilepsia 2003; 44(5):677–87.

6. Houser CR. Do structural changes in GABA neurons give rise to the epileptic state? Adv Exp Med Biol 2014;813:151–60.

7. Liu YQ, Yu F, Liu WH, et al. Dysfunction of hippo-campal interneurons in epilepsy. Neurosci Bull 2014;30(6):985–98.

8. Shetty AK, Upadhya D. GABA-ergic cell therapy for epilepsy: Advances, limitations and challenges. Neurosci Biobehav Rev 2016;62:35–47.

9. Li D, Wu Q, Han X. Application of Medial Ganglionic Eminence Cell Transplantation in Diseases Associ-ated With Interneuron Disorders. Front Cell Neurosci 2022;16:939294.

10. Zhu Q, Naegele JR, Chung S. Cortical GABAergic Interneuron/Progenitor Transplantation as a Novel Therapy for Intractable Epilepsy. Front Cell Neurosci 2018;12:167.

11. Hunt RF, Baraban SC. Interneuron Transplantation as a Treatment for Epilepsy. Cold Spring Harb Perspect Med 2015;5(12). https://doi.org/10.1101/cshperspect.a022376.

12. Southwell DG, Nicholas CR, Basbaum AI, et al. Inter-neurons from embryonic development to cell-based therapy. Science 2014;344(6180):1240622.

13. Tyson JA, Anderson SA. GABAergic interneuron transplants to study development and treat disease. Trends Neurosci 2014;37(3):169–77.

14. Anderson SA, Baraban SC. Cell therapy for epilepsy using GABAergic neural progenitors. Epilepsia 2010;51:94.

15. Sebe JY, Baraban SC. The promise of an interneuron-based cell therapy for epilepsy. Dev Neurobiol 2011; 71(1):107–17.

16. Maisano X, Carpentino J, Becker S, et al. Embryonic stem cell-derived neural precursor grafts for treat-ment of temporal lobe epilepsy. Neurotherapeutics 2009;6(2):263–77.

17. Richardson RM, Barbaro NM, Alvarez-Buylla A, et al. Developing cell transplantation for temporal lobe ep-ilepsy. Neurosurg Focus 2008;24(3–4):E17.

18. Džaja D, Hladnik A, Bičanić I, et al. Neocortical cal-retinin neurons in primates: increase in proportion and microcircuitry structure. Front Neuroanat 2014; 8:103.

19. Pelkey KA, Chittajallu R, Craig MT, et al. Hippocam-pal GABAergic inhibitory interneurons. Physiol Rev 2017;97(4):1619–747.

20. Markram H, Toledo-Rodriguez M, Wang Y, et al. In-terneurons of the neocortical inhibitory system. Nat Rev Neurosci 2004;5(10):793–807.

21. Huang ZJ, Paul A. The diversity of GABAergic neu-rons and neural communication elements. Nat Rev Neurosci 2019;20(9):563–72.

22. Freund TF, Buzsáki G. Interneurons of the hippo-campus. Hippocampus 1996;6(4):347–470.

23. Molnár Z, Clowry GJ, Šestan N, et al. New insights into the development of the human cerebral cortex. J Anat 2019;235(3):432–51.

24. Rudy B, Fishell G, Lee S, et al. Three groups of interneurons account for nearly 100% of neocortical

25. Pfeffer CK, Xue M, He M, et al. Inhibition of inhibition in visual cortex: the logic of connections between molecularly distinct interneurons. Nat Neurosci 2013;16(8):1068–76.

26. Pi HJ, Hangya B, Kvitsiani D, et al. Cortical interneu-rons that specialize in disinhibitory control. Nature 2013;503(7477):521–4.

27. Urrutia-Piñones J, Morales-Moraga C, Sanguinetti-González N, et al. Long-Range GABAergic Projec-tions of Cortical Origin in Brain Function. Front Syst Neurosci 2022;16:841869.

28. Kepecs A, Fishell G. Interneuron cell types are fit to function. Nature 2014;505(7483):318–26.

29. Bartos M, Vida I, Jonas P. Synaptic mechanisms of synchronized gamma oscillations in inhibitory inter-neuron networks. Nat Rev Neurosci 2007;8(1): 45–56.

30. Dupret D, Pleydell-Bouverie B, Csicsvari J. Inhibitory interneurons and network oscillations. Proc Natl Acad Sci U S A 2008;105(47):18079–80.

31. Sohal VS, Zhang F, Yizhar O, et al. Parvalbumin neu-rons and gamma rhythms enhance cortical circuit performance. Nature 2009;459(7247):698–702.

32. Katsarou AM, Li Q, Liu W, et al. Acquired parvalbumin-selective interneuronopathy in the multiple-hit model of infantile spasms: A putative basis for the partial responsiveness to vigabatrin analogs? Epilepsia Open 2018;3(Suppl 2):155–64.

33. Wichterle H, Garcia-Verdugo JM, Herrera DG, et al. Young neurons from medial ganglionic eminence disperse in adult and embryonic brain. Nat Neurosci 1999;2(5):461–6.

34. Simeone CA, Andrews JP, Johnson SP, et al. Xeno-transplantation of porcine progenitor cells in an epileptic California sea lion (Zalophus californianus): illustrative case. J Neurosurg Case Lessons 2022; 3(12). https://doi.org/10.3171/CASE21417.

35. Catherine Priest, Mansi Parekh, Whitney Blankenberger, et al. Preclinical-Development of NRTX 1001, an Inhibi-tory Interneuron Cellular Therapeutic for the Treatment of Chronic Focal Epilepsy. In: American Epilepsy Soci-ety. 2022. https://aesnet.org/abstractslisting/preclinical-development-of-nrtx-1001–an-inhibitory-interneuron-cellular-therapeutic-for-the-treatment-of-chronic-focal-epilepsy; 2022.

36. Casalia ML, Li T, Ramsay H, et al. Interneuron origins in the embryonic porcine medial ganglionic eminence. J Neurosci 2021;41(14):3105–19.

37. Alvarez-Dolado M, Calcagnotto ME, Karkar KM, et al. Cortical inhibition modified by embryonic neu-ral precursors grafted into the postnatal brain. J Neurosci 2006;26(28):7380–9.

38. Martínez-Cerdeño V, Noctor SC, Espinosa A, et al. Embryonic MGE precursor cells grafted into adult rat striatum integrate and ameliorate motor

GABAergic neurons. Dev Neurobiol 2011;71(1): 45–61.

symptoms in 6-OHDA-lesioned rats. Cell Stem Cell 2010;6(3):238–50.

39. Yang WZ, Liu TT, Cao JW, et al. Fear Erasure Facilitated by Immature Inhibitory Neuron Transplantation. Neuron 2016;92(6):1352–67.

40. Larimer P, Spatazza J, Espinosa JS, et al. Caudal Ganglionic Eminence Precursor Transplants Disperse and Integrate as Lineage-Specific Interneurons but Do Not Induce Cortical Plasticity. Cell Rep 2016; 16(5):1391–404.

41. Larimer P, Spatazza J, Stryker MP, et al. Development and long-term integration of MGE-lineage cortical interneurons in the heterochronic environment. J Neurophysiol 2017;118(1):131–9.

42. Hsieh JY, Baraban SC. Medial ganglionic eminence progenitors transplanted into hippocampus integrate in a functional and subtype-appropriate manner. eNeuro 2017;4(2). ENEURO.0359-16.2017.

43. Juarez-Salinas DL, Braz JM, Etlin A, et al. GABAergic cell transplants in the anterior cingulate cortex reduce neuropathic pain aversiveness. Brain 2019; 142(9):2655–69.

44. Zheng X, Salinas KJ, Velez DXF, et al. Host interneurons mediate plasticity reactivated by embryonic inhibitory cell transplantation in mouse visual cortex. Nat Commun 2021;12(1):862.

45. Frankowski JC, Tierno A, Pavani S, et al. Brain-wide reconstruction of inhibitory circuits after traumatic brain injury. Nat Commun 2022;13(1):3417.

46. Southwell DG, Froemke RC, Alvarez-Buylla A, et al. Cortical plasticity induced by inhibitory neuron transplantation. Science 2010;327(5969):1145–8.

47. Baraban SC, Southwell DG, Estrada RC, et al. Reduction of seizures by transplantation of cortical GABAergic interneuron precursors into Kv1.1 mutant mice. Proc Natl Acad Sci U S A 2009; 106(36):15472–7.

48. Zhu Q, Mishra A, Park JS, et al. Human cortical interneurons optimized for grafting specifically integrate, abort seizures, and display prolonged efficacy without over-inhibition. Neuron 2022. https://doi.org/10.1016/j.neuron.2022.12.014.

49. Henderson KW, Gupta J, Tagliatela S, et al. Long-term seizure suppression and optogenetic analyses of synaptic connectivity in epileptic mice with hippocampal grafts of GABAergic interneurons. J Neurosci 2014;34(40):13492–504.

50. Gupta J, Bromwich M, Radell J, et al. Restrained Dendritic Growth of Adult-Born Granule Cells Innervated by Transplanted Fetal GABAergic Interneurons in Mice with Temporal Lobe Epilepsy. eNeuro 2019;6(2). https://doi.org/10.1523/ENEURO.0110-18.2019.

51. Davis MF, Figueroa Velez DX, Guevarra RP, et al. Inhibitory Neuron Transplantation into Adult Visual Cortex Creates a New Critical Period that Rescues Impaired Vision. Neuron 2015;86(4):1055–66.

52. Howard MA, Rubenstein JLR, Baraban SC. Bidirectional homeostatic plasticity induced by interneuron cell death and transplantation in vivo. Proc Natl Acad Sci U S A 2014;111(1):492–7.

53. Martinez-Losa M, Tracy TE, Ma K, et al. Nav1.1-Overexpressing Interneuron Transplants Restore Brain Rhythms and Cognition in a Mouse Model of Alzheimer's Disease. Neuron 2018;98(1):75–89.e5.

54. Hammad M, Schmidt SL, Zhang X, et al. Transplantation of GABAergic interneurons into the neonatal primary visual cortex reduces absence seizures in Stargazer mice. Cereb Cortex 2015;25(9):2970–9.

55. Calcagnotto ME, Ruiz LP, Blanco MM, et al. Effect of neuronal precursor cells derived from medial ganglionic eminence in an acute epileptic seizure model. Epilepsia 2010;51(Suppl 3):71–5.

56. De la Cruz E, Zhao M, Guo L, et al. Interneuron progenitors attenuate the power of acute focal ictal discharges. Neurotherapeutics 2011;8(4):763–73.

57. Zhu B, Eom J, Hunt RF. Transplanted interneurons improve memory precision after traumatic brain injury. Nat Commun 2019;10(1):5156.

58. Hunt RF, Girskis KM, Rubenstein JL, et al. GABA progenitors grafted into the adult epileptic brain control seizures and abnormal behavior. Nat Neurosci 2013;16(6):692–7.

59. Arshad MN, Oppenheimer S, Jeong J, et al. Hippocampal transplants of fetal GABAergic progenitors regulate adult neurogenesis in mice with temporal lobe epilepsy. Neurobiol Dis 2022;174:105879.

60. Casalia ML, Howard MA, Baraban SC. Persistent seizure control in epileptic mice transplanted with gamma-aminobutyric acid progenitors. Ann Neurol 2017;82(4):530–42.

61. Cunningham M, Cho JH, Leung A, et al. hPSC-derived maturing GABAergic interneurons ameliorate seizures and abnormal behavior in epileptic mice. Cell Stem Cell 2014;15(5):559–73.

62. Liu Y, Liu H, Sauvey C, et al. Directed differentiation of forebrain GABA interneurons from human pluripotent stem cells. Nat Protoc 2013;8(9):1670–9.

63. Nicholas CR, Chen J, Tang Y, et al. Functional Maturation of hPSC-Derived Forebrain Interneurons Requires an Extended Timeline and Mimics Human Neural Development. Cell Stem Cell 2013;12(5):573–86.

64. Kim TG, Yao R, Monnell T, et al. Efficient specification of interneurons from human pluripotent stem cells by dorsoventral and rostrocaudal modulation. Stem Cell 2014;32(7):1789–804.

65. Sun AX, Yuan Q, Tan S, et al. Direct induction and functional maturation of forebrain GABAergic neurons from human pluripotent stem cells. Cell Rep 2016;16(7):1942–53.

66. Yang N, Chanda S, Marro S, et al. Generation of pure GABAergic neurons by transcription factor programming. Nat Methods 2017;14(6):621–8.

67. Germain ND, Banda EC, Becker S, et al. Derivation and Isolation of NKX2.1-Positive Basal Forebrain Progenitors from Human Embryonic Stem Cells. Stem Cells Dev 2013;22(10):1477–89.

68. Goulburn AL, Stanley EG, Elefanty AG, et al. Generating GABAergic cerebral cortical interneurons from mouse and human embryonic stem cells. Stem Cell Res 2012;8(3):416–26.

69. Maroof AM, Keros S, Tyson Ja, et al. Directed differentiation and functional maturation of cortical interneurons from human embryonic stem cells. Cell Stem Cell 2013;12(5):559–72.

70. Ni P, Noh H, Shao Z, et al. Large-Scale Generation and Characterization of Homogeneous Populations of Migratory Cortical Interneurons from Human Pluripotent Stem Cells. Mol Ther Methods Clin Dev 2019;13:414–30.

71. Chen CY, Plocik A, Anderson NC, et al. Transcriptome and in Vitro Differentiation Profile of Human Embryonic Stem Cell Derived NKX2.1-Positive Neural Progenitors. Stem Cell Rev Rep 2016;12(6):744–56.

72. Upadhya D, Hattiangady B, Castro OW, et al. Human induced pluripotent stem cell-derived MGE cell grafting after status epilepticus attenuates chronic epilepsy and comorbidities via synaptic integration. Proc Natl Acad Sci U S A 2019;116(1):287–96.

73. Waloschková E, Gonzalez-Ramos A, Mikroulis A, et al. Human Stem Cell-Derived GABAergic Interneurons Establish Efferent Synapses onto Host Neurons in Rat Epileptic Hippocampus and Inhibit Spontaneous Recurrent Seizures. Int J Mol Sci 2021;22(24). https://doi.org/10.3390/ijms222413243.

74. Gonzalez-Ramos A, Waloschková E, Mikroulis A, et al. Human stem cell-derived GABAergic neurons functionally integrate into human neuronal networks. Sci Rep 2021;11(1):22050.

75. Liu Y, Weick JP, Liu H, et al. Medial ganglionic eminence–like cells derived from human embryonic stem cells correct learning and memory deficits. Nat Biotechnol 2013;31(5):440–7.

76. Shrestha S, Anderson NC, Grabel LB, et al. Development of electrophysiological and morphological properties of human embryonic stem cell-derived GABAergic interneurons at different times after transplantation into the mouse hippocampus. PLoS One 2020;15(8). e0237426.

77. Doss MX, Sachinidis A. Current Challenges of iPSC-Based Disease Modeling and Therapeutic Implications. Cells 2019;8(5). https://doi.org/10.3390/cells8050403.

78. Bershteyn M, Broer S, Parekh M, et al. Human pallial MGE-type GABAergic interneuron cell therapy for chronic focal epilepsy, *Cell Stem Cell* (in press).

79. Blum D, Parekh M, Hampel P, et al. NRTX-1001: first-in-class human inhibitory neuron cell therapy for phase I/II clinical investigation in chronic focal epilepsy. American Epilepsy Society; 2022. https://aesnet.org/abstractslisting/nrtx-1001–first-in-class-human-inhibitory-neuron-cell-therapy-for-phase-i/ii-clinical-investigation-in-chronic-focal-epilepsy.

80. Babu H, Beach R, Burchiel K, et al. First-in-human trial of NRTX-1001 GABAergic interneuron cell therapy for treatment of focal epilepsy - Emerging clinical results. Nashville, TN: American Academy of Neurology; 2023. https://www.aan.com/MSA/Public/Events/AbstractDetails/55221.

81. Hodge RD, Bakken TE, Miller JA, et al. Conserved cell types with divergent features in human versus mouse cortex. Nature 2019;573(7772):61–8.

82. Boldog E, Bakken TE, Hodge RD, et al. Transcriptomic and morphophysiological evidence for a specialized human cortical GABAergic cell type. Nat Neurosci 2018;21(9):1185–95.

83. Krienen FM, Goldman M, Zhang Q, et al. Innovations present in the primate interneuron repertoire. Nature 2020;586(7828):262–9.

84. Khoshkhoo S, Vogt D, Sohal VS. Dynamic, Cell-Type-Specific Roles for GABAergic Interneurons in a Mouse Model of Optogenetically Inducible Seizures. Neuron 2017;93(2):291–8.

85. Huberfeld G, Blauwblomme T, Miles R. Hippocampus and epilepsy: Findings from human tissues. Rev Neurol 2015;171(3):236–51.

86. Handreck A, Backofen-Wehrhahn B, Bröer S, et al. Anticonvulsant Effects by Bilateral and Unilateral Transplantation of GABA-Producing Cells into the Subthalamic Nucleus in an Acute Seizure Model. Cell Transplant 2014;23(1):111–32.

87. Löscher W, Ebert U, Lehmann H, et al. Seizure suppression in kindling epilepsy by grafts of fetal GABAergic neurons in rat substantia nigra. J Neurosci Res 1998;51(2):196–209.

88. Overstreet-Wadiche LS, Bromberg Da, Bensen AL, et al. Seizures accelerate functional integration of adult-generated granule cells. J Neurosci 2006;26(15):4095–103.

89. Raijmakers M, Clynen E, Smisdom N, et al. Experimental febrile seizures increase dendritic complexity of newborn dentate granule cells. Epilepsia 2016;57(5):717–26.

90. Lentini C, d'Orange M, Marichal N, et al. Reprogramming reactive glia into interneurons reduces chronic seizure activity in a mouse model of mesial temporal lobe epilepsy. Cell Stem Cell 2021;28(12):2104–21.e10.

91. Southwell DG, Paredes MF, Galvao RP, et al. Intrinsically determined cell death of developing cortical interneurons. Nature 2012;491(7422):109–13.

Moving?

Make sure your subscription moves with you!

To notify us of your new address, find your **Clinics Account Number** (located on your mailing label above your name), and contact customer service at:

Email: journalscustomerservice-usa@elsevier.com

800-654-2452 (subscribers in the U.S. & Canada)
314-447-8871 (subscribers outside of the U.S. & Canada)

Fax number: 314-447-8029

Elsevier Health Sciences Division
Subscription Customer Service
3251 Riverport Lane
Maryland Heights, MO 63043

Printed and bound by CPI Group (UK) Ltd, Croydon, CR0 4YY

13/05/2025

01870195-0001